Experimental Acupuncturology

Jaung-Geng Lin
Editor

Experimental Acupuncturology

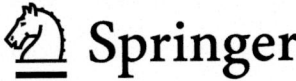 Springer

Editor
Jaung-Geng Lin
China Medical University
Taichung
Taiwan

ISBN 978-981-13-0970-0   ISBN 978-981-13-0971-7   (eBook)
https://doi.org/10.1007/978-981-13-0971-7

Library of Congress Control Number: 2018955934

This Springer imprint is published by Springer Nature, under the registered company Springer Nature Singapore Pte Ltd.
The registered company address is: 152 Beach Road, #21-01/04 Gateway East, Singapore 189721, Singapore

Foreword

I am honored to provide a foreword to this book, *Experimental Acupuncturology*. I congratulate Professor Jaung-Geng Lin and his team of experts on successfully completing this compilation of scientific evidence corroborating the clinical effects of acupuncture in various physiological and psychological conditions.

Formal recognition by the WHO and UNESCO as to the use and efficacy of acupuncture science in modern medicine has encouraged significant investment into the research and development of acupuncture science among top-ranking health science research institutions in China, Taiwan, Japan, Korea, France, and the USA.

This book features the use of acupuncture as a scientifically verifiable treatment for significant health-related issues including analgesia, drug addiction, depression, cognitive deficits, chronic itch, peripheral nerve regeneration, stroke, diabetes mellitus, sleep regulation, and gastrointestinal function. In this book, authors of chapters describe the mechanisms underlying the therapeutic effects of acupuncture in each condition, verifying the millennium-long and subjective experience. Discussions of preclinical experimental results in this book offer indisputable evidence as to how acupuncture modulates various aspects of the mammalian system, often leading to dramatic, measurable, and sustained improvements in disease-related symptoms. This book provides a new direction and guidance as to how the medical community can proceed with acupuncturology in modern prevention and precision medicine.

The editor of this book, Professor Lin, is the first Taiwanese scholar to ever receive a PhD in Acupuncture Science. In 1980, he received the Highest Golden Burnoose Award from the Kingdom of Saudi Arabia. Since then, he has received countless worldwide awards. His long-standing work in the clinic and laboratory has accrued abundant long-term experience in acupuncturology over many years. This wealth of experience places Dr. Lin in a unique position to effectively support the current and future medicinal community, both now and in the future. Indeed, since 2012, Dr. Lin has been recognized as an expert by the WHO and UNESCO; both organizations continue to seek his expertise and advice on acupuncture.

With yet more scientific evidence awaiting publications, I look forward to reading more chapters in future.

Taichung, Taiwan   Chancellor Wen-Hwa Lee

Editor's Preface

I am a medical doctor and also a Chinese medical doctor. I have always been passionate about general surgery, internal medicine, and Chinese medicine. My interest in acupuncture practice led me to work initially in Taipei Veterans General Hospital, where I was assigned to practice and provide medical service in Saudi Arabia from 1979 to 1980. Over my 40 years of practice, I have used acupuncture to successfully treat pain, anxiety, and insomnia and other disorders. Over that time, many worldwide national leaders and famous people have been treated with my acupuncture treatment.

From my understanding, the classic literature describes the effects of acupuncture according to personal experience only. The mechanisms underlying acupuncture effects have not yet been elucidated. Modern medicine needs animal studies to explore these mechanisms.

To answer this need, I encouraged my team of acupuncture research associates from China Medical University, National Taiwan University, and Da-Yeh University to contribute their clinical experience for this book. Their selected topics cover a brief history of acupuncture, how acupuncture affects analgesia, addiction, depression, itch, peripheral nerve regeneration, stroke, diabetes mellitus, cognitive deficits, and sleep disorders. In an effort to make this book even more useful, I also invited contributions from Professor Jen-Hwey Chiu at National Yang-Ming University, Professor Litscher Gerhard at the Medical University of Graz in Austria, and Professor Xinyan Gao at the Chinese Academy of Traditional Chinese Medicine, Beijing, China. These experts have added chapters covering details on moxibustion, laser acupuncture, and the effects of acupuncture in gastrointestinal function. This book has been proofread by Ms. Iona MacDonald, and I would like to extend my special appreciation and thanks to her.

This book aims to provide new direction and guidance on how the medical community can proceed with acupuncturology in the modern era of preventive and precision medicine. I hope that this book will prove to be an important reference for researchers devoted to the study of acupuncture and that it will serve as a textbook of experimental acupuncturology for medical students and clinicians.

Taichung, Taiwan   Jaung-Geng Lin

Contents

A Brief History of Acupuncture: From Traditional Acupuncturology to Experimental Acupuncturology

Chin-Yi Cheng and Jaung-Geng Lin

Abstract

The practice of acupuncture guided by the meridian theory is first mentioned in the *Yellow Emperor's Classic of Internal Medicine*. The basic theories and techniques of acupuncture were established in the Eastern Han Dynasty. The first book to combine the theories and practices of acupuncture was the *Systemic Classic of Acupuncture and Moxibustion*, written by Huangfu Mi. In the Song Dynasty, Wang Wei-Yi designed two life-size male bronze statues, which are recognized as the earliest bronze acupuncture models to be used for teaching purposes. During the Ming Dynasty, *The Great Compendium of Acupuncture and Moxibustion* by Yang Ji-Zhou had a huge influence on the development of modern acupuncture. In the early twentieth century, the development of acupuncture fell into neglect. However, much research subsequently explored acupuncture using modern scientific techniques and methods. From the 1950s to the 1980s, acupuncture gained new life through exploration of traditional theories and modern research. Scientific techniques explored the essence of meridians, acupuncture analgesia and anesthesia, the characteristics of *de qi*, and the phenomenon of propagated sensations along channels. At the same time, the launch of academic conferences greatly advanced the quality of experimental acupuncturology studies. The period from 1980 until now marks an important stage of development in experimental acupuncturology. Since the introduction of acupuncture in other countries including Japan, Korea, France, and the U.S.A.,

C.-Y. Cheng
School of Chinese Medicine, College of Chinese Medicine, China Medical University, Taichung, Taiwan

Department of Chinese Medicine, Hui-Sheng Hospital, Taichung, Taiwan

J.-G. Lin (✉)
School of Chinese Medicine, College of Chinese Medicine, China Medical University, Taichung, Taiwan
e-mail: jglin@mail.cmu.edu.tw

© Springer Nature Singapore Pte Ltd. 2018
J.-G. Lin (ed.), *Experimental Acupuncturology*,
https://doi.org/10.1007/978-981-13-0971-7_1

acupuncture has become more popular, developed rapidly, and has undergone systematic research.

Accumulating evidence reveals the benefits of acupuncture in treating various pathological conditions including pain, cardio-cerebrovascular diseases, neuro-psychological disorders, drug addictions, itchy skin conditions, immune disorders, and diabetes. Further analysis into the mechanisms of acupuncture is needed to determine future clinical applications for acupuncture.

Keywords

Acupuncture · Meridian · Acupuncture analgesia · Experimental acupuncturology

1.1   Historical Events of Traditional Acupuncturology

According to the *Yellow Emperor's Classic of Internal Medicine*, which was written over 2000 years ago, acupuncture comprises an important part of traditional Chinese medicine (TCM) and has been used to treat a variety of illnesses, under guidance of the meridian theory (Zhou and Benharash 2014a; White and Ernst 2004). The meridian theory believes that the *qi* (vital energy) and blood flow continuously through the meridians, which connect with corresponding organs. Acupuncture stimulation corrects the imbalance of *qi*-blood-yin-yang in the meridians and the target organs, and activates the regulatory functions to restore a healthier balance, thereby relieving suffering from disorders (Kong et al. 2007; Yang et al. 2014). In the Eastern Han Dynasty, the famous medical doctor Zhang Zhong-Jing used acupuncture and moxibustion methods under Nanjing guidance to treat various diseases, as described in his book *Treatise on Febrile Disease* (Zhang and Li 1999). During this period, the basic theories and fundamental techniques of acupuncture and moxibustion were established, but the precise location of acupuncture points remained unclear. Later, the renowned medical doctor Huangfu Mi wrote the *Systemic Classic of Acupuncture and Moxibustion* (256–282 A.D.), consisting of 12 volumes with 128 chapters and describing 349 acupoints (Zhang and Li 1999; Jiang 1985). This book details each of the organic meridians, the exact location of acupoints, gives detailed indications and methods of manipulation, and is recognized as being the first book to combine the theories and practices of acupuncture and moxibustion. It is also one of the most influential works available on acupuncture and moxibustion (Zhang et al. 2013). In the Tang Dynasty, the famous physician Sun Si-Miao compiled *Prescriptions Worth a Thousand Gold for Emergencies* (Bei Ji Qian Jin Yao Fang), in which a great deal of clinical experience in acupuncture treatment was recorded (Huang and Huang 2001). Subsequently, acupuncture was established over time as a special branch of medicine and continued to be developed and practiced, eventually becoming one of the most common types of therapy used in China (White and Ernst 2004). In the Song Dynasty, the famous acupuncturist Wang Wei-Yi was ordered by the government to revise the acupuncture classics, with emphasis on acupoint locations and their related meridians. Wang Wei-Yi compiled the *Illustrated Manual of the Bronze Man Showing Acupuncture and Moxibustion Points* (1026 A.D.) and designed two life-size male bronze sculptures, with 354 acupoints recorded on their surfaces. These are recognized to be the earliest bronze acupuncture models for teaching and examination purposes (White and Ernst 2004; Lehmann 2013). At this time, the meridian theory becomes more practical for use. During the Ming Dynasty, *The Great Compendium of Acupuncture and Moxibustion*, written by Yang Ji-Zhou, was published. This book serves as the basis of modern acupuncture, containing clear descriptions of the functions of 365 acupoints represented on the 14 meridians, and has greatly influenced the development of acupuncture (White and Ernst 2004). From the early period of the Qing Dynasty (around the 1640s) to the Opium Wars (1839–60), medical doctors demonstrated the superiority of herbal medicine over acupuncture, which became more and more neglected. Two publications that were released during this time are worth mentioning: the *Golden Mirror of Medicine*, written by Wu Qian in 1742, describes acupuncture in the practical form (Hanson 2003). In addition, Li Xue-Chuan compiled *The Source of Acupuncture and Moxibustion* in 1817 (Soldan et al. 2013), emphasizing the specificity of acupoints and systematically classifying the 361 acupoints on the 14 meridians.

1.2   Historical Events of Experimental Acupuncturology

With an increasing acceptance of Western medicine in China at the beginning of the twentieth century, governmental policies imposed a ban on traditional medicine and forbade its development, leading to the demise of TCM including acupuncture (White and Ernst 2004). However, the enormous need of the Chinese people for healthcare services meant that acupuncture was given a chance to develop and grow once more. At this time, many acupuncturists strove to elucidate the theories of acupuncture using modern science and technology. In 1934, Tang Shi-Cheng and his colleagues published a paper entitled *The Technique and Principles of Electroacupuncture and the Study of Electroacupuncture*, which proposed that electroacupuncture with pulsed current could be used in clinical practice (Fang et al. 2012). This is the first study to combine acupuncture with electric stimulation techniques. In the 1950s, acupuncture gained new life, as modern research began to investigate traditional theories. Acupuncture research institutes were established throughout China and acupuncture treatment became an integrated complementary therapy in hospital care. In addition, the Chinese government launched basic and clinical trials in acupuncture research (Wang et al. 2013). During this period, the study of the physical foundations of meridian channels was listed among key projects for Natural Science Development in China and acupuncture anesthesia was developed on the foundation of acupuncture analgesia (Dong 2013). A new subject was introduced–experimental acupuncturology–a method designed to probe acupuncture meridians and TCM points through the use of modern scientific techniques and experimental methods (Tang 1991). From the late 1950s to the 1960s,

Western medicine theories began to integrate Chinese medicine. Multidisciplinary projects employed modern experimental techniques to investigate the principles of acupuncture therapy, including acupuncture analgesia. During this period, the study of acupuncture analgesia developed into acupuncture anesthesia, which has since been widely applied (Liu et al. 2007; Hu et al. 2009). Meanwhile, research began to use modern techniques to investigate the essence of meridian channels (Ma et al. 2003). In 1965, acupuncture analgesia was selected as a key issue in national scientific studies by the Health Department in China and Professor Han Ji-Sheng began his lengthy exploration of the principles of acupuncture analgesia and acupuncture treatments for drug addiction (Han 2009). This period is therefore recognized as the founding stage of experimental acupuncturology. In the 1970s, numerous laboratory and clinical studies confirmed that acupuncture treatment could be used to reduce levels of acute and chronic pain (Strauss 1987). Furthermore, the discovery of endorphins and natural opiate-like molecules provided evidence of acupuncture analgesia (Strauss 1987). Research has shown that acupuncture needle sensation, known as *de qi*, resulting in numbness, soreness, distension, heaviness, dull or sharp pain during acupuncture stimulation, is closely related to the action of analgesia and anesthesia (Kong et al. 2007; Zhou and Benharash 2014b). Research has also demonstrated that the qualities of *de qi* including speed, intensity and type can influence the effect of acupuncture treatment (Hu et al. 2014). Simultaneously, studies on propagated sensation along channels (PSC) received substantial attention in China (Beissner and Marzolff 2012). A group of "meridian channel-sensitive subjects" were discovered, which generated a moving sensation along the meridian channel in response to stimulation of an acupoint, termed the PSC phenomenon (Beissner and Marzolff 2012). From the 1950s through the 1970s, numerous investigations explored acupuncture, acupoints and meridian systems with use of modern scientific methods, such as acupoint injection (isotope), magnetic therapy, acupoint laser irradiation, measurement of electric impedance, infrared spectrum analysis, and infrared thermal imaging (Yang et al. 2007). In June 1979, the First National Symposium of Acupuncture and Moxibustion and Acupuncture Anaesthesia was held in Beijing (Ballegaard et al. 1986), marking the birth of a new academic discipline, experimental acupuncturology. This period is recognized as being the maturing stage of experimental acupuncturology. After 1982, leading higher education institutes for Chinese medicine in Tianjin, Shanghai, Nanjing, Liaoning, and Shaanxi began to offer courses in experimental acupuncturology. In October 1986, the China Association of Acupuncture and Moxibustion was established in Shanghai, promoting the establishment and development of the experimental acupuncturology discipline. The First World Conference on Acupuncture and Moxibustion in Beijing in 1987 provided a significant advancement in the content and quality of experimental acupuncturology studies (Wang and Liu 1989). The period from 1980 until today is recognized as the developmental stage of experimental acupuncturology.

Ever since the introduction of Chinese acupuncture to Korea and Japan in the sixth century, acupuncture has formed a very important part of their traditional medicine (White and Ernst 2004). Between the 1940s and 1950s, Japanese researchers explored the essence of meridians. Yoshio Nagahama first discovered the phenomenon of PSC in 1946 and reported his findings in 1950 (Zhuang et al. 2013; Li et al. 2012). In 1952, Rokuro Fujita studied the electrical activity of acupoints and meridians and proposed that the main cause of the meridian phenomenon is the transmission of changes elicited by muscle contraction. In 1955, Kazuo Nakatani and colleagues published their findings on "well-transmit sub-meshwork (Ryodoraku)" in the *Journal of the Autonomic Nervous System* and developed the renowned Ryodoraku adjustment therapy (Schmidt et al. 2002; Buts'ka 2006). In 1963, the North Korean scientist Bong-Han Kim declared that the novel threadlike structures (Bonghan ducts) exist on the surfaces of internal organs and could serve as the anatomical basis of acupuncture meridians in human and animals (Shin et al. 2005; Lee et al. 2005). However, Bong-Han Kim's discovery could not be reproduced (Shin et al. 2005).

Acupuncture was first introduced into Europe during the sixteenth century. France was the first country to accept acupuncture and the practice of acupuncture became more popular there after the late 1920s (Lu and Lu 2013; White and Ernst 2004). In 1970, the France scientist Jean Borsarello used infrared thermal imaging to delineate meridians and acupoints in the human body (Wang et al. 2012). In 1984, Hungarian explorations found that meridian channels and acupoints have a higher metabolic rate and carbon dioxide release (Eöry 1984). In 1985, the French researcher Pierre de Vernejoul injected radioactive isotopes into specific meridian acupoints in patients and observed that the isotopes traveled the meridian pathway (de Vernejoul et al. 1985).

In the early 1800s, U.S. research demonstrated that acupuncture was an effective pain-management technique (Lu and Lu 2013). However, the pain-relieving effect of acupuncture did not attract significant interest in the U.S. and acupuncture remained virtually unknown in the U.S.A. until former President Nixon's visit to China in 1972 (Lu and Lu 2013), which sparked a renewed interest in acupuncture in the U.S.A. (Turnbull and Patel 2007). In 1973, the U.S. Food and Drug Administration approved acupuncture equipment as a class III medical device, which could be used only under appropriate research protocols (Medical assistance programs: sterilization procedures—1973). In 1974, the American Medical Association declared that acupuncture belonged within medical treatment modalities (Schwartz 1981). Since then, numerous studies have been conducted in the U.S.A. and other countries exploring the effects and mechanisms of acupuncture under various pathological conditions. The findings that acupuncture stimulation causes the release of neurotransmitters, peptides and endorphins, clearly explained the effects of acupuncture from a modern biomedical and pharmacological basis (Lu and Lu 2013). In the face of increasing recognition and widespread uptake of acupuncture activities, the World Health Organization (WHO) conducted a symposium on acupuncture in June 1979 in Beijing, China and the participants drew up a list of 43 suitable diseases that can be treated with acupuncture (Ma et al. 2006). In 1996, the WHO Consultation on acupuncture was held in Cervia, Italy and selection criteria were developed in a review of clinical studies, and participants listed 64 medical problems considered suitable for acupuncture treatment (Lin et al. 2009).

In recognition of the great usefulness of acupuncture in pain relief, the U.S. National Institutes of Health 1997 Consensus Statement on acupuncture declared that there was sufficient evidence to expand acupuncture intervention into conventional medicine (Lu and Lu 2013).

1.3   Published Literature on Acupuncture

Nowadays, much research seeks to evaluate the effectiveness of acupuncture and the underlying mechanisms of acupuncture treatment. Accumulating evidence reveals the benefits of acupuncture in treating various pathological conditions and its mechanisms are being clarified (Zhuang et al. 2013). In general, acupuncture studies are divided into specific research areas including meridian channels, acupoints, clinical acupuncture, and basic acupuncture. An extensive published literature exists on clinical and basic acupuncture; systemic PubMed searches identify thousands of clinical and basic research papers with "acupuncture" in the title (Hempel et al. 2014). The top three categories of acupuncture, ranked using published clinical and basic acupuncture research, are pain and analgesia, cardio-cerebrovascular diseases, and neuropsychological disorders (Cai et al. 2012). Moreover, there is an ever-growing literature on the efficacy of acupuncture in the treatment of addiction, the role of acupuncture in immunomodulation, and on its benefits in treating itching of the skin, and diabetes. Further analysis is required to clarify the effects and mechanisms of acupuncture in these conditions, to better determine future clinical applications.

Acknowledgment   This study was supported by grants from China Medical University Hospital (DMR-105-007), Taichung, Taiwan.

References

Ballegaard S, Jensen G, Pedersen F, Nissen VH. Acupuncture in severe, stable angina pectoris: a randomized trial. Acta Med Scand. 1986;220:307–13.

Beissner F, Marzolff I. Investigation of acupuncture sensation patterns under sensory deprivation using a geographic information system. Evid Based Complement Alternat Med. 2012;2012:591304.

Buts'ka LV. Analysis of obtained data after electropuncture diagnostics in sportsmen with different professional qualification. Lik Sprava. 2006;(5-6):43–9.

Cai Y, Shen J, Zhong D, Li Y, Wu T. Status quo, issues, and challenges for acupuncture research evidence: an overview of clinical and fundamental studies. J Evid Based Med. 2012;5:12–24.

de Vernejoul P, Albarede P, Darras JC. Study of acupuncture meridians using radioactive tracers. Bull Acad Natl Med. 1985;169:1071–5.

Dong J. The relationship between traditional Chinese medicine and modern medicine. Evid Based Complement Alternat Med. 2013;2013:153148.

Eöry A. In-vivo skin respiration (CO_2) measurements in the acupuncture loci. Acupunct Electrother Res. 1984;9:217–23.

Fang Z, Ning J, Xiong C, Shulin Y. Effects of electroacupuncture at head points on the function of cerebral motor areas in stroke patients: a PET study. Evid Based Complement Alternat Med. 2012;2012:902413.

Han JS. Acupuncture research is part of my life. Pain Med. 2009;10:611–8.

Hanson M. The golden mirror in the imperial court of the Qianlong emperor, 1739-1742. Early Sci Med. 2003;8:111–47.

Hempel S, Taylor SL, Solloway MR, Miake-Lye IM, Beroes JM, Shanman R, Booth MJ, Siroka AM, Shekelle PG. Evidence map of acupuncture. Evid Based Synth Program. 2014; 1–47.

Hu WL, Chang CH, Hung YC, Shieh TY. Acupuncture anesthesia for complicated dental extractions in patients with lidocaine allergy. J Altern Complement Med. 2009;15:1149–52.

Hu NJ, Lin C, Li J, Zhang P, Yuan HW, Qi DD, Hao J, Xin SY, Liu YQ, Li CH, et al. Remarks on the relationship between deqi and effect of acupuncture. Zhongguo Zhen Jiu. 2014;34:413–6.

Huang Y, Huang L. New evidences for adapting Qian Jin Yao Fang (thousand golden essential prescriptions) by Office of Revising Medical Books of the Song dynasty. Zhonghua Yi Shi Za Zhi. 2001;31:78–80.

Jiang Y. Texture research on Zhu Na, the native place of the renowned acupuncturist Huangfu Mi (Chi). Zhonghua Yi Shi Za Zhi. 1985;15:24–8.

Kong J, Gollub R, Huang T, Polich G, Napadow V, Hui K, Vangel M, Rosen B, Kaptchuk TJ. Acupuncture de qi, from qualitative history to quantitative measurement. J Altern Complement Med. 2007;13:1059–70.

Lee BC, Yoo JS, Baik KY, Kim KW, Soh KS. Novel threadlike structures (Bonghan ducts) inside lymphatic vessels of rabbits visualized with a Janus Green B staining method. Anat Rec B New Anat. 2005;286:1–7.

Lehmann H. Acupuncture in ancient China: how important was it really? J Integr Med. 2013;11:45–53.

Li J, Wang Q, Liang H, Dong H, Li Y, Ng EH, Wu X. Biophysical characteristics of meridians and acupoints: a systematic review. Evid Based Complement Alternat Med. 2012;2012:793841.

Lin ZP, Lan LW, He TY, Lin SP, Lin JG, Jang TR, Ho TJ. Effects of acupuncture stimulation on recovery ability of male elite basketball athletes. Am J Chin Med. 2009;37:471–81.

Liu TY, Yang HY, Chu LX, Kuai L, Gao M. The present situation and analysis of acupuncture anesthesia. Zhongguo Zhen Jiu. 2007;27:914–6.

Lu DP, Lu GP. An historical review and perspective on the impact of acupuncture on U.S. medicine and society. Med Acupunct. 2013;25:311–6.

Ma W, Tong H, Xu W, Hu J, Liu N, Li H, Cao L. Perivascular space: possible anatomical substrate for the meridian. J Altern Complement Med. 2003;9:851–9.

Ma T, Kao MJ, Lin IH, Chiu YL, Chien C, Ho TJ, Chu BC, Chang YH. A study on the clinical effects of physical therapy and acupuncture to treat spontaneous frozen shoulder. Am J Chin Med. 2006;34:759–75.

Schmidt J, Sparenberg C, Fraunhofer S, Zirngibl H. Sympathetic nervous system activity during laparoscopic and needlescopic cholecystectomy. Surg Endosc. 2002;16:476–80.

Schwartz R. Yin, Yang and the right to privacy: acupuncture and expertise: a challenge to physician control. Hast Cent Rep. 1981;11:5–7.

Shin HS, Johng HM, Lee BC, Cho SI, Soh KS, Baik KY, Yoo JS. Feulgen reaction study of novel threadlike structures (Bonghan ducts) on the surfaces of mammalian organs. Anat Rec B New Anat. 2005;284:35–40.

Soldan J, Ren YL, Zou P, Liang FR. Textual research of existing block-printed edition of source of acupuncture and moxibustion (Zhenjiu Fengyuan). Zhongguo Zhen Jiu. 2013;33:759–64.

Strauss S. The scientific basis of acupuncture. Aust Fam Physician. 1987;16:166–7, 169

Tang D. Experimental acupuncturology and its role in acupuncture education—suggestion offering the course of experimental acupuncture in acupuncture education. Zhen Ci Yan Jiu. 1991;16:76–8, 68

Turnbull F, Patel A. Acupuncture for blood pressure lowering: needling the truth. Circulation. 2007;115:3048–9.

U.S. Social and Rehabilitation Service. Medical assistance programs: sterilization procedures. Fed Regist. 1973;38:26460–1.

Wang K, Liu J. Needling sensation receptor of an acupoint supplied by the median nerve—studies of their electro-physiological characteristics. Am J Chin Med. 1989;17:145–55.

Wang X, Zhou S, Yao W, Wan H, Wu H, Wu L, Liu H, Hua X, Shi P. Effects of moxibustion stimulation on the intensity of infrared radiation of Tianshu (ST25) acupoints in rats with ulcerative colitis. Evid Based Complement Alternat Med. 2012;2012:704584.

Wang Y, Yin LM, Xu YD, Lui YY, Ran J, Yang YQ. The research of acupuncture effective biomolecules: retrospect and prospect. Evid Based Complement Alternat Med. 2013;2013:608026.

White A, Ernst E. A brief history of acupuncture. Rheumatology (Oxford). 2004;43:662–3.

Yang HQ, Xie SS, Liu SH, Li H, Guo ZY. Differences in optical transport properties between human meridian and non-meridian. Am J Chin Med. 2007;35:743–52.

Yang JW, Li QQ, Li F, Fu QN, Zeng XH, Liu CZ. The holistic effects of acupuncture treatment. Evid Based Complement Alternat Med. 2014;2014:739708.

Zhang Y, Li Z. Discussions on acute pharyngo - laryngeal diseases treated with acupuncture by physicians of successive ages. Zhonghua Yi Shi Za Zhi. 1999;29:166–7.

Zhang S, Mu W, Xiao L, Zheng WK, Liu CX, Zhang L, Shang HC. Is deqi an indicator of clinical efficacy of acupuncture? A systematic review. Evid Based Complement Alternat Med. 2013;2013:750140.

Zhou W, Benharash P. Effects and mechanisms of acupuncture based on the principle of meridians. J Acupunct Meridian Stud. 2014a;7:190–3.

Zhou W, Benharash P. Significance of "Deqi" response in acupuncture treatment: myth or reality. J Acupunct Meridian Stud. 2014b;7:186–9.

Zhuang Y, Xing JJ, Li J, Zeng BY, Liang FR. History of acupuncture research. Int Rev Neurobiol. 2013;111:1–23.

Acupuncture Analgesia for Animals

2

Yi-Wen Lin and Jaung-Geng Lin

Abstract

Acupuncture is part of Chinese traditional medicine (TCM), and is an ancient system of healing that is well documented for its therapeutic effects in pain management. In ancient Chinese medical text, acupuncture is described as the primary treatment for several clinical problems, especially in pain management. In early times, acupuncture was practiced with primitive sharp stones or bamboo that have been replaced over time with ultra-fine needles. Acupuncture is the art of inserting fine needles into specific points on the skin, called acupoints, to initiate a phenomenon such as *de-qi*. *De-qi* is a crucial indicator during acupuncture treatments, marked by some obvious feelings such as soreness, heaviness, fullness, numbness, migration. There are over 360 acupoints located along 14 main body meridians traversing the head, arms, legs and trunk. All meridians are symmetrical, traversing both sides of the body, except for the single meridians known as the Conception and Governor Vessels, which run along the body's midline. In general, it is difficult to associate meridians with any anatomical or physiological structures. However, virtually all acupoints are located in deep tissues with abun-

Y.-W. Lin
Graduate Institute of Acupuncture Science, College of Chinese Medicine, China Medical University, Taichung, Taiwan

School of Post-Baccalaureate Chinese Medicine, College of Chinese Medicine, China Medical University, Taichung, Taiwan

Research Center for Chinese Medicine & Acupuncture, China Medical University, Taichung, Taiwan

J.-G. Lin (✉)
School of Chinese Medicine, College of Chinese Medicine, China Medical University, Taichung, Taiwan
e-mail: jglin@mail.cmu.edu.tw

© Springer Nature Singapore Pte Ltd. 2018
J.-G. Lin (ed.), *Experimental Acupuncturology*,
https://doi.org/10.1007/978-981-13-0971-7_2

dant sensory nerve terminals, suggesting that a strong relationship exists between the meridian points and viscera in relation to nerve connection. It is thought that peripheral A and C fibers may mediate the afferent transmission of the acupuncture signals and ameliorate painful sensation. Recently, the World Health Organization (WHO) reported on the efficacy and safety of acupuncture treatment in over 30 effective symptoms, conditions and diseases. Acupuncture is most often used for pain relief, although it is also used for many other conditions.

Keywords

Acupuncture · Chinese medicine · Inflammatory pain · Fibromyalgia pain · Neuropathic pain

2.1   Introduction

The effectiveness of acupuncture in the relief of pain was first reported in the 1970s by Johnson and colleagues (Johnson 1973). In ancient times, acupuncturists used manual manipulation methods to achieve clinical benefits. Today, electroacupuncture has become more popular, especially in pain management. Recently, several studies have suggested that acupuncture increases the release of endogenous opiates (Han 2003), serotonin (Chang et al. 2004) and adenosine (Goldman et al. 2010) and thereby produces its anti-nociceptive effect. The major mechanism underlying acupuncture analgesia is the release of opiates in the CNS. Transcutaneous electric stimulation of acupoints can reduce opioid intake and opioid adverse effects after intraabdominal surgery (Wang et al. 1997). Pretreatment with EA can reliably reduce postoperative analgesic requirements and side effects of analgesics in patients undergoing lower abdominal surgery (Lin et al. 2002). Manual acupuncture can increase pain threshold accompanied by releasing morphine-like factor and further blocked by opioid receptor antagonist naloxone (Han 2003). Chen and Han indicate that EA analgesia at 2 Hz is elicited in rats by activating μ opioid receptors (Chen and Han 1992). In contrast, EA at 100 Hz can release dynorphins that bind to κ opioid receptors in the spinal cord of rats (Chen and Han 1992). Moreover, injection of κ opioid receptor antagonist reliably attenuates analgesia elicited by EA 2 Hz, whereas the analgesic effect of EA 100 Hz is alleviated by κ-opioid receptor antagonist treatment. Subsequently, mixed-frequency stimulation (2 and 100 Hz) has been used to reduce acupuncture tolerance and increase the curative effect over that produced by single-frequency stimulation (Hamza et al. 1999). Ankle joint mobilization has been found to attenuate postoperative pain by activating the peripheral opioid system (Martins et al. 2012). Opiate receptors not only exist in the brain and spinal cord but also in peripheral sensory neurons (Stein 2003). Paradoxically, chronic opiate administration in humans has been associated with hyperalgesia associated with hyperexcitability and functional remodeling of tetrodotoxin-resistant (TTX-R) Na^+ and transient receptor potential vanilloid 1 (TRPV1) channels of sensory neurons (Ross et al. 2012). In clinical medicine, opiates are the most commonly used and most powerful analgesics available for severe acute and chronic pain. Opiate use is associated with a significant risk of systemic side effects including addiction, tolerance, respiratory depression, nausea, and more. As mentioned earlier, a novel and curative generation of opiates that target the peripheral site, is emerging. Opiates that have a peripheral site of action in inflamed tissue selectively activate peripheral opioid receptors and avoid centrally-mediated side effects. Acupuncture has important advantages over opiates in the treatment of pain, including convenience, low costs, curative ability, and a lower risk of side effects.

Acupuncture has been reported to increase the release of adenosine at peripheral sites (Goldman et al. 2010). Needling can trigger a widespread increase in purines including adenosine and adenosine 5′-triphosphate (ATP), which is consistent with an elevation in adenosine levels after tissue damage. The anti-nociceptive effects of adenosine A1 receptors in both peripheral and central regions are well documented, but these agents are associated with dramatic site effects, especially in relation to the heart. Adenosine A1 receptor agonists reportedly reduce inflammatory and neurogenic pain. Evidence suggests that acupuncture reliably increases both ATP and adenosine at peripheral sites and thereby attenuates inflammatory and neuropathic pain (Goldman et al. 2010). These mechanisms indicate that the adenosine A1 receptor (A1R) is crucial for acupuncture analgesia. Prostatic acid phosphatase (PAP) is expressed in nociceptive neurons and functions as an ectonucleotidase to increase adenosine concentrations adenosine at the peripheral level. PAP reportedly exists in skeletal muscle located near the Zusanli acupoint, and serves as a rate-limiting ectonucleotidase that increases adenosine concentrations (Goldman et al. 2010; Quintero et al. 2007). As a result of this activation, painful peripheral neuropathy is eliminated in mice. Intravenous injection of adenosine can usually relieve postoperative pain and reduce opiate use (Gan and Habib 2007). The antinociceptive effects of PAP were evaluated in preclinical investigations to determine whether PAP sustains A1R activation followed by depletion of phosphatidylinositol 4,5-bisphosphate (PIP2) (Gan and Habib 2007). Intrathecal injection of human PAP (hPAP) can induce A1R-dependent antinociception in preclinical models of inflammatory pain and neuropathic pain (Sowa et al. 2010). The increase in adenosine levels induced by acupuncture has a short antinociceptive effect, peaking at 30 min (Goldman et al. 2010). We urgently need to find a way of achieving prolonged biologic effects from acupuncture. Some researchers have suggested that injection of hPAP at BL40 acupoints provides a novel way of generating longer-lasting antinociception (Hurt and Zylka 2012).

The clinical use of acupuncture is associated with several advantages such as convenience, low cost, and fewer side effects, compared with pharmacologic therapy. In particular, acupuncture has demonstrated high efficacy in the relief of pain-related symptoms. Electroacupuncture (EA) has demonstrated improvements in several spinal cord injury (SCI) parameters: neurologic recovery scores; application of high-frequency EA at 75 Hz to the BL-62 and SI-3 acupoints limits SCI-related damage to spinal cord neurons and axons (Wong et al. 2003); and enhances recovery of bladder function in acute SCI (Liu et al. 2013). In a small study, manual acupuncture at the BL-33 acupoint reduced urinary incontinence in 15% of 13 patients with chronic SCI and improved incontinence by at least 50% in another 46% (Honjo et al. 2000). Almost all patients with SCI will suffer from pain symptoms, especially neuropathic and musculoskeletal pain (Cardenas and Jensen 2006; Widerstrom-Noga et al. 2001). The evidence in these studies suggests the effectiveness of acupuncture for SCI and its complications. Animal experimental models suggest that several potential mechanisms explain the beneficial clinical effects of acupuncture, including a reduction in glial fibrillary acidic protein (GFAP) in the injured cord, thereby inhibiting reactive astrocyte proliferation and reducing glial scar formation (Politis and Korchinski 1990), and a reduction in epidermal growth factor receptor (EGFR) levels, suggesting less scar formation Politis and Korchinski 1990. EA also reduces free radical formation, and down-regulates AQP-4 (aquaporin) expression after SCI, thereby inhibiting spinal cord edema that can produce secondary spinal cord damage. In addition, acute SCI models in animals have shown that EA reduces spinal cord atrophy, with a two-third reduction of anterior horn neuron loss, and reduces the acute stress response as measured by serum cortisol levels (Politis and Korchinski 1990). EA has also shown the potential to enhance spinal cord regeneration, with earlier and higher levels of laminin expression in the injured cord in EA-treated animals (Zhu 2002). Notably, Wu et al. reported that acupuncture reverses elevations in acetylcholinesterase and succinate dehydrogenase and reductions of acid phosphatase in the anterior horn of the spinal cord observed in experimental SCI, which could inhibit or delay the deterioration of those anterior horn cell neurons (Wu et al. 1999). High-frequency EA causes release of dynorphins (Han 2003). In SCI patients with moderate to severe pain, acupuncture improved pain intensity and SCI-related sequelae (Nayak et al. 2001).

Rheumatoid arthritis (RA) treatment includes disease-modifying antirheumatic drugs (DMARDs), which have proven to be beneficial in the treatment of RA. However, DMARDs can have a wide range of side effects, depending on the drug used, such as suppression of the immune system, leading to an increased risk of side effect (Galarza-Delgado et al. 2017; Nam et al. 2017). Acupuncture avoids these side effects and can effectively relieve RA-elicited symptoms and enhance the patient's quality of life, especially in regard to pain management. Acupuncture is noticed to expand joint motion and improve emotion by modulating of immune system, nerve system, endocrine system, etc. The adjuvant uses of auricular EA resulted in significant short- and long-term treatment effects in the treatment of patients with RA (Bernateck et al. 2008).

2.2   Inflammatory Pain

Inflammatory pain is disabling, and difficult to treat clinically. A number of animal models reproduce human inflammatory processes, such as the model of carrageenan-induced paw edema, via complete Freund's adjuvant (CFA)-induced paw edema, capsaicin, collagen-induced arthritis (CIA), amongst others. Inflammatory pain is often associated with peripheral tissue damage, ischemia, hypoxia, acidosis, and aggregation of inflammatory mediators that can further increase pain sensitivity and lower the pain threshold (Steen et al. 1996; Walder et al. 2010). Damaged tissue also releases endogenous inflammatory factors that activate nociceptive fibers or nearby non-neural cells (mast cells, macrophages, platelets, and immune cells). Nerve terminals are induced by the inflammatory mediators to deliver painful signals (Julius and Basbaum 2001).

CFA and carrageenan are most often used to initiate a mice inflammatory pain by injecting into the peripheral site for inducing either cell immune or non-cell immune inflammatory pain (Ikeuchi et al. 2009; Chen et al. 2011; Huang et al. 2013). Increased painful response was induced successfully and can be further divided into two pain subtypes. Painful sensation to harmful stimuli at original injection site is defined as primary hyperalgesia. For example, inflammatory pain sensation can be induced with carrageenan injected into the origin knee joint (Ikeuchi et al. 2009). In contrast, inflammatory mediators induced hyperalgesia to noxious stimuli maybe also induced outside of the injection site and often considered as secondary hyperalgesia. With this issue, both mechanical and thermal hyperalgesia of the hindpaw was induced in mice after carrageenan inflammation in the muscle (Sluka et al. 2007). Both acute and chronic inflammatory pain can be induced and further maintained for 30 days. Pain is not only a single phenomenon but can be separated into different directions. Accordingly, emotional dimension from pain induction can also been associated with the feelings of unpleasantness that can infect unpleasant emotions secondary effects (Price et al. 2001). Pain can be further separated to at least four categories: nociceptive, inflammatory, neuropathic and idiopathic pain. Nociceptive and inflammatory pains are often acute and short-term effect. In contrast, neuropathic and idiopathic pains can be maintained for at least for several months to years. Inflammatory pain models can now also be initiated for a longer time. Investigator can induce different duration of inflammatory pain according to which mediators they injected. Formalin test can be used to induce both inflammatory and non-inflammatory pain at different phase (Hunskaar and Hole 1987), and injection of carrageenan or CFA into the peripheral tissue to induce inflammatory pain. Neuropathic pain is more complicated with multiple etiological factors that caused by damage to nerve fibers by different manipulation. The manipulation can further affect the somatosensory system with a long-term effect. Bennett and colleagues have developed a partial nerve injury animal model by loose ligation of the nerve for the first time (Bennett and Xie 1988). Accordingly, several surgical strategies have been used by using cuts, ligations, freezing to induce neuropathic pain (Shields et al. 2003).

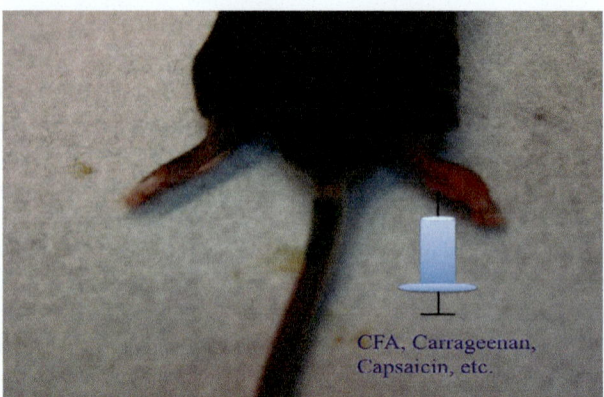

Induction of inflammatory pain by injection of CFA, carrageenan or capsaicin into hindpaw

In acupuncture research, CFA injection is the animal model most commonly used to induce peripheral inflammatory pain (Chen et al. 2011; Huang et al. 2013). Advantages of the CFA model include its high rate of success in the induction of inflammatory pain, convenience, and low cost. The acupoints that are selected for inflammatory pain relief are GB30 and ST36 (as shown in Table 2.1, permit no. 2017-061). Accurately locating those acupoints that are usually used in mice or rats is crucial for EA research. As shown in Fig. 2.1, GB30, GB34, ST36, SP6, and BL60 are usually selected for pain relief as according to advice given in the human's atlas and ancient Chinese medicine.

2.3   Potential Mechanisms Underlying the Effects of Acupuncture in Inflammatory Pain

Recent articles have suggested that EA can reduce pain through a mechanism that reduces phosphorylation of N-Methyl-D-aspartate (NMDA) receptor (Ryu et al. 2008). Other researchers have found that 2 Hz EA at the Zusanli and Sanyinjiao acupoints reduces thermal hypersensitivity of the hind paw induced by CFA injection (Jang et al. 2011). The same result can be achieved by injecting dizocilpine, an NMDAR antagonist. The antinociceptive effects of these single agents may be increased by the combined administration of EA and dizocilpine. Notably, phosphorylation of ERK is increased during the inflammatory process and can be decreased by both dizocilpine and EA delivered to the spinal cord (Jang et al. 2011).

Central sensitization of nociceptive transmission may be initiated in inflammatory, neuropathic, and postoperative pain syndromes, and NMDAR activation may further increase Ca^{2+} influx and activation of second messenger pathways underlying painful sensations. Jung et al. reported that intracellular Ca^{2+} is a crucial target in analgesia associated with 2 Hz EA, and can be modulated through spinal NMDAR (Jung et al. 2010). NMDARs can also be regulated by several protein kinases and phosphatases, and it has been suggested that protein phosphatases 1 and 2A have a crucial role in EA-mediated analgesia through the regulation NMDA receptor phosphorylation in the spinal cord (Ryu et al. 2008).

Table 2.1 Acupoints GB30 and ST36 are most often used for EA manipulation

Injection	Type	Frequency	Amplitude	Acupoints	Behavior	Source
CFA	EA	10 100	3 mA	GB30	T	Zhang et al. (2005)
		10	3 mA	GB30	T	Zhang et al. (2005)
		10	3 mA	GB30	PPC	
		30	2 mA	GB30	T	Zhang et al. (2005)
		60 4	1	GB30-34	T	
		2 100	1	GB30-34	M and T	
		2 100	1	GB30-34		
		60 2	<1	GB30-34	T	
		4 16	0.5–1–1.5 V	GB30-34	T	Wang et al. (2006)
		2 100 alt	1 2	ST36 BL60	M	
		100-4 alt	1	ST36 BL60	T	
		2	1	ST36 SP6	T	Jang et al. (2011)
		1 15 100		ST36 SP6	M	
		100	0.5–1–1.5 mA	ST36 SP6	M and T	
		100	1 1.2 1.5	ST36 SP6	TF	
	MA			ST36	T	
				ST36	M and T	Goldman et al. (2010)
				ST36	FF	

PPC pain-paired compartment

TF tail flick

(continued)

Table 2.1 (continued)

Carrageenan	EA				*M* mechanical
	10	1	ST36 SP6	M	*T* thermal
	2	0.5 1 3	ST36 SP6	T	*FF* flinching frequency
	4	0.6–0.8	ST36 SP6		
	2 15 120	1 2 3	ST36 SP6	T	
	3	1–3 mA	ST36	M	
	1 120	1 3	ST36	T	
	100	2	ST36 SP9	M	
	60 2	1 2 3	ST36 BL60	T	
	10	1.2 3	GB30	T	
			SP6	M	

Fig. 2.1 EA manipulation with steel needles inserted into the ST36 and ST37 acupoints

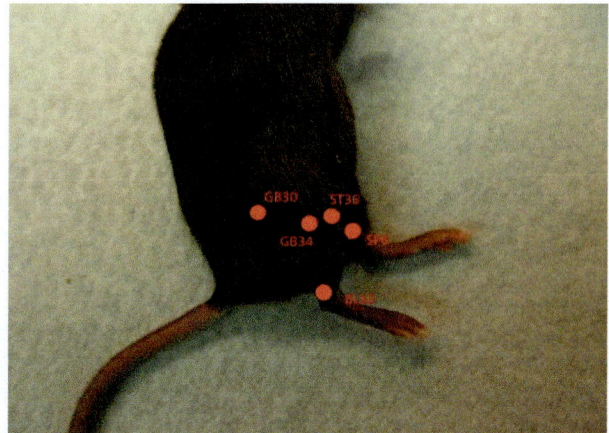

Fig. 2.2 Pharmacological injection of drugs into acupoint

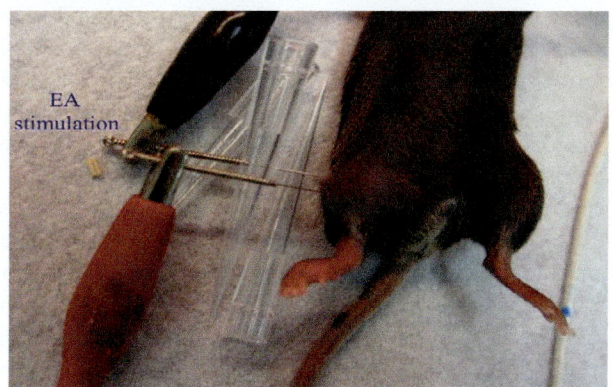

Wang et al. used immunohistochemistry to demonstrate that DRG neurons expressing both IB4 and NR1 are dramatically increased after CFA-mediated inflammatory pain. This increase can be reversed by EA treatment, suggesting a specific role of NMDARs in IB4-positive nociceptive neurons (Wang et al. 2006). Furthermore, medium-to-high frequency EA (10 and 100 Hz) reliably reduced CFA-initiated inflammatory pain, and when EA was used simultaneously with a sub-effective dose of MK-801, the antinociceptive effect was prolonged (Zhang et al. 2005). Improved knowledge about the mechanisms of pain signaling has resulted in the technique of acupoint pharmacological injection, whereby pharmacological agents may be injected directly into acupoints for increased pain relief (Fig. 2.2).

2.4   Fibromyalgia Pain

Fibromyalgia (FM) is a puzzling muscle pain syndrome with chronic widespread and mechanical pain. The prevalence of this debilitating condition is approximated to be 2–8% of the population (five million adults in the U.S.) (English 2014; Clauw

2014). FM is characterized by pain that is spread throughout the body, accompanied by fatigue, depression, memory problems, anxiety, sleep disturbances, and headaches. Chronic symptoms may affect the whole body, and the underlying disease mechanisms are unclear. Research indicates that FM results from an imbalance of several neurotransmitters in the central nervous system, including serotonin, dopamine, and norepinephrine (Riva et al. 2012; Valim et al. 2013). Decreased levels of serotonin have been reported in the cerebrospinal fluid of FM patients, which suggests that central inhibition of pain is reduced (Dadabhoy et al. 2008). Mental traumatic syndromes reduced hypothalamic-pituitary-adrenal (HPA) function, and long-lasting stress have also been associated with FM (Parker et al. 2001). Both peripheral nerve activation and central sensitization may play crucial roles in the development of FM, a chronic pain syndrome that is defined by widespread pain for more than 3 months and the presence of more than 11 trigger points in 18 specialized points (Gerwin 2011). Given the lack of understanding of the disease etiology and the multitude of possible mechanisms, the treatment of FM is complex and many controversial approaches have been adopted, such as drug therapy, exercise, and dietary changes. Currently, there is no cure for FM, but clinicians usually prescribe supporting therapy to ease pain symptoms and improve quality of life. Such treatment includes muscle relaxants, analgesics, antidepressants, and sedatives. Three medications commonly used in clinics for the treatment of FM are supported by the U.S. Food and Drug Administration (FDA): (1) pregabalin, a presynaptic voltage-gated calcium channel blocker that reduces synaptic transmission and thereby attenuates FM-related pain and sleep disturbances (Roth et al. 2014; Smith and Moore 2012); duloxetine, another agent that can ameliorate some FM symptoms, but is not universally effective and is associated with serious side effects (Häuser et al. 2014); and milnacipran, a serotonin-norepinephrine reuptake inhibitor (SNRI) that was designed to treat FM has had moderate success but is accompanied by adverse events, most commonly nausea (Trugman et al. 2014).

The development of treatment for FM has been limited and understanding remains poor as to the mechanisms underlying persistent pain signaling (Vierck Jr. 2006; DeSantana and Sluka 2008). Many animal studies have used a model of FM induced by repeated acidic saline injections into the gastrocnemius muscle (GM). This chronic muscle pain model produces symptoms similar to those experienced in FM patients, with long-lasting, spreading mechanical hyperalgesia, fatigue, sympathetic predominance, and altered central sensitization (Sluka et al. 2001; Pratt et al. 2013; DeSantana et al. 2013). These FM animals are sensitive to antidepressants and anticonvulsants, but not to non-steroidal anti-inflammatory drugs (NSAIDS) (DeSantana and Sluka 2008). FM may result from activation of acid sensing ion channels (ASICs), vanilloid receptor 1 (TRPV1), or others. ASIC3 and TRPV1 are voltage-insensitive cationic channels that are gated by extracellular protons. Interestingly, decreases in tissue pH have been observed in animals with FM, ischemia, arthritis, tumors, or brain trauma, and protons have been shown to activate the terminals of nociceptors *in situ*. Recordings of peripheral dorsal root ganglion (DRG) neurons have shown that extracellular acidification induces inward currents with differing kinetics, ion selectivity, and pH dependence. Although much is known about how ion channels give rise to peripheral sensation and central sensitization leading to FM pain, less is known about the mechanisms involved in FM pain signaling.

Several different physiological mechanisms may contribute to FM pain. NMDA receptors, ASIC3, TRPV1, calcium channels (Cav), and substance P (SP) have all been implicated as having roles (Sluka et al. 2003; Chen et al. 2010, 2014; Chen and Chen 2014). Dual acid saline injections activate the cAMP pathway in the spinal cord (Hoeger-Bement and Sluka 2003). Activation of ERK, a member of the MAPK family, has also been reported in the anterior paraventricular nucleus of the thalamus (Chen et al. 2010). Administration of neurotrophin-3 reduces acid-induced chronic muscle pain (Gandhi et al. 2004), while pregabalin and the M-type voltage gated potassium channel activator flupirtine have also proven effective in treating muscle pain (Yokoyama et al. 2007; Nielsen et al. 2004). The development and maintenance of this type of chronic muscle hyperalgesia is associated with changes in the amygdala and thalamus (Cheng et al. 2011; Chen et al. 2010). However, information about the detailed mechanisms underlying FM remains very limited.

Controversy surrounds the efficacy and safety of opioids for treating FM pain syndromes. Much evidence suggests that opioids offer little help to FM patients suffering from widespread pain, but some FM patients feel relief following opioid administration. In contrast, in an animal model, FM can be reduced by administering μ- or δ-opioid receptor agonists (Sluka et al. 2002), or glutamate receptor antagonists at the spinal cord level (Skyba et al. 2002). However, opioid use is not ideal in humans, due to the potential for tolerance and addiction. Acupuncture may be advantageous in treating complicated FM syndromes, as it has the ability to reduce pain, anxiety, depression, and sleep disturbance (Chen et al. 2011, 2012; Sniezek and Siddiqui 2013; Li et al. 2014; Mao et al. 2014).

2.5   Possible Mechanisms Underlying FM in Mice

Moderate-intensity aerobic exercise successfully attenuates mechanical hyperalgesia induced in mice by acidic saline injection and increases neurotrophin-3 (NT-3) synthesis in skeletal muscle, and thus is an ideal model for FM. The increase of NT-3 is similar to that observed in humans (Sharma et al. 2010). These researchers also describe a significantly greater increase in NT-3 protein in the GM compared with soleus muscle, which indicates that exercise can concisely induce NT-3 synthesis in a specific muscle target (Sharma et al. 2010). Other researchers have indicated that low-intensity exercise alleviates mechanical hyperalgesia in the FM model through activation of the endogenous opioid system (Bement and Sluka 2005). This aligns with clinical phenomena showing a reduction in FM following low-intensity exercise or morphine injection (Hoeger-Bement and Sluka 2003). Furthermore, a recent study demonstrated that injecting acidic saline (pH 4.0) into the GM in rats induces a bilateral mechanical hyperalgesia similar to that observed with FM in humans (ref). These researchers used

EA at 15 or 100 Hz for 20 min on 5 consecutive days at the ST36 and SP6 acupoints. They suggest that there was a significant reduction of mechanical hyperalgesia in response to EA at 15 or 100 Hz.

2.6   Neuropathic Pain

Neuropathic pain is a physiological and pathological process of the somatosensory system that may originates from either the peripheral or central nervous system (Magrinelli et al. 2013). This pain state is characterized by a persistent stressor that can induce biological, physiological, and pathological alterations that further initiate multiple neuropsychiatric disorders. Neuropathic pain can be very difficult to treat, with around 40–60% of patients achieving only partial relief. Moreover, with a prevalence rate of around 6.9–10% and associated high insurance costs, this disorder is a legitimate health concern (van Hecke et al. 2014). Sodium channel blockers, including carbamazepine and lamotrigine, are often used to relieve neuropathic pain such as trigeminal neuropathic pain (Di Stefano et al. 2014; Lauria et al. 2012). In animal studies, sciatic nerve ligation (SNL), sciatic nerve incision (SNI), and chronic constriction injury (CCI) are usually used in neuropathic pain studies (Fig. 2.3). Several different drug classes are used in the clinical situation, including antidepressants, opiates, and GABAergic drugs, all of which are accompanied by several side effects. Acupuncture offers an alternative therapy that is convenient, cheap, and with few side effects.

The threshold for LTP induction in C-fibers in spinal cord dorsal horn is lower in a rat model of neuropathic pain, and the amplitude of field potentials is higher in these rats (Xing et al. 2007). Interestingly, 2 Hz EA delivered at the ST 36 and SP 6 acupoints can reliably reduce neuropathic pain by inducing LTD in C-fibers (Xing et al. 2007), and the analgesic effect is increased by administration of the NMDAR antagonist MK-801 or the opioid receptor antagonist naloxone. Li and colleagues reported that EA has antidepressive and anxiolytic effects in the neuropathic pain model in rats, accompanied by restoration of NR1 phosphorylation in the

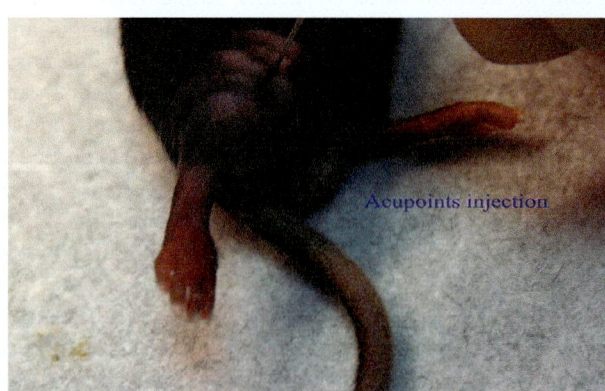

Fig. 2.3 Acupoints that are always used in animal EA experiments

Fig. 2.4 Methods to induce neuropathic pain

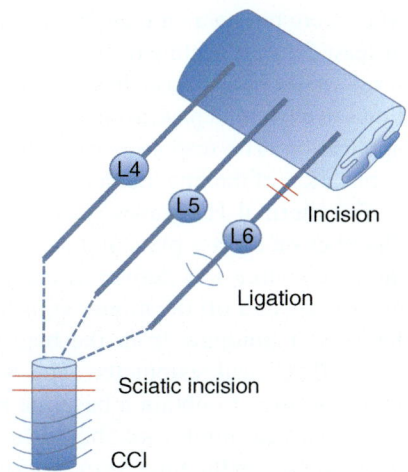

hippocampus (Li et al. 2014). Another study demonstrated that 2 and 15 Hz EA reduces CCI-induced neuropathic pain, accompanied by reductions in TRPV4 levels in the cortex instead of the spinal cord (Hsu et al. 2014). Low-frequency EA attenuates cold hypersensitivity (allodynia) in rats that is mediated by the endogenous opioid, but not noradrenergic, system (Moon et al. 2014). The antinociceptive effect of EA is partly mediated by inhibiting glial cell proliferation (Gim et al. 2011). EA can reduce mechanical and thermal hyperalgesia by simultaneously attenuating the expression of P2X3 receptors in DRG neurons from rats suffering from CCI induction. Evidence has also demonstrated that the analgesic effect of EA on chronic neuropathic pain is mediated by P2X3 receptors in rat dorsal ganglion neurons (Tu et al. 2012). The methodology of neuropathic pain is shown in Fig. 2.4. The most commonly used models for inducing neuropathic pain include sciatic nerve incision, ligation, and CCI. The CCI model reliably induces neuropathic pain by setting 4 loose ligatures around the sciatic nerve. The rats were administered isoflurane anesthesia and the sciatic nerve was exposed. A four 4–0 chromic gut sutures were tied loosely to the sciatic nerve to induce CCI model.

2.7 Animal Behavior for Pain Investigation

Animal behavior analysis is used to evaluate painful responses in animals. The von Frey filaments test and mechanical devices are used for measuring mechanical pain thresholds, the plantar thermal sensitivity (Hargreaves) test, tail-flick test, and the hot/cold plate for evaluating thermal analgesia (Mogil 2009; Langford et al. 2010), locomotor activity testing for fatigue, the open-field and forced-swimming tests for detecting depression.

Mechanical hyperalgesia of allodynia can be measured by testing the number of responses to stimulation with 3–5 applications of von Frey filaments. Furthermore, the electronic von Frey test can be used to record withdrawal force units in grams.

Mice were put on a wire mesh platform fixed in a plexi-glass chamber and allowed at least 30 min acclimatization. A von Frey filament of 0.02 g for mice bending force would be used as a basal stimulation. Fine filaments were briefly applied 3–5 times to each hind paw, average as pain threshold, with a 30-s interval between each application. The responses were then considered valid with an abrupt foot lift on application of the fine filament.

For thermal Hargraves' test, the experimental mice were moved to a small chamber on a glass plate and calm down for more than 30 min. The accrue radiant heat source was deliver directly to the hindpaw surface of mice through the clear glass and till the mouse significantly withdrew the hindpaw. The withdraw latency of hindpaw from the beginning of stimulation could be measured by using IITC analgesiometer. The radiant light intensity was set according to breed of mice to obtain a baseline response with a time approximately 10 s. To avoid harmful injury, we should turn down to machine within 30 s to minimize heat damage to the mice skin. Thermal hyperalgesia was measured 3–5 trials for average. Between trials a 10 min recovery period should be held. The thermal responses were measured and defined as the mean from 3 to 5 trials at each measure time point.

Alternatively, both hot and cold plate can be used for high and low thermal induced pain behavior. After induction of pain, animals were placed and measured parameters using a hot/cold plate (IITC Life Sciences, Woodland Hills, CA, USA). Five minutes of animal behavior were recorded by using a digital camera and were further analyzed offline using a personal computer. For hot and cold plate, we can analyze the duration of forepaw licking, the number of jumping instances, the latency for first jump, paw withdraw latency, paw withdraw number, rearing time and number. The tail flick test is often used in pain research, which is similar to hot plate test, by recording the responses to ho on the mice tail. The light beam is located and focused on the mice's tail and record the tail withdraw latency. When the mice feel the high thermal and flick its tail, the time was recorded as its pain threshold. All pain experiments were tested prior to different kind of pain induction at different timing following injections. All tests should be performed at constant room temperature, and all stimuli should be applied since the mice were calm but not sleeping or grooming.

Conclusions

In summary, based on introduction from this section, we conclude that Acupuncture is effective in treating pain syndrome including inflammatory, fibromyalgia, and neuropathic pain. Here we collective most therapeutic effect acupoints for treatment of different pain. We also introduce several approaches to induce animal pain model such as inflammatory, fibromyalgia, and neuropathic pain. This section further describes the detail mechanisms underlying these pain syndromes. This knowledge will further helpful for doctors and researchers to address pain issue for drug development, acupuncture science, and novel technique investigations.

References

Bement MK, Sluka KA. Low-intensity exercise reverses chronic muscle pain in the rat in a naloxone-dependent manner. Arch Phys Med Rehabil. 2005;86:1736–40.

Bennett GJ, Xie YK. A peripheral mononeuropathy in rat that produces disorders of pain sensation like those seen in man. Pain. 1988;33:87–107.

Bernateck M, Becker M, Schwake C, Hoy L, Passie T, Parlesak A, Fischer MJ, Fink M, Karst M. Adjuvant auricular electroacupuncture and autogenic training in rheumatoid arthritis: a randomized controlled trial. Auricular acupuncture and autogenic training in rheumatoid arthritis. Forsch Komplementmed. 2008;15:187–93.

Cardenas DD, Jensen MP. Treatments for chronic pain in persons with spinal cord injury: a survey study. J Spinal Cord Med. 2006;29:109–17.

Chang FC, Tsai HY, Yu MC, Yi PL, Lin JG. The central serotonergic system mediates the analgesic effect of electroacupuncture on ZUSANLI (ST36) acupoints. J Biomed Sci. 2004;11:179–85.

Chen WN, Chen CC. Acid mediates a prolonged antinociception via substance P signaling in acid-induced chronic widespread pain. Mol Pain. 2014;10:30.

Chen XH, Han JS. Analgesia induced by electroacupuncture of different frequencies is mediated by different types of opioid receptors: another cross-tolerance study. Behav Brain Res. 1992;47:143–9.

Chen WK, Liu IY, Chang YT, Chen YC, Chen CC, Yen CT, Shin HS, Chen CC. Ca(v)3.2 T-type Ca^{2+} channel-dependent activation of ERK in paraventricular thalamus modulates acid-induced chronic muscle pain. J Neurosci. 2010;30:10360–8.

Chen WH, Hsieh CL, Huang CP, Lin TJ, Tzen JT, Ho TY, Lin YW. Acid-sensing ion channel 3 mediates peripheral anti-hyperalgesia effects of acupuncture in mice inflammatory pain. J Biomed Sci. 2011;18:82.

Chen WH, Tzen JT, Hsieh CL, Chen YH, Lin TJ, Chen SY, Lin YW. Attenuation of TRPV1 and TRPV4 expression and function in mouse inflammatory pain models using electroacupuncture. Evid Based Complement Alternat Med. 2012;2012:636848.

Chen WN, Lee CH, Lin SH, Wong CW, Sun WH, Wood JN, Chen CC. Roles of ASIC3, TRPV1, and NaV1.8 in the transition from acute to chronic pain in a mouse model of fibromyalgia. Mol Pain. 2014;10:40.

Cheng SJ, Chen CC, Yang HW, Chang YT, Bai SW, Chen CC, Yen CT, Min MY. Role of extracellular signal-regulated kinase in synaptic transmission and plasticity of a nociceptive input on capsular central amygdaloid neurons in normal and acid-induced muscle pain mice. J Neurosci. 2011;31:2258–70.

Clauw DJ. Fibromyalgia: a clinical review. JAMA. 2014;311:1547–55.

Dadabhoy D, Crofford LJ, Spaeth M, Russell IJ, Clauw DJ. Biology and therapy of fibromyalgia. Evidence-based biomarkers for fibromyalgia syndrome. Arthritis Res Ther. 2008;10:211.

DeSantana JM, Sluka KA. Central mechanisms in the maintenance of chronic widespread noninflammatory muscle pain. Curr Pain Headache Rep. 2008;12:338–43.

DeSantana JM, da Cruz KM, Sluka KA. Animal models of fibromyalgia. Arthritis Res Ther. 2013;15:222.

Di Stefano G, La Cesa S, Truini A, Cruccu G. Natural history and outcome of 200 outpatients with classical trigeminal neuralgia treated with carbamazepine or oxcarbazepine in a tertiary centre for neuropathic pain. J Headache Pain. 2014;15:34.

English B. Neural and psychosocial mechanisms of pain sensitivity in fibromyalgia. Pain Manag Nurs. 2014;15:530–8.

Galarza-Delgado DA, Azpiri-Lopez JR, Colunga-Pedraza IJ, Cardenas-de la Garza JA, Vera-Pineda R, Serna-Pena G, Arvizu-Rivera RI, Martinez-Moreno A, Wah-Suarez M, Garza Elizondo MA. Assessment of six cardiovascular risk calculators in Mexican mestizo patients with rheumatoid arthritis according to the EULAR 2015/2016 recommendations for cardiovascular risk management. Clin Rheumatol. 2017;36(6):1387–93.

Gan TJ, Habib AS. Adenosine as a non-opioid analgesic in the perioperative setting. Anesth Analg. 2007;105:487–94.

Gandhi R, Ryals JM, Wright DE. Neurotrophin-3 reverses chronic mechanical hyperalgesia induced by intramuscular acid injection. J Neurosci. 2004;24:9405–13.

Gerwin RD. Fibromyalgia tender points at examination sites specified by the American College of Rheumatology criteria are almost universally myofascial trigger points. Curr Pain Headache Rep. 2011;15:1–3.

Gim GT, Lee JH, Park E, Sung YH, Kim CJ, Hwang WW, Chu JP, Min BI. Electroacupuncture attenuates mechanical and warm allodynia through suppression of spinal glial activation in a rat model of neuropathic pain. Brain Res Bull. 2011;86:403–11.

Goldman N, Chen M, Fujita T, Xu Q, Peng W, Liu W, Jensen TK, Pei Y, Wang F, Han X, et al. Adenosine A1 receptors mediate local anti-nociceptive effects of acupuncture. Nat Neurosci. 2010;13:883–8.

Hamza MA, White PF, Ahmed HE, Ghoname EA. Effect of the frequency of transcutaneous electrical nerve stimulation on the postoperative opioid analgesic requirement and recovery profile. Anesthesiology. 1999;91:1232–8.

Han JS. Acupuncture: neuropeptide release produced by electrical stimulation of different frequencies. Trends Neurosci. 2003;26:17–22.

Häuser W, Walitt B, Fitzcharles MA, Sommer C. Review of pharmacological therapies in fibromyalgia syndrome. Arthritis Res Ther. 2014;16:201.

Hoeger-Bement MK, Sluka KA. Phosphorylation of CREB and mechanical hyperalgesia is reversed by blockade of the cAMP pathway in a time-dependent manner after repeated intramuscular acid injections. J Neurosci. 2003;23:5437–45.

Honjo H, Naya Y, Ukimura O, Kojima M, Miki T. Acupuncture on clinical symptoms and urodynamic measurements in spinal-cord-injured patients with detrusor hyperreflexia. Urol Int. 2000;65:190–5.

Hsu HC, Tang NY, Lin YW, Li TC, Liu HJ, Hsieh CL. Effect of electroacupuncture on rats with chronic constriction injury-induced neuropathic pain. Sci World J. 2014;2014:129875.

Huang CP, Chen HN, Su HL, Hsieh CL, Chen WH, Lai ZR, Lin YW. Electroacupuncture reduces carrageenan- and CFA-induced inflammatory pain accompanied by changing the expression of Nav1.7 and Nav1.8, rather than Nav1.9, in mice dorsal root ganglia. Evid Based Complement Alternat Med. 2013;2013:312184.

Hunskaar S, Hole K. The formalin test in mice: dissociation between inflammatory and non-inflammatory pain. Pain. 1987;30:103–14.

Hurt JK, Zylka MJ. PAPupuncture has localized and long-lasting antinociceptive effects in mouse models of acute and chronic pain. Mol Pain. 2012;8:28.

Ikeuchi M, Kolker SJ, Sluka KA. Acid-sensing ion channel 3 expression in mouse knee joint afferents and effects of carrageenan-induced arthritis. J Pain. 2009;10:336–42.

Jang JY, Kim HN, Koo ST, Shin HK, Choe ES, Choi BT. Synergistic antinociceptive effects of N-methyl-D-aspartate receptor antagonist and electroacupuncture in the complete Freund's adjuvant-induced pain model. Int J Mol Med. 2011;28:669–75.

Johnson E. CDA assists in oral surgery performed under acupuncture anesthesia. Dent Assist. 1973;42:16.

Julius D, Basbaum AI. Molecular mechanisms of nociception. Nature. 2001;413:203–10.

Jung TG, Lee JH, Lee IS, Choi BT. Involvement of intracellular calcium on the phosphorylation of spinal N-methyl-D-aspartate receptor following electroacupuncture stimulation in rats. Acta Histochem. 2010;112:127–32.

Langford DJ, Bailey AL, Chanda ML, Clarke SE, Drummond TE, Echols S, Glick S, Ingrao J, Klassen-Ross T, Lacroix-Fralish ML, et al. Coding of facial expressions of pain in the laboratory mouse. Nat Methods. 2010;7:447–9.

Lauria G, Faber CG, Merkies IS, Waxman SG. Diagnosis of neuropathic pain: challenges and possibilities. Expert Opin Med Diagn. 2012;6:89–93.

Li Q, Yue N, Liu SB, Wang ZF, Mi WL, Jiang JW, Wu GC, Yu J, Wang YQ. Effects of chronic electroacupuncture on depression- and anxiety-like behaviors in rats with chronic neuropathic pain. Evid Based Complement Alternat Med. 2014;2014:158987.

Lin JG, Lo MW, Wen YR, Hsieh CL, Tsai SK, Sun WZ. The effect of high and low frequency electroacupuncture in pain after lower abdominal surgery. Pain. 2002;99:509–14.

Liu Z, Wang W, Wu J, Zhou K, Liu B. Electroacupuncture improves bladder and bowel function in patients with traumatic spinal cord injury: results from a prospective observational study. Evid Based Complement Alternat Med. 2013;2013:543174.

Magrinelli F, Zanette G, Tamburin S. Neuropathic pain: diagnosis and treatment. Pract Neurol. 2013;13:292–307.

Mao JJ, Farrar JT, Bruner D, Zee J, Bowman M, Seluzicki C, DeMichele A, Xie SX. Electroacupuncture for fatigue, sleep, and psychological distress in breast cancer patients with aromatase inhibitor-related arthralgia: a randomized trial. Cancer. 2014;120:3744–51.

Martins DF, Bobinski F, Mazzardo-Martins L, Cidral-Filho FJ, Nascimento FP, Gadotti VM, Santos AR. Ankle joint mobilization decreases hypersensitivity by activation of peripheral opioid receptors in a mouse model of postoperative pain. Pain Med. 2012;13:1049–58.

Mogil JS. Animal models of pain: progress and challenges. Nat Rev Neurosci. 2009;10:283–94.

Moon HJ, Lim BS, Lee DI, Ye MS, Lee G, Min BI, Bae H, Na HS, Kim SK. Effects of electroacupuncture on oxaliplatin-induced neuropathic cold hypersensitivity in rats. J Physiol Sci. 2014;64:151–6.

Nam JL, Takase-Minegishi K, Ramiro S, Chatzidionysiou K, Smolen JS, van der Heijde D, Bijlsma JW, Burmester GR, Dougados M, Scholte-Voshaar M, et al. Efficacy of biological disease-modifying antirheumatic drugs: a systematic literature review informing the 2016 update of the EULAR recommendations for the management of rheumatoid arthritis. Ann Rheum Dis. 2017;76:1113.

Nayak S, Shiflett SC, Schoenberger NE, Agostinelli S, Kirshblum S, Averill A, Cotter AC. Is acupuncture effective in treating chronic pain after spinal cord injury? Arch Phys Med Rehabil. 2001;82:1578–86.

Nielsen AN, Mathiesen C, Blackburn-Munro G. Pharmacological characterisation of acid-induced muscle allodynia in rats. Eur J Pharmacol. 2004;487:93–103.

Parker AJ, Wessely S, Cleare AJ. The neuroendocrinology of chronic fatigue syndrome and fibromyalgia. Psychol Med. 2001;31:1331–45.

Politis MJ, Korchinski MA. Beneficial effects of acupuncture treatment following experimental spinal cord injury: a behavioral, morphological, and biochemical study. Acupunct Electrother Res. 1990;15:37–49.

Pratt D, Fuchs PN, Sluka KA. Assessment of avoidance behaviors in mouse models of muscle pain. Neuroscience. 2013;248:54–60.

Price MP, McIlwrath SL, Xie J, Cheng C, Qiao J, Tarr DE, Sluka KA, Brennan TJ, Lewin GR, Welsh MJ. The DRASIC cation channel contributes to the detection of cutaneous touch and acid stimuli in mice. Neuron. 2001;32:1071–83.

Quintero IB, Araujo CL, Pulkka AE, Wirkkala RS, Herrala AM, Eskelinen EL, Jokitalo E, Hellstrom PA, Tuominen HJ, Hirvikoski PP, Vihko PT. Prostatic acid phosphatase is not a prostate specific target. Cancer Res. 2007;67:6549–54.

Riva R, Mork PJ, Westgaard RH, Okkenhaug Johansen T, Lundberg U. Catecholamines and heart rate in female fibromyalgia patients. J Psychosom Res. 2012;72:51–7.

Ross GR, Gade AR, Dewey WL, Akbarali HI. Opioid-induced hypernociception is associated with hyperexcitability and altered tetrodotoxin-resistant Na+ channel function of dorsal root ganglia. Am J Physiol Cell Physiol. 2012;302:C1152–61.

Roth T, Arnold LM, Garcia-Borreguero D, Resnick M, Clair AG. A review of the effects of pregabalin on sleep disturbance across multiple clinical conditions. Sleep Med Rev. 2014;18:261–71.

Ryu JW, Lee JH, Choi YH, Lee YT, Choi BT. Effects of protein phosphatase inhibitors on the phosphorylation of spinal cord N-methyl-D-aspartate receptors following electroacupuncture stimulation in rats. Brain Res Bull. 2008;75:687–91.

Sharma NK, Ryals JM, Gajewski BJ, Wright DE. Aerobic exercise alters analgesia and neurotrophin-3 synthesis in an animal model of chronic widespread pain. Phys Ther. 2010;90:714–25.

Shields SD, Eckert WA III, Basbaum AI. Spared nerve injury model of neuropathic pain in the mouse: a behavioral and anatomic analysis. J Pain. 2003;4:465–70.

Skyba DA, King EW, Sluka KA. Effects of NMDA and non-NMDA ionotropic glutamate receptor antagonists on the development and maintenance of hyperalgesia induced by repeated intramuscular injection of acidic saline. Pain. 2002;98:69–78.

Sluka KA, Kalra A, Moore SA. Unilateral intramuscular injections of acidic saline produce a bilateral, long-lasting hyperalgesia. Muscle Nerve. 2001;24:37–46.

Sluka KA, Rohlwing JJ, Bussey RA, Eikenberry SA, Wilken JM. Chronic muscle pain induced by repeated acid injection is reversed by spinally administered mu- and delta-, but not kappa-, opioid receptor agonists. J Pharmacol Exp Ther. 2002;302:1146–50.

Sluka KA, Price MP, Breese NM, Stucky CL, Wemmie JA, Welsh MJ. Chronic hyperalgesia induced by repeated acid injections in muscle is abolished by the loss of ASIC3, but not ASIC1. Pain. 2003;106:229–39.

Sluka KA, Radhakrishnan R, Benson CJ, Eshcol JO, Price MP, Babinski K, Audette KM, Yeomans DC, Wilson SP. ASIC3 in muscle mediates mechanical, but not heat, hyperalgesia associated with muscle inflammation. Pain. 2007;129:102–12.

Smith MT, Moore BJ. Pregabalin for the treatment of fibromyalgia. Expert Opin Pharmacother. 2012;13:1527–33.

Sniezek DP, Siddiqui IJ. Acupuncture for treating anxiety and depression in women: a clinical systematic review. Med Acupunct. 2013;25:164–72.

Sowa NA, Street SE, Vihko P, Zylka MJ. Prostatic acid phosphatase reduces thermal sensitivity and chronic pain sensitization by depleting phosphatidylinositol 4,5-bisphosphate. J Neurosci. 2010;30:10282–93.

Steen KH, Steen AE, Kreysel HW, Reeh PW. Inflammatory mediators potentiate pain induced by experimental tissue acidosis. Pain. 1996;66:163–70.

Stein C. Opioid receptors on peripheral sensory neurons. Adv Exp Med Biol. 2003;521:69–76.

Trugman JM, Palmer RH, Ma Y. Milnacipran effects on 24-hour ambulatory blood pressure and heart rate in fibromyalgia patients: a randomized, placebo-controlled, dose-escalation study. Curr Med Res Opin. 2014;30:589–97.

Tu WZ, Cheng RD, Cheng B, Lu J, Cao F, Lin HY, Jiang YX, Wang JZ, Chen H, Jiang SH. Analgesic effect of electroacupuncture on chronic neuropathic pain mediated by P2X3 receptors in rat dorsal root ganglion neurons. Neurochem Int. 2012;60:379–86.

Valim V, Natour J, Xiao Y, Pereira AF, Lopes BB, Pollak DF, Zandonade E, Russell IJ. Effects of physical exercise on serum levels of serotonin and its metabolite in fibromyalgia: a randomized pilot study. Rev Bras Reumatol. 2013;53:538–41.

van Hecke O, Austin SK, Khan RA, Smith BH, Torrance N. Neuropathic pain in the general population: a systematic review of epidemiological studies. Pain. 2014;155:654–62.

Vierck CJ Jr. Mechanisms underlying development of spatially distributed chronic pain (fibromyalgia). Pain. 2006;124:242–63.

Walder RY, Rasmussen LA, Rainier JD, Light AR, Wemmie JA, Sluka KA. ASIC1 and ASIC3 play different roles in the development of hyperalgesia after inflammatory muscle injury. J Pain. 2010;11:210–8.

Wang B, Tang J, White PF, Naruse R, Sloninsky A, Kariger R, Gold J, Wender RH. Effect of the intensity of transcutaneous acupoint electrical stimulation on the postoperative analgesic requirement. Anesth Analg. 1997;85:406–13.

Wang L, Zhang Y, Dai J, Yang J, Gang S. Electroacupuncture (EA) modulates the expression of NMDA receptors in primary sensory neurons in relation to hyperalgesia in rats. Brain Res. 2006;1120:46–53.

Widerstrom-Noga EG, Felipe-Cuervo E, Yezierski RP. Chronic pain after spinal injury: interference with sleep and daily activities. Arch Phys Med Rehabil. 2001;82:1571–7.

Wong AM, Leong CP, Su TY, Yu SW, Tsai WC, Chen CP. Clinical trial of acupuncture for patients with spinal cord injuries. Am J Phys Med Rehabil. 2003;82:21–7.

Wu Y, Liu C, Chen Q. Effect of acupuncture on enzymology of motor neuron of anterior horn of experimental spinal cord injury in rats. Zhongguo Zhong Xi Yi Jie He Za Zhi. 1999;19:740–2.

Xing GG, Liu FY, Qu XX, Han JS, Wan Y. Long-term synaptic plasticity in the spinal dorsal horn and its modulation by electroacupuncture in rats with neuropathic pain. Exp Neurol. 2007;208:323–32.

Yokoyama T, Maeda Y, Audette KM, Sluka KA. Pregabalin reduces muscle and cutaneous hyperalgesia in two models of chronic muscle pain in rats. J Pain. 2007;8:422–9.

Zhang RX, Wang L, Wang X, Ren K, Berman BM, Lao L. Electroacupuncture combined with MK-801 prolongs anti-hyperalgesia in rats with peripheral inflammation. Pharmacol Biochem Behav. 2005;81:146–51.

Zhu Z. Effects of electroacupuncture on laminin expression after spinal cord injury in rats. Zhongguo Zhong Xi Yi Jie He Za Zhi. 2002;22:525–7.

Electroacupuncture for the Treatment of Morphine and Cocaine Addiction

3

Yi-Hung Chen and Jaung-Geng Lin

Abstract

Opiate and cocaine are two major drugs of addiction. The first report to verify the success of electroacupuncture (EA) in the treatment of opiate addiction was published in 1972. It stated that in opiate addicts, the application of EA to 4 body points and 2 ear points relieved the symptoms of opioid withdrawal. Dr. Wen's method was subsequently modified in 1985 by the US National Acupuncture Detoxification Association (NADA). The so-called "NADA" protocol consists of a 5-point auricular acupuncture. In 2012, we systematically reviewed the evidence from randomized clinical trials published in Chinese and English from 1970 onwards. Most of these trials agreed that acupuncture was an effective strategy for the treatment of opiate addiction. The conditioned place preference (CPP) paradigm assesses the rewarding effects of a variety of drugs. Animal models have demonstrated that acupuncture affects the reinforcing effects of morphine and cocaine. Several animal studies have demonstrated that EA at 2 and 100 Hz facilitates the recovery of ventral tegmental area (VTA) dopaminergic neurons damaged by chronic morphine administration and up-regulates BDNF protein levels in the VTA. In addition, EA has been found to reduce cocaine-induced seizures and death in basic studies. According to the evidence, EA effectively modulates mesolimbic dopamine neurons and thus reduces the effects of positive and negative reinforcement involved in opiate addiction.

Y.-H. Chen
Graduate Institute of Acupuncture Science, College of Chinese Medicine, China Medical University, Taichung, Taiwan

J.-G. Lin (✉)
School of Chinese Medicine, College of Chinese Medicine, China Medical University, Taichung, Taiwan
e-mail: jglin@mail.cmu.edu.tw

© Springer Nature Singapore Pte Ltd. 2018
J.-G. Lin (ed.), *Experimental Acupuncturology*,
https://doi.org/10.1007/978-981-13-0971-7_3

Keywords

Addiction · Cocaine · Morphine · Acupuncture

3.1   Opioid Addiction

Opioid addiction is a chronic, relapsing brain disease that requires long-term chronic disease management and takes a huge toll on society at many levels, directly or indirectly resulting in lost productivity, disrupted relationships, crime and violence, HIV and other infective diseases, and death (Hser et al. 2001; McLellan et al. 2000). Methadone maintenance therapy has been used since the mid-1960s for the treatment of opioid addiction (Dole and Nyswander 1965, 1966a, b; Riordan et al. 1994) and is effective in the long-term treatment of severe opiate dependence (Ward et al. 1999). However, patients on methadone maintenance programs report a wide range of side effects, including constipation, dizziness, drowsiness, dry mouth, headache, increased sweating, itching, lightheadedness, nausea, vomiting and weakness.

3.2   Cocaine Addiction

Cocaine is heavily abused for its psychomotor stimulant properties (Haasen et al. 2004). In 2015, it was estimated that 246 million people—around 5% of all people aged 15–64 years worldwide—used an illicit drug in 2013 (UNODC World Drug Report 2015). The global prevalence of cocaine use is currently estimated at ~0.4% of the adult population. Cocaine use remains high in Western and Central Europe, North America and Oceania (Australia), although there appears to have been a decline in use overall since 2010. In contrast, there has been a worldwide increase in the non-medical use of pharmaceutical opioids. Whereas patients with opioid use disorder who successfully manage to become abstinent through medically supervised withdrawal or other means are offered medication options for long-term maintenance treatment, no pharmacological option has as yet proven effective for cocaine dependence (EMCDDA 2015).

3.3   Acupuncture Treating Drug Addiction: Clinical Evidence

3.3.1   Early Studies

The first report to verify the success of electroacupuncture in the treatment of opiate addiction was published in 1972. Dr. H. L. Wen stated that in opiate addicts, the application of electroacupuncture to 4 body points and 2 ear points relieved the symptoms of opioid withdrawal (Cui et al. 2008).

3.3.2 A Protocol in Western Countries: NADA

Dr. Wen's method was modified in 1985 by the US National Acupuncture Detoxification Association (NADA). The so-called "NADA" protocol consists of a 5-point auricular acupuncture, in which needles are inserted with no electrical stimulation bilaterally into the outer ear or auricle at the sympathetic, shenmen, kidney, lung, and liver points. The NADA protocol relieves withdrawal symptoms and prevents symptoms of craving (McLellan et al. 1993). Auricular acupuncture is used in substance misuse treatment centers worldwide (D'Alberto 2004; Margolin 2003).

In 2005, a protocol was published that describes how to place self-sticking electrodes to the skin at various acupoints, which are then subjected to electrical stimulation to ameliorate the signs of opiate withdrawal and prevent a heroin relapse. This device is called the Han's acupoint nerve stimulator (HANS) (Cui et al. 2008).

3.3.3 Acupuncture Effectively Treats Opiate Addiction: Clinical Study Evidence

In 2012, we systematically reviewed the evidence from randomized clinical trials published in Chinese and English from 1970 onwards (Lin et al. 2012). Most of these trials agreed that acupuncture was an effective strategy for the treatment of opiate addiction. Our analysis groups the most frequently used points or sites for the treatment of opiate addiction according to their locations: points on the extremities: ST36 (Zusanli, 足三里), SP6 (Sanyinjiao, 三陰交), LI4 (Hegu, 合谷), and PC6 (Neiguan, 內關); points and areas on the trunk: EX-B2 (Jiaji, 夾脊), BL23 (Shenshu, 腎俞), EX-HN1 (Sishencong, 四神聰), GV20 (Baihui, 百會), and GV14 (Dazhui, 大椎); and points on the ear: Sympathetic, Shenman, Kidney, and Lung.

3.3.4 Acupuncture for the Treatment of Cocaine Addiction: Clinical Study Evidence

Acupuncture has also been used in the treatment of cocaine addiction (Avants et al. 1995; Lipton et al. 1994; Mansvelder 2005; Margolin et al. 2002), although results have been equivocal, since not all of the research findings were positive (Margolin et al. 2002). Further research is needed into the effects of acupuncture on cocaine addiction, particularly in view of the fact that as yet, no medications provide effective treatment for cocaine dependence (Benavidez et al. 2013).

3.4   Conditioned Place Preference (CPP): Assessment of Rewarding Effects

3.4.1   History

The conditioned place preference (CPP) paradigm assesses the rewarding effects of a variety of drugs (Carr et al. 1989; Schechter and Calcagnetti 1993; Tzschentke 1998). Different designs and apparatuses are used by different laboratories. The basic characteristics of a typical CPP experiment involve the repeated pairing of environmental cues (i.e., the conditioned stimulus) with the stimulus of interest (e.g., drug, food), i.e., the unconditioned stimulus. These conditioned–unconditioned stimulus pairings are inter-mixed with a similar exposure to the other environmental cue without the unconditioned stimulus. Over time, the conditioned stimulus will elicit responses similar to that with the unconditioned stimulus. Following this conditioning, animals undergo choice testing, in which they are given unrestricted exposure to both contexts without the unconditioned stimulus. Increased time spent in the paired environment relative to a control value is considered as evidence that the unconditioned stimulus was rewarding. A wide array of stimuli can condition an increase in preference, including access to "natural" appetitive stimuli of food (Spyraki et al. 1982), water (Agmo et al. 1993), sweet fluids (Agmo and Marroquin 1997), conspecific interaction (Calcagnetti and Schechter 1992), wheel running (Antoniadis et al. 2000), copulation (Meisel et al. 1996), and novel stimuli (Bevins and Bardo 1999). Under the appropriate conditions, cocaine and opiates have a rewarding effect, as indexed by the CPP (Bardo and Bevins 2000).

3.5   Possible Mechanisms for Drug Addiction and the Interaction with Acupuncture

3.5.1   The Ventral Tegmental Area and the Nucleus Accumbens (NAc)

The mesolimbic dopamine system, or mesolimbic pathway, has strong associations with the development of drug addiction. Originating in the ventral tegmental area (VTA) in the midbrain, the pathway projects to regions in the brain, including the NAc and prefrontal cortex (Yang et al. 2008). Drugs of abuse increase dopamine levels in the NAc, resulting in feelings of well-being and pleasure, which positively reinforce the drugtaking (Peoples et al. 1998; Weiss et al. 1992). Conversely, opioid withdrawal reduces dopamine outflow in the NAc (Diana et al. 1996; Rossetti et al. 1999), causing dysphoria and significant distress, which is negatively reinforcing (Weiss and Porrino 2002; Wise et al. 1995).

It is well known that opioids bind with specific opioid receptors in the nervous system to achieve their pharmacological effects. Three principal classes of opioid receptors exist; μ, κ, δ (mu, kappa, and delta), although as many as 17 have been reported, including the ε, ι, λ, and ζ (epsilon, iota, lambda and zeta) receptors. Activation of μ- and κ-opioid receptors affects dopamine neuron activity differently in the mesolimbic dopamine system (Mansvelder 2005; Margolis et al. 2003; Yang et al. 2008). μ-Opioid receptors are expressed upon inhibitory GABA interneurons in the VTA, so the activation of μ-receptors can hyperpolarize GABAergic neurons and disinhibit dopaminergic neurons (Johnson and North 1992), leading to increased dopamine release from the NAc. In contrast, the κ-receptors are expressed in pre-synaptic dopaminergic nerve terminals in the NAc. Activation of the κ-receptor inhibits the dopaminergic neuron, leading to decreased accumbal dopamine release (Spanagel et al. 1992).

By binding to the dopamine transporter, cocaine inhibits catecholamine reuptake and increases synaptic dopamine levels in the mesocorticolimbic system, leading to increased activation of type 1 and type 2 dopamine receptors. The behavioral effects of cocaine are primarily due to the blockade of dopamine reuptake, although cocaine also blocks the reuptake of norepinephrine and serotonin. Psychoactive drugs that lead to addiction generally increase dopamine release within the nucleus accumbens (Yu et al. 2011).

3.5.2   Effects of Acupuncture on Drug Addiction

Manual acupuncture (MA) and EA are capable of triggering a chain of events that has been illustrated by preclinical data. Early studies focused on the effects of MA or EA on the opiate withdrawal syndrome. In a rat experimental model of morphine addiction, 100 Hz EA profoundly suppressed the opiate withdrawal syndrome, reducing wet shakes, teeth chattering, escape attempts, weight loss, and penile licking ($p < 0.05$), while 2 Hz EA resulted in a milder yet still significant suppression of escape attempts and wet shakes (Han and Zhang 1993). EA may suppress the opiate withdrawal syndrome by activating δ- and κ-opioid receptors and accelerating the release of dynorphin (Cui et al. 2000; Green and Lee 1998; Han and Zhang 1993; Wen and Ho 1982; Wu et al. 1999).

3.5.3   EA Reduces Morphine-Induced CPP

Further studies in animal models have demonstrated that acupuncture affects the reinforcing effects of morphine (see Table 3.1). Wang et al. reported that morphine-induced place preference in rats is significantly suppressed by 2 Hz EA and 2/100 Hz, but not by 100 Hz (Wang et al. 2000). Other research has shown that 100 Hz EA significantly attenuates morphine-induced CPP, and that this effect is completely blocked by δ- and κ-opioid receptor antagonists, which suggests that the activation of δ- and κ-opioid receptors mediates the anti-craving effects induced by 100 Hz EA (Shi et al. 2003).

EA at 2 Hz increased preproenkephalin mRNA levels (Spanagel et al. 1992), whereas EA 100 Hz increased preprodynorphin (PPD) mRNA levels in the NAc

Table 3.1 Recent studies investigating the effects of acupuncture/EA on morphine or cocaine-induced CPP

Addiction drug/animal model	Acupoints	Major findings	Conclusion	Reference
Cocaine/CPP in rats	ST36 and SP6 acupoints	• EA at 100 Hz, but not 2 Hz, significantly attenuated the expression of cocaine-induced CPP • EA did not influence the natural place preference in rats • EA 100 Hz inhibition of cocaine-induced CPP was reversed by pretreatment with naloxone 10 mg/kg, but not at lower doses	The effect of EA is mediated by an endogenous κ-opioid mechanism	Ren et al. (2002)
Morphine/CPP in rats	ST36 and SP6 acupoints	• EA of 2 and 2/100 Hz significantly decreased morphine-induced CPP • EA of 100 Hz had no effects on CPP • EA inhibition of morphine-induced CPP was reversed by pretreatment with naloxone 1 mg/kg, s.c.	Low-frequency EA (2 Hz) inhibits the expression of morphine-induced CPP, presumably via activation of opioid receptors	Wang et al. (2000)
Morphine/CPP in rats	ST36 and SP6 acupoints	• EA 100 Hz significantly attenuated morphine-induced CPP • Injection (i.c.v.) of the δ-opioid receptor antagonist naltrindole (NTI) or the κ-antagonist norbinaltorphimine (nor-BNI), but not the μ-antagonist, completely blocked the inhibitory effect of EA 100 Hz in the expression of morphine-induced CPP	Inhibition of morphine-craving induced by repeated EA100 Hz is mediated by the activation of supra-segmental δ- and κ-opioid receptors	Shi et al. (2003)
Morphine/CPP in rats	ST36 and SP6 acupoints	• EA at 2 Hz and 100 Hz suppressed the expression of morphine-induced CPP • EA at 2 Hz increased preproenkephalin mRNA levels, whereas EA at 100 Hz increased preprodynorphin mRNA levels in the NAc	Enkephalin and dynorphin in NAc may play important roles in the mechanisms underlying the inhibitory effect of EA on the expression and reinstatement of morphine-induced CPP in rats	Shi et al. (2004)
Morphine/CPP in rats	ST36 and SP6 acupoints	• Morphine-induced CPP was inhibited by 3 or 5 consecutive sessions, but not by a single session of 2 Hz EA • A test of spatial learning and memory ability using the Morris water maze task revealed that 2 Hz EA exhibited a promoting rather than a deteriorating effect on the ability of spatial memory • 2 Hz EA alone produced a moderate yet significant CPP	Low-frequency EA can produce a rewarding effect. The suppressive effect of EA on morphine-induced CPP is not due to a deteriorating effect on the ability of spatial memory	Chen et al. (2005)

Table 3.1 (continued)

Model	Acupoints	Findings		Reference
Morphine/CPP in rats	ST36 and SP6 acupoints	• In immunohistochemical observations, VTA dopaminergic neuron cell size was significantly reduced in rats treated with chronic morphine, with a concomitant decrease in the number of BDNF-positive cells, compared to saline-treated rats. A much milder morphological change, accompanied by an increased number of BDNF-positive cells, was observed in dopaminergic neurons in the rats that received repeated 100 Hz EA after morphine withdrawal • Enzyme-linked immunosorbent assay (ELISA) confirmed a significant up-regulation of BDNF protein levels in the VTA in rats treated with 100 Hz EA after morphine abstinence	Activation of endogenous BDNF by PES may play a role in the recovery of the injured dopaminergic neurons in the morphine-addicted rats	Chu et al. (2007)
Morphine/CPP in rats	ST36 and SP6 acupoints	• Morphine induced CPP and increased levels of dopamine and its metabolites in the NAc • These effects were reversed by EA	The mesolimbic dopaminergic system appears to play an important role in the mechanisms underlying EA-induced suppression of the rewarding effect of drug-associated environmental cues in the rat	Ma et al. (2008)
Morphine/CPP in rats	ST36 and SP6 acupoints	• In rats treated with morphine for 14 days, a small dose of morphine failed to induce a CPP response. Sensitivity to morphine was reinstated by EA treatments given for 10 consecutive days. The electrophysiological response of VTA dopamine neurons to morphine was markedly reduced in chronic morphine-treated rats compared to saline-treated controls. A substantial recovery of the reactivity of VTA dopamine neurons to morphine was observed in rats that received 100 Hz EA for 10 days	100 Hz EA normalizes the activity of VTA dopamine neurons and has potential for the treatment of opiate addiction	Hu et al. (2009)

(continued)

Table 3.1 (continued)

Morphine/CPP in rats	ST36 and SP6 acupoints	• A single session of 2 Hz EA significantly increased enkephalin levels in the NAc of morphine-induced CPP rats; three consecutive sessions of EA induced stronger effects • Intracerebroventricular injection of the μ-opioid receptor antagonist CTAP or δ-opioid receptor antagonist NTI, but not κ-opioid receptor antagonist nor-BNI, dose-dependently reversed the inhibitory effects of 2 Hz EA on the expression of morphine-induced CPP • Three consecutive sessions of 2 Hz EA up-regulated preproenkephalin mRNA levels in the NAc	The inhibitory effects of 2 Hz EA on the expression of the morphine CPP is mediated by μ- and δ-, but not κ-opioid receptors, possibly via accelerating both the release and synthesis of enkephalin in the NAc	Liang et al. (2010)
Morphine/CPP in rats	ST36 and SP6 acupoints	• A significant preference to the 2 Hz EA-paired compartment • This rewarding effect of EA was prevented by pretreatment with the opioid receptor antagonist naloxone, the CB_1 cannabinoid antagonist AM251, and the D_1 dopamine receptor antagonist SCH23390	2 Hz EA is capable of inducing CPP in the rat via the activation of the endogenous opioid, cannabinoid and dopamine systems	Xia et al. (2011)

(Shi et al. 2004). Enzyme-linked immunosorbent assay (ELISA) confirmed a significant up-regulation of brain-derived neurotrophic factor (BDNF) protein levels in the VTA in rats treated with 100 Hz EA after morphine abstinence (Chu et al. 2007). Morphine has been found to induce CPP and increase tissue contents of dopamine and its metabolites in the NAc; both effects are reversible with the use of EA (Ma et al. 2008).

The inhibitory effects of 2 Hz EA on the expression of morphine-induced CPP are mediated by the μ- and δ-opioid receptors but not the κ-opioid receptor, possibly via acceleration of both the release and synthesis of enkephalin in the NAc (Liang et al. 2010).

3.5.4   Low-Frequency EA Can Induce a Rewarding Effect

Several animal studies (Chu et al. 2007, 2008; Hu et al. 2009) have demonstrated that EA at 2 and 100 Hz facilitates the recovery of VTA dopaminergic neurons damaged by chronic morphine administration and up-regulates BDNF protein levels in the VTA. This suggests that using EA to treat opiate addiction activates endogenous BDNF. CCP testing has also suggested that low-frequency EA produces a rewarding effect (Xia et al. 2011). This rewarding effect of EA is prevented by pretreatment with the opioid receptor antagonist naloxone, the CB_1 cannabinoid antagonist AM251, and the D_1 dopamine receptor antagonist SCH23390, suggesting the involvement of their respective receptors (Xia et al. 2011).

3.6   Acupuncture Reduces Cocaine-Induced Behavioral Sensitization

As mentioned earlier, acupuncture treats cocaine addiction. However, the mechanism of acupuncture in drug addiction remains unclear. In basic research, EA 100 Hz inhibition of cocaine-induced CPP was reversed by pretreatment with naloxone 10 mg/kg, but not at lower doses. The results suggest that the effect of EA on cocaine addiction is mediated by an endogenous k-opioid mechanism (Ren et al. 2002).

A recent study performed immunohistochemical analyses to examine the influence of acupuncture upon locomotor activity and brain tyrosine hydroxylase (TH) expression in rats administered repeated injections of cocaine hydrochloride (15 mg/kg, i.p. for 10 consecutive days) followed by one challenge injection on the fourth day after the last daily injection (Lee et al. 2009). Cocaine challenge substantially increased locomotor activity and TH expression in the VTA. Bilateral acupuncture treatment at the HT7 (Shenman, 神門) point for 1 min significantly inhibited these cocaine-induced effects (Lee et al. 2009).

Mechanical stimulation of HT7 suppresses cocaine-induced locomotor activity in a stimulus-, time-dependent manner, which is blocked by severance of the ulnar nerve or local anesthesia (Kim et al. 2013). Cocaine-induced locomotor activity is suppressed after HT7 stimulation at frequencies of either 50 Hz or 200 Hz. No such effect is apparent through the blocking of C/Aδ-fibers in the ulnar nerve with resiniferatoxin, nor by direct stimulation of C/Aδ-fiber afferents with capsaicin. Kim et al. concluded that A-fiber activation of ulnar nerves originating from both superficial and deep tissue is responsible for the effects of MA at HT7 on cocaine-induced locomotion. Acupuncture has been found to prevent stress-induced relapse of cocaine-seeking (Yoon et al. 2012). Acupuncture at HT7, but not at the control acupoint (LI5), reduced reinstatement of cocaine-seeking and c-Fos expression in the NAc. This study suggests that acupuncture can regulate neuronal activation in the NAc shell to attenuate stress-induced relapse.

3.6.1 Acupuncture Reduces Cocaine-Induced Seizures and Death

Generalized tonic-clonic seizures and status epilepticus are common sequelae of cocaine abuse. Cocaine at higher doses can cause sudden death. Acupuncture is becoming ever more popular as a treatment modality for an array of ailments. We have previously characterized the protective profile of EA on cocaine-induced seizures and mortality in mice (Chen et al. 2013). In that study, we treated mice with EA (2 Hz, 50 Hz, 100 Hz), or performed needle insertion without anesthesia at the Dazhui (GV14) and Baihui (GV20) acupoints before administering cocaine. Following a single intraperitoneal dose of cocaine (75 mg/kg), EA at 50 Hz applied to GV14 and GV20 significantly reduced the severity of cocaine-induced seizures. Moreover, needle insertion at GV14 and GV20 combined with EA at 2 Hz and 50 Hz at both acupoints significantly reduced the mortality rate after a single lethal dose of cocaine (125 mg/kg). In the sham control group, EA at 50 Hz applied to the bilateral SI11 (Tianzong) acupoints did not protect the animals against cocaine-induced effects. In addition, EA at 50 Hz applied to GV14 and GV20 failed to protect against seizures and lethality induced by local anesthesia with procaine. An immunohistochemistry study that investigated c-fos expression examined four brain regions: the paraventricular thalamus, the lateral hypothalamic area, the amygdala and the caudoputamen (Chen et al. 2013). Cocaine 75 mg/kg provoked c-fos expression in each region, while pretreatment with EA at 50 Hz at GV14 and GV20 decreased cocaine-induced c-fos expression in the paraventricular thalamus and lateral hypothalamic areas. Subcutaneous administration of the dopamine D_3 receptor antagonist SB-277011-A (30 mg/kg) failed to affect the severity of cocaine-induced seizures and prevented the effects of EA on cocaine-induced seizures.

This is the first report to show that EA reduces seizure severity and death caused by cocaine. We found evidence for involvement of the D_3 receptor in the anticonvulsant effects of EA. Future research is needed to determine whether intra-anterior paraventricular thalamus injection of a D_3 receptor antagonist prevents EA-induced anticonvulsive effects and antagonizes EA-induced c-Fos expression in the paraventricular thalamus or reduces mortality induced by cocaine.

3.7   Future Directions

Much evidence shows that acupuncture effectively modulates mesolimbic dopamine neurons to reduce the effects of positive and negative reinforcement involved in opiate addiction. Neurotransmitter systems involving opioids and GABA have been implicated in this modulation. However, much remains unclear regarding the action of acupuncture in addiction and this warrants future studies.

References

Agmo A, Marroquin E. Role of gustatory and postingestive actions of sweeteners in the generation of positive affect as evaluated by place preference conditioning. Appetite. 1997;29:269–89.

Agmo A, Federman I, Navarro V, Padua M, Velazquez G. Reward and reinforcement produced by drinking water: role of opioids and dopamine receptor subtypes. Pharmacol Biochem Behav. 1993;46:183–94.

Antoniadis EA, Ko CH, Ralph MR, McDonald RJ. Circadian rhythms, aging and memory. Behav Brain Res. 2000;111:25–37.

Avants SK, Margolin A, Chang P, Kosten TR, Birch S. Acupuncture for the treatment of cocaine addiction. Investigation of a needle puncture control. J Subst Abus Treat. 1995;12:195–205.

Bardo MT, Bevins RA. Conditioned place preference: what does it add to our preclinical understanding of drug reward? Psychopharmacology. 2000;153(1):31–43.

Benavidez DC, Flores AM, Fierro I, Alvarez FJ. Road rage among drug dependent patients. Accid Anal Prev. 2013;50:848–53.

Bevins RA, Bardo MT. Conditioned increase in place preference by access to novel objects: antagonism by MK-801. Behav Brain Res. 1999;99:53–60.

Calcagnetti DJ, Schechter MD. Place conditioning reveals the rewarding aspect of social interaction in juvenile rats. Physiol Behav. 1992;51:667–72.

Carr GD, Fibiger HC, Phillips AG. Conditioned place preference as a measure of drug reward. In: Liebman JM, Cooper SJ, editors. The neuropharmacological basis of reward. Oxford: Clarendon Press; 1989. p. 264–319.

Chen JH, Liang J, Wang GB, Han JS, Cui CL. Repeated 2 Hz peripheral electrical stimulations suppress morphine-induced CPP and improve spatial memory ability in rats. Exp Neurol. 2005;194:550–6.

Chen YH, Ivanic B, Chuang CM, Lu DY, Lin JG. Electroacupuncture reduces cocaine-induced seizures and mortality in mice. Evid Based Complement Alternat Med. 2013;2013:134610.

Chu NN, Zuo YF, Meng L, Lee DY, Han JS, Cui CL. Peripheral electrical stimulation reversed the cell size reduction and increased BDNF level in the ventral tegmental area in chronic morphine-treated rats. Brain Res. 2007;1182:90–8.

Chu NN, Xia W, Yu P, Hu L, Zhang R, Cui CL. Chronic morphine-induced neuronal morphological changes in the ventral tegmental area in rats are reversed by electroacupuncture treatment. Addict Biol. 2008;13:47–51.

Cui CL, Wu LZ, Han JS. Spinal kappa-opioid system plays an important role in suppressing morphine withdrawal syndrome in the rat. Neurosci Lett. 2000;295:45–8.

Cui CL, Wu LZ, Luo F. Acupuncture for the treatment of drug addiction. Neurochem Res. 2008;33:2013–22.

D'Alberto A. Auricular acupuncture in the treatment of cocaine/crack abuse: a review of the efficacy, the use of the National Acupuncture Detoxification Association protocol, and the selection of sham points. J Altern Complement Med. 2004;10:985–1000.

Diana M, Pistis M, Muntoni A, Gessa G. Mesolimbic dopaminergic reduction outlasts ethanol withdrawal syndrome: evidence of protracted abstinence. Neuroscience. 1996;71:411–5.

Dole VP, Nyswander M. A medical treatment for diacetylmorphine (heroin) addiction. A clinical trial with methadone hydrochloride. JAMA. 1965;193:646–50.

Dole VP, Nyswander M. Study of methadone as an adjunct in rehabilitation of heroin addicts. IMJ Ill Med J. 1966a;130:487–9.

Dole VP, Nyswander ME. Rehabilitation of heroin addicts after blockade with methadone. N Y State J Med. 1966b;66:2011–7.

EMCDDA. European Monitoring Centre for Drugs and Drug Addiction [website on the Internet] Drug profiles. 2015.

Green PG, Lee NM. Dynorphin (1-13) attenuates withdrawal in morphinedependent rats: effect of route of administration. Eur J Pharmacol. 1998;145:267–72.

Haasen C, Prinzleve M, Zurhold H, Rehm J, Guttinger F, Fischer G, Jagsch R, Olsson B, Ekendahl M, Verster A, et al. Cocaine use in Europe—a multi-centre study. Methodology and prevalence estimates. Eur Addict Res. 2004;10:139–46.

Han JS, Zhang RL. Suppression of morphine abstinence syndrome by body electroacupuncture of different frequencies in rats. Drug Alcohol Depend. 1993;31:169–75.

Hser YI, Hoffman V, Grella CE, Anglin MD. A 33-year follow-up of narcotics addicts. Arch Gen Psychiatry. 2001;58:503–8.

Hu L, Chu NN, Sun LL, Zhang R, Han JS, Cui CL. Electroacupuncture treatment reverses morphine-induced physiological changes in dopaminergic neurons within the ventral tegmental area. Addict Biol. 2009;14:431–7.

Johnson SW, North RA. Opioids excite dopamine neurons by hyperpolarization of local interneurons. J Neurosci. 1992;12:483–8.

Kim SA, Lee BH, Bae JH, Kim KJ, Steffensen SC, Ryu YH, Leem JW, Yang CH, Kim HY. Peripheral afferent mechanisms underlying acupuncture inhibition of cocaine behavioral effects in rats. PLoS One. 2013;8:e81018.

Lee B, Han SM, Shim I. Acupuncture attenuates cocaine-induced expression of behavioral sensitization in rats: possible involvement of the dopaminergic system in the ventral tegmental area. Neurosci Lett. 2009;449:128–32.

Liang J, Ping XJ, Li YJ, Ma YY, Wu LZ, Han JS, Cui CL. Morphine-induced conditioned place preference in rats is inhibited by electroacupuncture at 2 Hz: role of enkephalin in the nucleus accumbens. Neuropharmacology. 2010;58:233–40.

Lin JG, Chan YY, Chen YH. Acupuncture for the treatment of opiate addiction. Evid Based Complement Alternat Med. 2012;2012:739045.

Lipton DS, Brewington V, Smith M. Acupuncture for crack-cocaine detoxification: experimental evaluation of efficacy. J Subst Abus Treat. 1994;11:205–15.

Ma YY, Shi XD, Han JS, Cui CL. Peripheral electrical stimulation-induced suppression of morphine-induced CCP in rats: a role for dopamine in the nucleus accumbens. Brain Res. 2008;1212:63–70.

Mansvelder HD. Yin and yang of VTA opioid signaling. Focus on "both kappa and mu opioid agonists inhibit glutamatergic input to ventral tegmental area neurons". J Neurophysiol. 2005;93:3046–7.

Margolin A. Acupuncture for substance abuse. Curr Psychiatry Rep. 2003;5:333–9.

Margolin A, Kleber HD, Avants SK, Konefal J, Gawin F, Stark E, Sorensen J, Midkiff E, Wells E, Jackson TR, et al. Acupuncture for the treatment of cocaine addiction: a randomized controlled trial. JAMA. 2002;287:55–63.

Margolis EB, Hjelmstad GO, Bonci A, Fields HL. Kappa-opioid agonists directly inhibit midbrain dopaminergic neurons. J Neurosci. 2003;23:9981–6.

McLellan AT, Grossman DS, Blaine JD, Haverkos HW. Acupuncture treatment for drug abuse: a technical review. J Subst Abus Treat. 1993;10:569–76.

McLellan AT, Lewis DC, O'Brien CP, Kleber HD. Drug dependence, a chronic medical illness: implications for treatment, insurance, and outcomes evaluation. JAMA. 2000;284:1689–95.

Meisel RL, Joppa MA, Rowe RK. Dopamine receptor antagonists attenuate conditioned place preference following sexual behavior in female Syrian hamsters. Eur J Pharmacol. 1996;309:21–4.

Peoples LL, Uzwiak AJ, Guyette FX, West MO. Tonic inhibition of single nucleus accumbens neurons in the rat: a predominant but not exclusive firing pattern induced by cocaine self-administration sessions. Neuroscience. 1998;86:13–22.

Ren YH, Wang B, Luo F, Cui CL, Zheng JW, Han JS. Peripheral electric stimulation attenuates the expression of cocaine-induced place preference in rats. Brain Res. 2002;957:129–35.

Riordan C, Frances R, Isbell P, Khantzian E, Kosten T, Meyer R, Cabaj R, Blume S, Fullilove M, Greenfield S. Position statement on methadone maintenance treatment. Am J Psychiatry. 1994;151:792–4.

Rossetti ZL, Isola D, De Vry J, Fadda F. Effects of nimodipine on extracellular dopamine levels in the rat nucleus accumbens in ethanol withdrawal. Neuropharmacology. 1999;38:1361–9.

Schechter MD, Calcagnetti DJ. Trends in place preference conditioning with a cross-indexed bibliography; 1957-1991. Neurosci Biobehav Rev. 1993;17:21–41.

Shi XD, Ren W, Wang GB, Luo F, Han JS, Cui CL. Brain opioid-receptors are involved in mediating peripheral electric stimulation-induced inhibition of morphine conditioned place preference in rats. Brain Res. 2003;981:23–9.

Shi XD, Wang GB, Ma YY, Ren W, Luo F, Cui CL, Han JS. Repeated peripheral electrical stimulations suppress both morphine-induced CPP and reinstatement of extinguished CPP in rats: accelerated expression of PPE and PPD mRNA in NAc implicated. Brain Res Mol Brain Res. 2004;130:124–33.

Spanagel R, Herz A, Shippenberg TS. Opposing tonically active endogenous opioid systems modulate the mesolimbic dopaminergic pathway. Proc Natl Acad Sci U S A. 1992;89:2046–50.

Spyraki C, Fibiger HC, Phillips AG. Attenuation by haloperidol of place preference conditioning using food reinforcement. Psychopharmacology. 1982;77:379–82.

Tzschentke TM. Measuring reward with the conditioned place preference paradigm: a comprehensive review of drug effects, recent progress and new issues. Prog Neurobiol. 1998;56:613–72.

UNODC World Drug Report 2015. United Nations Office on Drugs and Crime, Vienna, Austria; 2015.

Wang B, Luo F, Xia YQ, Han JS. Peripheral electric stimulation inhibits morphine-induced place preference in rats. Neuroreport. 2000;11:1017–20.

Ward J, Hall W, Mattick RP. Role of maintenance treatment in opioid dependence. Lancet. 1999;353:221–6.

Weiss F, Porrino LJ. Behavioral neurobiology of alcohol addiction: recent advances and challenges. J Neurosci. 2002;22:3332–7.

Weiss F, Paulus MP, Lorang MT, Koob GF. Increases in extracellular dopamine in the nucleus accumbens by cocaine are inversely related to basal levels: effects of acute and repeated administration. J Neurosci. 1992;12:4372–80.

Wen HL, Ho WK. Suppression of withdrawal symptoms by dynorphin in heroin addicts. Eur J Pharmacol. 1982;82:183–6.

Wise RA, Newton P, Leeb K, Burnette B, Pocock D, Justice JB Jr. Fluctuations in nucleus accumbens dopamine concentration during intravenous cocaine self-administration in rats. Psychopharmacology. 1995;120:10–20.

Wu LZ, Cui CL, Tian JB, Ji D, Han JS. Suppression of morphine withdrawal by electroacupuncture in rats: dynorphin and kappa-opioid receptor implicated. Brain Res. 1999;851:290–6.

Xia W, Chu NN, Liang J, Li YJ, Zhang R, Han JS, Cui CL. Electroacupuncture of 2 Hz has a rewarding effect: evidence from a conditioned place preference study in rats. Evid Based Complement Alternat Med. 2011;2011:730514.

Yang CH, Lee BH, Sohn SH. A possible mechanism underlying the effectiveness of acupuncture in the treatment of drug addiction. Evid Based Complement Alternat Med. 2008;5:257–66.

Yoon SS, Yang EJ, Lee BH, Jang EY, Kim HY, Choi SM, Steffensen SC, Yang CH. Effects of acupuncture on stress-induced relapse to cocaine-seeking in rats. Psychopharmacology. 2012;222:303–11.

Yu JS, Shen KH, Chen WC, Her JS, Hsieh CL. Effects of electroacupuncture on benign prostate hyperplasia patients with lower urinary tract symptoms: a single-blinded, randomized controlled trial. Evid Based Complement Alternat Med. 2011;2011:303198.

Acupuncture Treatment in Depression

4

Kuan-Pin Su, Li-Wei Chou, Mao-Feng Sun, and Jaung-Geng Lin

Abstract

Clinical evidence increasingly supports acupuncture treatment for depression. However, efficacy evaluations are beset by many critical challenges relating to the limited range of study designs and important conceptual differences between Chinese and Western medical systems. Recently, clinical researchers have attempted to overcome these problems by using a standard research approach for acupuncture designed to be appropriate for use in randomized controlled trials (RCTs) and also within the conceptual framework that is used in traditional Chinese medicine (TCM). This review summarizes and discusses the existing evidence-based medicine. The analysis examined data from 26 RCTs (involving a total of 2618 patients) that investigated the effectiveness of

K.-P. Su
Graduate Institute of Neural and Cognitive Sciences, School of Medicine, China Medical University, Taichung, Taiwan

Department of Psychiatry and Mind-Body Research Center, China Medical University Hospital, Taichung, Taiwan

L.-W. Chou
Department of Physical Medicine and Rehabilitation, China Medical University Hospital, Taichung, Taiwan

Graduate Institute of Acupuncture Science, College of Chinese Medicine, China Medical University, Taichung, Taiwan

M.-F. Sun
School of Chinese Medicine, College of Chinese Medicine, China Medical University, Taichung, Taiwan

Department of Chinese Medicine, China Medical University Hospital, Taichung, Taiwan

J.-G. Lin (✉)
School of Chinese Medicine, College of Chinese Medicine, China Medical University, Taichung, Taiwan
e-mail: jglin@mail.cmu.edu.tw

© Springer Nature Singapore Pte Ltd. 2018
J.-G. Lin (ed.), *Experimental Acupuncturology*,
https://doi.org/10.1007/978-981-13-0971-7_4

manual, laser or electroacupuncture treatment, used as monotherapy or as augmentation therapy in patients with depression. The evidence supports the use of acupuncture as a safe and promising therapy. The antidepressant effects of acupuncture can be explained biologically in terms of regulating functions and effects upon monoamine neurotransmitters, anti-inflammation, and neuroplasticity. However, significant placebo effects exist in all of the included studies. In order to decrease the placebo effect, a more appropriate study design for comparing verum and sham acupunctures might be to compare active and inactive stimulation with laser acupuncture and with electroacupuncture. Depression is a heterogeneous disorder. For future research, it is important that clinical trials include TCM personalized medicine and that they identify subtypes of depressed patients that would best suit specific styles and techniques of acupuncture.

Keywords

Acupuncture · Depression · Randomized controlled trials · Traditional Chinese medicine · Psychiatric disorder · Biological mechanism

4.1   Introduction

Major depressive disorder (MDD) is a serious psychiatric illness with a high lifetime prevalence rate of up to one-tenth or one-fifth and a disease that causes significant loss of productivity, functional decline, and higher risk of mortality (WHO 1999; Wittchen 2012). The growing burden of MDD is as evidenced by the projection that depression will become a leading cause of disease or injury worldwide by 2020 (Murray and Lopez 1997). Importantly, depression has been identified as being the leading cause of disability worldwide and a major contributor to the overall global burden of disease (WHO 2016). Despite the availability of numerous antidepressants with different mechanisms of action, their clinical efficacy in the treatment of MDD remains poor for clinicians and patients alike (Su 2012; Su et al. 2013), which makes this illness very difficult to treat and burdensome to patients and their families. Current conventional antidepressant treatments fail to meet clinical needs in the real world and are limited by their reliance upon pharmacotherapy. Depression is highly heterogeneous, marked by inconsistent responses to treatment and very small therapeutic effects. It is critically important that novel and alternative treatments are developed for depression (Chen et al. 2011; Chiu et al. 2008; Su et al. 2013).

While there is increasing clinical evidence in support of the use of acupuncture in the treatment of depression, efficacy evaluations pose many critical challenges due to inherent limitations in study designs and important conceptual differences between Chinese and Western medical systems. Recent attempts to overcome these problems include the introduction of a standard research approach that is designed for adaptation into RCTs while still respecting the acupuncture conceptual framework that is part of traditional Chinese medicine (TCM). The purpose of this review is to summarize and discuss the existing evidence on the effectiveness and mechanisms of acupuncture therapy for depression.

4.2   Major Depressive Disorder

4.2.1   Clinical Manifestations

The term depression encompasses a wide spectrum of conditions, ranging from a functional emotional reaction to an incapacitating clinical status. It can be differentiated from a normal status of a transient sad mood response, to a symptom of various psychiatric disorders. Whereas classic severe depression is seldom associated with an external precipitating cause, other forms of depression are often related to stressful life events. Furthermore, clinical depression does not usually remit when the external cause of these emotions dissipates and the mood is disproportionate to the cause. However, it is difficult to draw clear distinctions between depressive states associated with or without precipitating psychosocial factors.

A clinical definition of depression requires patients to have the following manifestation: (1) strong sad feelings or no strong feelings, (2) guilty, helpless or hopeless feelings, or (3) a loss of interest in life. The diagnosis of depression is based on a mental status examination performed by experienced psychiatrists. Confirmation of the pathological state cannot be relied upon using evidence from self-rating scales or nonprofessionals (Chang et al. 2014b). The diagnosis of MDD requires a distinct change of mood that is accompanied by at least several psychophysiological changes, such as loss of interest or pleasure in activities, disturbances in sleep, appetite, or sexual desire, loss of the ability to experience pleasure in work or with friends; suicidal thoughts, and slowing of speech and action (American Psychiatric Association 1994).

4.2.2   Biological Mechanisms

Depression is a highly heterogeneous disorder with a variable course, inconsistent response to treatment, and no clearly established pathological mechanism. Several etiological hypotheses have been proposed that are supported by both preclinical and clinical evidence (Belmaker and Agam 2008; Krishnan and Nestler 2008). The most widely accepted hypothesis is the monoamine theory, supported by the finding that many antidepressant agents produced their antidepressant effects by inhibiting reuptake of monoamine neurotransmission (Berton and Nestler 2006). The serotonergic and noradrenergic systems originate in the nuclei raphes and locus coeruleus, respectively, and project over almost the entire brain, suggesting that they are capable of modulating many areas of feeling, thinking, and behaviors (Stahl and Briley 2004). No specific biomarkers are available for clinical application for diagnosis of serotonin dysregulation in patients with depression. However, several studies have shown that the common polymorphic variant of the serotonin transporter–linked polymorphic region (5-HTTLPR) causes reduced uptake of the neurotransmitter serotonin into the presynaptic cells in the brain and confers a predisposition to depression (Pezawas et al. 2005). In a well-known representative birth cohort study, the 5-HTTLPR was found to moderate the influence of stressful life events upon depression. Individuals with one or two copies of the short allele of the 5-HTTLPR exhibited more depressive symptoms, were more likely to be diagnosed with depression, and be suicidal in relation to stressful life events than individuals homozygous for the long allele (Caspi et al. 2003). This epidemiological study provides evidence of a gene-by-environment interaction, in which an individual's response to environmental insults is moderated by his or her genetic makeup.

A second commonly investigated theory suggests that depression is associated with impaired neuroplasticity and hippocampal neurogenesis (Duman et al. 1999; Santarelli et al. 2003). Furthermore, animal studies suggest that the behavioral effects of chronic antidepressants may be mediated by an induction of neuroplasticity and neurogenesis in the brain (Santarelli et al. 2003). The hypothalamic-pituitary-adrenal (HPA) axis is involved in dysregulation of neuroplasticity and neurogenesis and pathogenesis of depression (Pariante and Miller 2001). Physical or psychological stress is perceived by the cortical brain and transmitted to the hypothalamus, where corticotropin-releasing hormone (CRH) is released onto pituitary receptors that then stimulate the secretion of corticotropin into plasma and activate the corticotropin receptors in the adrenal cortex to release the glucocorticoid cortisol. Evidence shows that cortisol and CRH are involved in depression (Belmaker and Agam 2008; Pariante and Miller 2001). Excess glucocorticoids reduce neurogenesis and induce atrophic changes in hippocampal subregions (Popoli et al. 2012), which contribute to the hippocampal volume reductions seen in depression (Duman and Charney 1999; Sapolsky 2000).

Accumulating evidence suggests that depression might be associated with activated inflammatory processes: e.g., depressed patients with elevated C-reactive protein (CRP), acute phase proteins, and pro-inflammatory cytokines (Maes et al. 2011; Raison et al. 2006; Su 2009, 2012). Children exposed to early-life adverse experiences display enduring low-grade systemic inflammation in adulthood (Danese et al. 2008), which is not only a risk factor for depression but also a feature of chronic physical diseases. The 'inflammation theory' explains the high comorbidity of physical illness in depression as a potential "interface between mind and body" (Su 2008). This theory is supported by the fact that interferon-alpha (IFN-α) induces clinical depression in up to 30% of patients with chronic hepatitis C virus infection (Su et al. 2010). Furthermore, our research has confirmed the notion that using an anti-inflammatory strategy such as omega-3 polyunsaturated fatty acids acts as an effective antidepressant in patients with depression (Chang et al. 2014a; Chen et al. 2008; Lin et al. 2010, 2012; Su et al. 2008, 2014). Several biological mechanisms potentially play a role in this clinical phenomenon. For example, microglia, the resident macrophages of the brain, up-regulate expression of detrimental factors of reactive oxygen species such as nitric oxide via inducible nitric oxide synthase (iNOS) and induce oxidative stress, thereby contributing to the pathogenesis of depression (Lu et al. 2013; Talarowska et al. 2014a, b). In contrast, anti-oxidative enzymes such as heme oxygenase-1 (HO-1) can reverse oxidative stress and may characterize antidepressant mechanisms (Gozzelino et al. 2010; Lu et al. 2010).

Interaction exists amongst the major dysfunctions in psycho-immuno-endocrinology in depression (Su 2012). For example, neuroinflammation reduces survival of serotonergic neurons (Hochstrasser et al. 2011) and decreases neurogenesis (Song and Wang 2011), while antidepressants exert neuroprotection against microglia-mediated neurotoxicity (Zhang et al. 2012a). Inflammation has been reported to predict development of depressive symptoms (Bonaccorso et al. 2001; Su 2012). Cerebrospinal fluid (CSF) concentrations of 5-hydroxyindoleacetic acid (5-HIAA) are associated with depressive symptoms induced by IFN-α (Raison et al. 2009). Other findings from studies investigating the inflammation theory provide mechanistic insights by examining biomarkers such as plasma adrenocorticotropic hormone (ACTH), cortisol (Capuron et al. 2003b), and serum tryptophan concentrations (Capuron et al. 2003a), and even alterations in brain function, as revealed in functional imaging (Capuron et al. 2005).

4.2.3 Current Antidepressant Treatments Fail to Meet Clinical Needs

Clinical features, biological markers, and treatment outcomes are heterogeneous in depression. Thus, current diagnostic schemas contribute to difficulties in finding any reliable biological marker (Su and Balanzá-Martínez 2013). The heterogeneity of depression could also be reflected by the current classification system of monoamine reuptake mechanisms for antidepressant agents. For example, the selective serotonin reuptake inhibitors (SSRIs) and serotonin-norepinephrine reuptake inhibitors (SNRIs) are the most commonly prescribed antidepressant agents. However, tianepine, which enhances serotonin reuptake, is also approved as an antidepressant treatment. Furthermore, other antidepressant agents have no involvement with serotonin reuptake, such as the norepinephrine-dopamine reuptake inhibitors (NDRIs) and second-generation antipsychotics (SGAs). The existing evidence surrounding serotonin, norepinephrine and dopamine implies that the 'monoamine hypothesis' fails to elucidate the etiology of depression (Su 2012).

Current conventional treatments for depression rely mainly on pharmacotherapy, but the outcomes from numerous large-scale clinical trials and meta-analytic reviews fail clinical needs in the real world. For example, SSRIs are considered to be the first-line pharmacotherapy for MDD. However, only 27% of MDD patients remitted after a 14-week, persistent and vigorous treatment regime in the Sequenced Treatment Alternatives to Relieve Depression (STAR*D) study (Rush 2007; Trivedi et al. 2006). In addition, one-third of patients remained significantly ill after 1-year-long, 4-stage, drug and non-drug treatments (Gaynes et al. 2008; Sinyor et al. 2010). Unfortunately, physicians still rely on "trial-and-error" when seeking the most appropriate medication for an individual patient (Santen et al. 2011). The current situation of under-treatment and under-effectiveness of available therapies is considered to be even worse in reality, because many patients refuse to take medications due to adverse effects and stigma relating to drug therapies.

The pathophysiology of depression is poorly understood, but is increasingly recognized as complex and multifactorial. According to the diagnostic criteria in the *Diagnostic and Statistical Manual of Mental Disorders*, 5th Edition (DSM-5), and the *International Statistical Classification of Diseases and Related Health Problems*, 10th Revision (ICD-10), individuals within the same diagnostic categories of MDD can have distinctly different clinical manifestations (Chang et al. 2014b). Furthermore, the diagnostic classification does not provide reliable or predictive effects as to treatment efficacy and/or occurrence of treatment-related adverse effects. Accordingly, unsatisfactory outcomes of all antidepressant therapies coupled with the small-to-moderate effect sizes from all biomarker studies and clinical trials makes it impossible to use a single hypothesis to explain the etiology of MDD. It is critically important that new treatments are developed for depression.

4.2.4 Chinese Medicine Theory in Depression

Traditional Chinese medicine (TCM) is based on individual patients' patterns of diagnoses. In TCM theory, eight major parameters, *yin (陰)* and *yang (陽)*, *external (表)* and *internal (裡)*, *cold (寒)* and *hot (熱)*, and *deficiency (虛)* and *excess (實)*, describe the patterns of bodily disharmony. Additional systems, such as *qi (氣)*, *blood (血)*, and *body fluid (津液)* differentiation and *zang fu (臟腑)* (organ) differentiation are also used. The onset of depression is often due to "damage" caused by extreme emotion. *Liver qi (肝氣)* is affected initially, followed by disharmony of the *qi* mechanism of the five viscera, particularly *liver*, *spleen*, and *heart*, resulting in a loss of regulation of the *qi* and *blood*. *Liver depression (肝鬱)* may repress the *spleen* and lead to consumption and damage of the *heart qi (心氣)*. If the *heart* loses its nourishment and restfulness, *heart shen (心神)* (spirit) occurs, resulting in an unstable and depressed mood. Prolonged *qi depression (氣鬱)* will accumulate and transform into *fire (火)* (Yeung et al. 2015).

In 2015, a systemic review of Chinese herbal medicine treatment for depression included a total of 61 studies, 2504 subjects, and 27 TCM patterns (Yeung et al. 2015). These researchers analyzed the top four commonly studied TCM patterns of *liver qi depression (肝氣鬱結), liver depression and spleen deficiency (肝鬱脾虛), dual deficiency of the heart and spleen (心脾兩虛),* and *liver depression and qi stagnation (肝鬱氣滯)*. According to TCM theory, *liver qi depression* is an impairment of the *liver* function, obstructing free movement of *qi* and resulting in stagnation of *qi* in the *liver*. *Liver depression and spleen deficiency* is a pathological change in which the transporting and transforming function of the *spleen* is affected by depressed *liver qi*, leading to *spleen* deficiency. *Dual deficiency of the heart and spleen* is a condition in which both *heart blood* and *spleen qi* are deficient, leading to disordered *heart* function and an impairment of the transporting and transforming function of the *spleen*. *Liver depression and qi stagnation* is a pathological change in which the *liver* is depressed, leading to impeded circulation of *qi* and stagnation of *qi* movement (WHO 2007).

Another RCT used acupuncture to treat depressed individuals after making a diagnosis based on the TCM patterns of differentiation (MacPherson et al. 2013). The primary and secondary *zang fu* syndromes were identified and the combined diagnoses revealed a predominant *Liver Qi Stagnation* cluster (66%) and a *Spleen Deficiency* cluster (34%). The typical symptoms of the *Liver Qi Stagnation* cluster along with depression might include irritability, frustration, restlessness, alternating moods, distension of the hypochondrium, and variations in muscle tension relating to stress, especially around the shoulders (Maciocia 1994). In *Spleen Qi Deficiency*, typical symptoms along with depression can include tiredness, loose stools, weakness, feeling bloated after eating, a heavy sensation in the limbs, and possible loss of appetite (Maciocia 1994). In this trial, men were more likely to be diagnosed with the *Liver Qi Stagnation* cluster and women with the *Spleen Qi Deficiency* cluster.

As no "gold standard" exists in the classification of TCM patterns, their criteria can differ between TCM practitioners and doctors. Future studies using both Western and Chinese medicine systems in diagnosis and severity assessment may facilitate a wider understanding of this disorder and lead to an improved treatment of depression.

4.3 Overview of Acupuncture in Depression

Acupuncture involves the insertion of fine needles into the skin at specific sites (acupoints). The technique is often considered to be "traditional Chinese medicine (TMC)," representing an ancient physiological system that believes health to be the result of harmony among bodily functions and between body and nature. In TMC, whole-body systems are thought to regulate through the normal flow of energy (*qi*). Disturbances in *qi* are thought to cause diseases. Acupuncture techniques are believed to cure disease by restoring *qi* (Wang and Wu 2014). Efforts have been made to characterize the effects of acupuncture in terms of the established principles of medical physiology upon which Western medicine is based (Berman et al. 2010).

Acupuncture has been used in a broad spectrum of health conditions, including clinical depression. Compared to conventional treatment, several potential advantages are associated with acupuncture, including its low cost, low number of complications, the ability to offer a personalized treatment program, and fewer adverse side effects (Consensus 1998). However, evaluation of the efficacy of acupuncture in the treatment of major depressive disorder (MDD) poses many challenges, in particular because of the conceptual differences between Chinese and Western medical diagnostic systems. Recent investigations have attempted to overcome these difficulties by introducing a standard research approach that could be successfully adopted by RCTs while also respecting the TCM conceptual framework of acupuncture (Schnyer et al. 2008). The main aim of this review is to summarize the evidence to determine whether or not acupuncture is effective in the treatment of depression.

4.4   Antidepressant Effects of Acupuncture

4.4.1   Methodology

This systematic review analysed evidence from published and unpublished RCTs comparing active acupuncture (manual, electrical, or laser) with control acupuncture, no treatment (wait-list), pharmacological treatment, or massage in the treatment of depression. Eligible studies included subjects aged over 18 years with MDD as defined by the *Diagnostic and Statistical Manual of Mental Disorders*, third or fourth Edition (DSM-III or IV).

The primary outcome measurements were reductions in severity of depression and improvements in depressive symptoms in clinician-rated and/or patient self-reported rating scales e.g., the Hamilton Rating Scale for Depression (HAMD), Beck Depression Inventory (BDI), Patient Health Questionnaire (PHQ-9), and/or Clinical Global Impression (CGI) scale.

The electronic literature search was conducted using PubMed a language filter to include all studies written in English. RCTs that satisfied the inclusion criteria were retrieved and read in full text. All 26 RCTs included in this review satisfied the specifications in the revised CONSORT and STRICTA guidelines (Allen et al. 2006; Andreescu et al. 2011; Chen et al. 2014; Chung et al. 2012; Gallagher et al. 2001; He et al. 2007; Luo et al. 1998; MacPherson et al. 2013; Man et al. 2014; Manber et al. 2004, 2010; Mischoulon et al. 2012; Qu et al. 2013; Quah-Smith et al. 2005, 2013a; Röschke et al. 2000; Song et al. 2007; Whiting et al. 2008; Yeung et al. 2011; Zhang 2005; Zhang et al. 2009, 2013).

4.4.2   Results

The trials contained a total of 2618 participants. Table 4.1 summarizes trial characteristics main results. The average number of participants was 101. Treatment interventions lasted between 2 and 12 weeks, with the majority lasting 6 or 8 weeks. The primary outcome measurement in 22 of the trials was the HAMD score. Manual acupuncture (MA) was applied in 11 trials, electroacupuncture (EA) in 9 trials, their combination in 2 trials, and laser acupuncture in 2 trials.

There was evidence of high heterogeneity in the trial designs and methodologies, reflected by choice of active acupoints, sham techniques, control groups, treatment durations, treatment frequency, monotherapy/augmentation, uncontrolled medications, outcome measurements and statistical methods. For our analyses, we grouped the trials by similarity of study design.

Table 4.1 Study details for the 26 randomized controlled trials of acupuncture for depression included in the review

Study	N	Intervention	Sessions/weeks	Acupoints	Sham acupuncture	Outcomes measurements	Results
Man et al. (2014)	43	Verum DCEAS + AD/sham DCEAS + AD	12/4	–	Sham EA (inactive)	HAMD	Verum DCEAS was significantly better than sham EA
Chen et al. (2014)	105	Verum MA + PRX/ Verum EA + PRX/ PRX alone	18/6	–	No	Symptom Checklist-90	No significant differences between verum MA and EA; Verum MA and EA were better than PRX alone
Zhang et al. (2013)	73	Verum DCEAS + FLX/sham EA + FLX	9/3	–	Sham EA (Streitberger needle)	HAMD	Verum DCEAS was significantly better than sham EA
Sun et al. (2013)	75	Verum EA/sham EA/ FLX alone	30/6	DU20, ST36, LR3, SP6, PC6, H7	Sham EA (inactive)	HAMD	No significant differences were reported among the three study groups. Verum and sham EA had significantly faster onset of effect compared with FLX
Quah-Smith et al. (2013a)	47	Verum LA/sham LA	12/8	LR14, CV14, LR8, HT7, KI3	Sham (inactive LA)	HAMD	Verum LA was significantly better than sham LA
MacPherson et al. (2013)	755	MA/ounseling/usual care	12/12	–	No	PHQ-9	MA and counseling were significantly better than usual care alone. No significant differences between MA and counseling groups
Qu et al. (2013)	160	Verum MA + PRX/ Verum EA + PRX/ PRX alone	18/6	GV20, DU20(EA), Yintang(EA), GV16, GV14, GB20, PC6, SP6	No	HAMD	PRX + MA and PRX + EA were significantly better than PRX alone. No significant differences were observed between the MA and EA groups

(continued)

Table 4.1 (continued)

Study	N	Intervention	Ratio	Acupoints	Sham/Control	Measure	Results
Chung et al. (2012)	20	Verum EA/sham EA	8/4	DU20, Yintang, Sishencong, GB15, GB8, Taiyang, ST8, SP6, LR3, HT7, PC6	Sham (inactive)	HAMD	No significant differences were observed between the two groups
Mischoulon et al. (2012)	30	Once-weekly MA + EA + AD/ twice-weekly MA + EA + AD	8(16)/8	H7, LI4, ST36, SP6, LR3, GV20, Yintang	No	HAMD	No significant differences were observed between the two groups
Duan et al. (2011)	75	Verum EA + FLX/ FLX alone	36/6	Sishencong, Anmian I, SP6, KI3, KI6, DU24, GB13, GB20, ST25, ST34, ST40, ST36, ST44, H7, PC6 and others	No	HAMD	No significant differences were observed between the two groups
Andreescu et al. (2011)	53	Verum EA/sham EA	12/6–8	DU20, Yintang	Sham (NSPEC)	HAMD	No significant differences were observed between the two groups
Yeung et al. (2011)	30	Once-weekly MA + AD/twice-weekly MA + AD	8(16)/8	H7, LI4, ST36, SP6, LR3, GV20(EA) Yintang(EA)	No	HAMD	No significant differences were observed between the two groups
Manber et al. (2010)	150 PD	Verum MA/sham MA/massage	12/8	–	Sham (NSPEC) Control (massage)	HAMD	Verum MA was significantly better than the sham MA and massage groups

Study	N	Intervention	Sessions/weeks	Acupoints	Sham	Scale	Results
Zhang et al. (2009)	80	Verum MA + low FLX/sham MA+ high FLX	30/6	GV20, Sishencong, Yintang, GV26, P6, H7, LR3, LI4	Sham (NSPEC)	HRDS	No significant reduction in HAMD scores in both groups, but verum MA was better in reduction of anxiety and FLX side-effects
Whiting et al. (2008)	19	Verum MA/sham MA	12/–	–	Sham (NSPEC)	BDI	No significant differences were observed between the two groups
Zhang et al. (2007)	42	Verum EA + PAX/ PAX alone	30/6	–	No	HAMD	Verum EA + PAX was significantly better than PAX alone
He et al. (2007)	61	Verum MA + TCM/ TCM alone	21/6	GV20, GV24, Yintang, GV26, Anmian, CV17, PC6, PC7, H7, LR3	No	HAMD	Verum MA + TCM was significantly better than TCM alone
Song et al. (2007)	90	FLX/Verum EA/sham EA	30/6	–	Sham (inactive)	HAMD	No significant differences were observed among the three groups
Allen et al. (2006)	151	Verum MA/sham MA/waiting list	8/4	–	Sham (NSPEC)	HAMD	No significant differences were observed between verum and sham MA; Verum and sham MA were better than waiting list
Zhang et al. (2005)	90 PSD	Verum MA/FLX	28/2	PC6, GV26, SP6, GV20, H7, H1, BL40, LU5	No	HAMD	No significant differences were observed between the two groups
Quah-Smith et al. (2005)	30	Verum LA/sham LA	8/4	LR14, CV15, CV14, HT7, LR8, KI10, LI4, SP6, GV20	Sham (inactive LA)	BDI	Verum LA was significantly better than sham LA at week 12 but not at week 4

(continued)

Table 4.1 (continued)

Manber et al. (2004)	61	Verum MA/sham MA/massage	12/8	L14, SP1, SP6, GB21, UB60, UB67, REN3, 4, 5, 6, ST36, ST45, UB23, UB32, KD4, GB44, all ear points, REN12	Sham (NSPEC) Control (massage)	HAMD	No significant differences were observed between verum and sham MA; Verum and sham MA were better than massage
Gallagher et al. (2001)	38	Verum MA/sham MA/waiting list	–/8	Individually tailored	Sham (NSPEC)	HAMD	No significant differences in HAMD scores were observed between all three groups
Röschke et al. (2000)	70	MIA + Verum MA/ MIA + sham MA/ MIA + control	12/4	UB 15, UB17, UB18, H7, P6, ST40, SP5, SP6, LU1	Sham (NSPEC) Control (routine clinical care)	HAMD	MIA + verum MA and MIA + sham MA were significantly better than MIA alone. No significant differences were observed between the verum and sham groups
Luo et al. (1998) phase 2	241	EA + placebo/AMP/ EA + AMP	36/6	Baihui, Yintang	No	HAMD	No significant differences were observed between the two groups; EA was better than AMP for anxiety somatization and cognitive disturbance
Luo et al. (1998) phase 1	29	EA + placebo/AMP/ EA + AMP	36/6	Baihui, Yintang	No	HAMD	No significant differences in HAMD scores were observed between the three groups

PSD post-stroke depression. *PD* pregnant women with depression, *HAMD* Hamilton rating scale for depression, *CGI* clinical global impression, *BDI* Beck depression inventory, *SF-36* 36-item short form health survey. *SDS* self directed support, *PHQ-9* patient health questionnaire, *Verum MA* active manual acupuncture at specific points, *Sham MA* manual acupuncture at non-specific locations, *EA* electroacupuncture, *DCEAS* dense cranial electroacupuncture stimulation, *SPEC/NSPEC* specific/non-specific acupoints for treatment of depression, *Verum LA* active laser acupuncture, *Sham MA* inactive laser acupuncture, *AMP* amitriptyline, *MIA* mianserin, *TCA* tricyclic antidepressant, *FLX* fluoxetine, *PRX* paroxetine, *BUP* bupropion, *AD* antidepressants not specified, *TCM* traditional Chinese medicine, *MA* manual acupuncture, *EA* electroacupuncture, *LA* laser acupuncture, *SPEC/NSPEC* specific/non-specific acupuncture for treatment of depression, *M* massage, *WL* wait list

4.4.2.1 Medication Versus Acupuncture

Four studies compared the effect of antidepressants versus acupuncture. There was no evidence of significant overall superiority for acupuncture over medication (Luo et al. 1998; Song et al. 2007; Sun et al. 2013; Zhang 2005). However, the onset of antidepressant effect with both verum and sham acupuncture was significantly faster than that of fluoxetine in one study (Sun et al. 2013). In another study, acupuncture was slightly more effective than amitriptyline in the alleviation of anxiety and cognitive disturbance (Luo et al. 1998).

4.4.2.2 Acupuncture Plus Medication Versus Medication Only

Seven studies compared medication only (Western or traditional Chinese medicine) with medication augmented by acupuncture (Chen et al. 2014; Duan et al. 2011; He et al. 2007; Luo et al. 1998; Qu et al. 2013; Röschke et al. 2000; Zhang et al. 2009). Five of these trials demonstrated greater improvements in depressive symptoms with augmentation treatment compared with medication alone (Chen et al. 2014; Duan et al. 2011; He et al. 2007; Qu et al. 2013; Röschke et al. 2000). One study also compared specific versus non-specific acupuncture; there was no significant difference between the verum and sham acupuncture groups (Röschke et al. 2000). In another study, there was no significant difference in antidepressive effects between verum acupuncture/low-dose fluoxetine and sham acupuncture/high-dose fluoxetine, indicating that augmenting antidepressant therapy with acupuncture enables a reduced dosage of medication without loss of efficacy (Zhang et al. 2009).

4.4.2.3 Verum Versus Sham Acupuncture

Two different study designs were used in the RCTs to compare verum and sham acupuncture. In the first design, six trials compared acupuncture using specific versus non-specific acupoints for treatment of depression; five used MA (Allen et al. 2006; Gallagher et al. 2001; Manber et al. 2004, 2010; Whiting et al. 2008) and one used EA (Andreescu et al. 2011). Only one study differentiated between the types of acupuncture and demonstrated the effectiveness of verum acupuncture (Manber et al. 2010). Possibly, even non-specific acupoints produce therapeutic effects. Future study designs should account for the possible confounding effects of control groups.

The second study design compared active and inactive stimulation with laser acupuncture (Quah-Smith et al. 2005, 2013a) and with EA (Chung et al. 2012; Man et al. 2014; Song et al. 2007; Sun et al. 2013; Zhang et al. 2013). Interestingly, four out of these seven trials revealed positive findings in favor of verum acupuncture (Man et al. 2014; Quah-Smith et al. 2005, 2013b; Zhang et al. 2013). In contrast to non-differentiation in specific/non-specific acupoint designs, active/inactive stimulation designs appear to offer a more appropriate way of providing a control group.

4.4.2.4 Adverse Effects

Adverse treatment effects were not mentioned in five out of 26 RCTs (Gallagher et al. 2001; Manber et al. 2004; Röschke et al. 2000; Song et al. 2007; Sun et al. 2013). Acupuncture was generally considered to be safe and well-tolerated in the remaining 19 RCTs, with some minor adverse effects including needle-related pain, bruising, mild bleeding and soreness at the site of needling. Six subjects reportedly discontinued study treatment because of needle-related pain or intolerability (Allen et al. 2006; Mischoulon et al. 2012; Yeung et al. 2011; Zhang et al. 2013). Four well-controlled studies failed to show any obvious differences between the treatment and control groups (Andreescu et al. 2011; Chung et al. 2012; He et al. 2007; Man et al. 2014). Non-specific adverse effects, including physical tiredness, headache, sleep problems, minimal transient fatigue and dizziness, were as likely to have been caused by depression as they were by acupuncture (Allen et al. 2006; Chen et al. 2014; Luo et al. 1998; Manber et al. 2010; Quah-Smith et al. 2005, 2013a). One trial reported skin erythema of the acupoints in 80 patients (Zhang et al. 2009). No serious adverse events relating to acupuncture were reported in the largest study that included 755 subjects (MacPherson et al. 2013).

4.4.2.5 Acupoints

Selected acupoints were well-defined in 16 RCTs and not in the remaining 10, where the acupuncturist examined each patient using TCM diagnostic assessments, and selected acupoints based on TCM theory. They reported their prescription of acupoints for each patient at each session. The selection of acupoints was based on the differentiation of symptoms.

The most frequently chosen acupoints in the RCTs were positioned in the meridians (channel) of the Du (governor vessel, GV), heart, spleen, pericardium and liver. The 10 most commonly used acupoints were DU20 (GV20, Baihui, 12 RCTs), HT7 (Shenmen, 11 RCTs), SP6 (Sanyinjiao, 11 RCTs), Yintang (Extra-ordinary points, 9 RCTs), PC6 (Neiguan, 8 RCTs), LR3 (Taichong, 6 RCTs), LI4 (Hegu, 5 RCTs), ST36 (Zusanli, 5 RCTs), Sishencong (Extra-ordinary points, 3 RCTs), and KI3 (Taixi, 2 RCTs). The wide variation in study design and inadequate methodological quality makes it difficult to conclude which acupoints have a higher efficacy and which TCM patterns respond better to regular antidepressant medication.

4.4.3 Discussion

In this review, 26 acupuncture RCTs investigated the effectiveness of acupuncture alone or in combination with manual, laser or EA in with the treatment of depression. Acupuncture was compared with active controls of medication or non-specific acupuncture, or with inactive controls of routine care or sham acupuncture. This review identified significant placebo effects in all 26 studies, which is consistent with clinical trials of depression in general. It is therefore very important to improve the design of the placebo (sham) arm, by for example using Streitberger non-invasive acupuncture needles (Zhang et al. 2013), to differentiate the effects of verum from those of sham acupuncture in future research.

In most of the head-to-head clinical trials, acupuncture and medication did not differ significantly in reducing depressive symptoms. Evidence suggests that acupuncture might be more effective than medication in the reduction of specific symptom clusters such as anxiety somatization and cognitive disturbance (Luo et al. 1998), and that the onset of antidepressant effects of acupuncture might be faster than that with antidepressant drugs (Sun et al. 2013). However, these findings should be interpreted with caution because they were not conducted under double-blind conditions. Conducting appropriate head-to-head comparisons between medication and acupuncture require the study design to have one arm with "verum acupuncture and placebo" and the other arm with "sham acupuncture and the compared drug."

Medication combined with acupuncture might produce additional benefits over medication alone. Five trials showed greater improvements in depressive symptoms when an acupuncture intervention was added to the medication treatment (Chen et al. 2014; Duan et al. 2011; He et al. 2007; Qu et al. 2013; Röschke et al. 2000). However, since both verum and sham acupuncture were better than medication alone, the placebo effect cannot be ruled out (Röschke et al. 2000).

The influence of placebo upon study outcomes can be reduced by comparing active and inactive stimulation with laser acupuncture (Quah-Smith et al. 2005, 2013a) and with EA (Chung et al. 2012; Man et al. 2014; Song et al. 2007; Sun et al. 2013; Zhang et al. 2013). Two studies that compared active and inactive laser acupuncture showed clear superiority with active treatment. EA was associated with positive antidepressant results in another couple of studies (Man et al. 2014; Zhang et al. 2012b). In comparisons between manual and EA interventions, between-group differences did not reach significance (Chen et al. 2014; Qu et al. 2013). In summary, active/inactive stimulation designs might be more appropriate than specific/non-specific acupoint designs for providing a control group in acupuncture research.

Significant adverse events relating to acupuncture are grouped under three categories: mechanical injuries, infections and other adverse events (Norheim 1996). The main reason as to why most clinical trials prefer acupuncture points placed on the limbs, rather than on the trunk, is to avoid the very severe event of pneumothorax. All of the RCTs included in this review applied acupuncture to acupoints on the head and limbs. Thus, there were no reports of pneumothorax. Acupuncture was generally reported to be safe and well-tolerated by the trials in this review, although five of them did not report adverse events (Gallagher et al. 2001; Manber et al. 2004; Röschke et al. 2000; Song et al. 2007; Sun et al. 2013). Adverse events were consistent with those of previous acupuncture studies, and included needle-related pain, bruising, mild bleeding and soreness. Subjects rarely discontinue acupuncture because of needle-related pain or intolerability. No serious adverse events relating to acupuncture treatment were reported in any of the studies in this review.

4.4.4 Methodology Problems and Limitations

The most significant problem facing generalization of clinical trial results is small sample size, which is often exacerbated by high dropout rates, preventing the ability to effectively detect minor differences between acupuncture and control treatments. Moreover, the significant placebo effect compounds the difficulty of detecting any small differences between active and control interventions. A small effect of antidepressant treatment is expected to be defined as being around 0.2–0.3. An adequately-sized study sample ensures that even small effects are detected and prevents false positive results. For the detection of antidepressant effects, an adequate sample size for double-blind RCTs is deemed to be between 100 and 200 patients with MDD (Gibertini et al. 2012). A higher number is needed if the control treatment is associated with large placebo effects. In this review, the average sample size was 101 patients, but this was significantly inflated by the one study that recruited 755 patients (MacPherson 2014); excluding this trial reduced the average sample size to 74 patients. Notably, a common problem encountered in acupuncture research is the availability of suitable control interventions. For example, sham acupuncture may demonstrate antidepressive efficacy despite being delivered into a non-specific location (i.e., needle insertion avoiding acupuncture points and meridians) (Birch 2004; Lewith et al. 2006; MacPherson et al. 2010).

Trials of acupuncture have often been criticized for providing insufficient details of the intervention. Such details are necessary for facilitating interpretation of the trial data and for making judgments regarding transferability and generalizability. The STandards for Reporting Interventions in Clinical Trials of Acupuncture (STRICTA) recommendations were included as part of the Consolidated Standards of Reporting Trials (CONSORT) family of reporting guidelines in 2010 and are now recommended as a framework for better reporting of interventions in clinical trials of acupuncture. Some studies use two active control treatment arms (head-to-head, superiority comparisons), which is strengthened by the convenience to replicate in clinical practice. The lack of inactive controls is usually challenged by the confounding placebo effects.

The issue of diagnostic frameworks is worth considering when assessing the relevance of these trials in clinical practice. TCM patterns of symptoms, signs and diagnoses do not fit within a Western framework. TCM pattern differentiation is a diagnostic conclusion of the pathological changes of a disease state based on an individual's symptoms, physical signs, appearance of the tongue, and form of pulse. Western medicine diagnoses of depression may be diagnosed differently within Chinese medicine, depending on the overall pattern. Although it is believed that pattern-based TCM treatment will provide better efficacy, scant study data exist as to the additional benefits of TCM pattern differentiation. Although we were able to report the pattern diagnoses used by the studies in this review, the procedure and quality of the diagnostic process remains unclear. Such uncertainties would inevitably lead to discrepancies in the selection of acupoints for antidepressant treatment. According to TCM principles, TCM practitioners and acupuncturists routinely individualize their treatments to match the inherent variations presented by their patients. Usually, treatments in pragmatic acupuncture trials usually allow practitioners to vary their treatments in this regard.

Meta-analysis was not possible in this review due to differences in study design and low methodological quality. Further studies are needed that are of better methodological quality to allow research to define the efficacy of acupuncture and ensure that acupoints are selected according to a pattern-based treatment in depression.

4.5   Biological Mechanisms for Acupuncture in Depression

Biological mechanisms underlying the antidepressant effects relating to acupuncture treatment remain unclear, for several reasons. First, the majority of studies have been conducted in animals; it is difficult to generalize animal findings to humans. Second, acupuncture activates peripheral nerve fibers in a non-specific way, which means that it is difficult to systematically study responses. Third, the acupuncture experience is dominated by a strong psychosocial context, which includes expectations, beliefs, and the therapeutic milieu (Berman et al. 2010). However, despite these limitations, some physiological phenomena associated with acupuncture have been identified.

Acupuncture indisputably alters levels of certain neurotransmitters, such as norepinephrine, serotonin, and dopamine, which play key roles in the neuropathogenesis of depression (Cabyoglu et al. 2006; Chein and Zakaria 1974; Han 1986; Kwon et al. 2012a, b; Park et al. 2012; Yu et al. 2013). For example, the regulation of the 5-hydroxyindole-3-acetic acid/serotonin (5-HIAA/5-HT) ratio and serotonin transporter expression by acupuncture stimulation were associated with acupuncture-induced benefits in an animal model of depression (Park et al. 2012). In a chronic depression model in mice, acupuncture produced antidepressant-like effects relating to its modulation of tryptophan-kynurenine and dopamine metabolism in the brain (Kwon et al. 2012b). In addition, acupuncture stimulation significantly reduced the 3,4-dihydroxyphenylacetic acid/dopamine (DOPAC/DA) ratio relating to maternal separation-induced depression-like behaviors in another animal model of depression (Kwon et al. 2012a), indicating that acupuncture plays an important role in the functional recovery of the prefrontal-limbic system in depressive illness.

Acupuncture enhances neurogenesis and neuroplasticity (Chung et al. 2014; Gao et al. 2011; Hwang et al. 2010; Luo et al. 2014; Nam et al. 2013; Sun et al. 2013; Witzel et al. 2011), a crucial determinant of antidepressant effects (Duman et al. 1999; Santarelli et al. 2003). For example, a review of preclinical studies found that acupuncture induces neurogenesis via up-regulation of brain-derived neurotrophic factor (BDNF), glial cell line-derived neurotrophic factor, basic fibroblast growth factor and neuropeptide Y, and activation of the function of the primo vascular system (Nam et al. 2013). In young rat brains, BrdU/NeuN double labeling revealed a significant increase in the number of newly differentiated neurons following EA treatment (Gao et al. 2011). EA also ameliorates reductions in proliferating cells and differentiated neuroblasts in the rat dentate gyrus induced by diabetes (Chung et al. 2014). In rats with focal ischemic injuries, acupuncture treatment was associated with neurogenesis and regulation of GSK3beta/PP2A expression (Luo et al. 2014). In humans, both fluoxetine and acupuncture treatment restored the normal concentration of glial cell line-derived neurotrophic factor (GDNF), which plays an important role in the pathogenesis of MDD (Sun et al. 2013). In addition, both EA and acupressure improved maladaptive neuroplasticity in humans, as measured by magnetoencephalography (Witzel et al. 2011).

Anti-inflammatory and antioxidative effects induced by acupuncture might be related to its antidepressant effects (Choi et al. 2010; Kwon et al. 2012b; Lao et al. 2001; Liu et al. 2004; Shiue et al. 2008; Song et al. 2009, 2014; Yu et al. 2013). In a chronic inflammation-induced depression model in murine, acupuncture has antidepressant-like effects due to its modulatory effects on trypto-phan-kynurenine metabolism and dopamine metabolism in the brain (Kwon et al. 2012b), indicating that anti-inflammatory effects from acupuncture. The neuroprotective effects of acupuncture may be partly mediated via inhibition of inflammation and microglial activation (Choi et al. 2010; Liu et al. 2004). In a rat model of persistent pain and inflammation, acupuncture delayed the onset and facilitated the recovery of inflammatory hyperalgesia and suppressed inflammation-induced spinal Fos expression in neurons (Lao et al. 2001). EA significantly reduced the release of pro-inflammatory cytokines and organ dys-function after LPS challenge by activating the cholinergic anti-inflammatory pathway in animal models (Song et al. 2014) and decreased levels of nitric oxide and leukotriene B4 (Carneiro et al. 2010). In humans, both EA and fluoxetine induced anti-inflammatory effects by reducing interleukin-1β, while EA treatment also restored the balance between Th1 and Th2 systems by increasing levels of tumor necrosis factor-α and decreasing levels of interleukin-4 (Song et al. 2009).

Conclusions

Acupuncture has been widely used as an alternative treatment for depression and offers a safe and effective promising therapy in future clinical applications. The biological mechanisms underlying acupuncture are relevant to its antidepressant effects. Supportive clinical evidence is accumulating, but evaluating the efficacy of acupuncture poses many critical challenges for study designs. Depression is heterogeneous and every intervention produces only small effects. Thus, it is important to identify those patients who will be most responsive to acupuncture treatment.

The use of acupuncture in the treatment of depression is supported by person-alized medicine inherited from TCM. Many different styles and manipulations exist for acupuncture; it is of great clinical interest to investigate specific acupuncture manipulations for specific subtypes of depression. In addition, there is much room for improvement in the clinical research methodological quality. More clinical evidence is needed to endorse the use of acupuncture as an alternative treatment for depression.

Acknowledgments This review includes works supported by the following grants: Ministry of Science and Technology (MOST) 104-2314-B-039-022-MY2, 103-2320-B-039-MY3, 103-2320-B-038-012-MY3, 103-2923-B-039-002-MY3, 102-2911-I-039-501, 101-2628-B-039-001-MY3 and 101-2320-B-038-020-MY2; NHRI-EX105-10528NI from the National Health Research Institutes; and CMU CMU104-S-1603, 104-S44, 103-S-03, DMR-103-078, 102-068 and 101-081 from the China Medical University in Taiwan. We would like to thank Dr. Ivana Kormanikova for reviewing the literature reviewing and data collection.

References

Allen JJ, Schnyer RN, Chambers AS, Hitt SK, Moreno FA, Manber R. Acupuncture for depression: a randomized controlled trial. J Clin Psychiatry. 2006;67:1665–73.

American Psychiatric Association. Diagnostic and statistical manual of mental disorders. 4th ed. Washington, DC: American Psychiatric Association; 1994.

Andreescu C, Glick RM, Emeremni CA, Houck PR, Mulsant BH. Acupuncture for the treatment of major depressive disorder: a randomized controlled trial. J Clin Psychiatry. 2011;72:1129–35.

Belmaker RH, Agam G. Major depressive disorder. N Engl J Med. 2008;358:55–68.

Berman BM, Langevin HM, Witt CM, Dubner R. Acupuncture for chronic low back pain. N Engl J Med. 2010;363:454–61.

Berton O, Nestler EJ. New approaches to antidepressant drug discovery: beyond monoamines. Nat Rev Neurosci. 2006;7:137–51.

Birch S. Clinical research on acupuncture. Part 2. Controlled clinical trials, an overview of their methods. J Altern Complement Med. 2004;10:481–98.

Bonaccorso S, Puzella A, Marino V, Pasquini M, Biondi M, Artini M, Almerighi C, Levrero M, Egyed B, Bosmans E, et al. Immunotherapy with interferon-alpha in patients affected by chronic hepatitis C induces an intercorrelated stimulation of the cytokine network and an increase in depressive and anxiety symptoms. Psychiatry Res. 2001;105:45–55.

Cabyoglu MT, Ergene N, Tan U. The mechanism of acupuncture and clinical applications. Int J Neurosci. 2006;116:115–25.

Capuron L, Neurauter G, Musselman DL, Lawson DH, Nemeroff CB, Fuchs D, Miller AH. Interferon-alpha-induced changes in tryptophan metabolism. Relationship to depression and paroxetine treatment. Biol Psychiatry. 2003a;54:906–14.

Capuron L, Raison CL, Musselman DL, Lawson DH, Nemeroff CB, Miller AH. Association of exaggerated HPA axis response to the initial injection of interferon-alpha with development of depression during interferon-alpha therapy. Am J Psychiatry. 2003b;160:1342–5.

Capuron L, Pagnoni G, Demetrashvili M, Woolwine BJ, Nemeroff CB, Berns GS, Miller AH. Anterior cingulate activation and error processing during interferon-alpha treatment. Biol Psychiatry. 2005;58:190–6.

Carneiro ER, Xavier RA, De Castro MA, Do Nascimento CM, Silveira VL. Electroacupuncture promotes a decrease in inflammatory response associated with Th1/Th2 cytokines, nitric oxide and leukotriene B4 modulation in experimental asthma. Cytokine. 2010;50:335–40.

Caspi A, Sugden K, Moffitt TE, Taylor A, Craig IW, Harrington H, McClay J, Mill J, Martin J, Braithwaite A, Poulton R. Influence of life stress on depression: moderation by a polymorphism in the 5-HTT gene. Science. 2003;301:386–9.

Chang JP, Chang SS, Yang HT, Palani M, Chen CP, Su KP. Polyunsaturated fatty acids (PUFAs) levels in patients with cardiovascular diseases (CVDs) with and without depression. Brain Behav Immun. 2014a;44:28–31.

Chang JP, Lin CC, Hwu HG, Su KP. View on DSM from Taiwan: transition from IV to 5. Acta Psychiatr Scand. 2014b;129:235.

Chein EY, Zakaria S. Letter: acupuncture for psychiatric disorders. JAMA. 1974;229:639.

Chen PJ, Hsieh CL, Su KP, Hou YC, Chiang HM, Lin IH, Sheen LY. The antidepressant effect of Gastrodia elata Bl. On the forced-swimming test in rats. Am J Chin Med. 2008;36:95–106.

Chen PJ, Liang KC, Lin HC, Hsieh CL, Su KP, Hung MC, Sheen LY. Gastrodia elata Bl. Attenuated learning deficits induced by forced-swimming stress in the inhibitory avoidance task and Morris water maze. J Med Food. 2011;14:610–7.

Chen J, Lin W, Wang S, Wang C, Li G, Qu S, Huang Y, Zhang Z, Xiao W. Acupuncture/electroacupuncture enhances anti-depressant effect of Seroxat: the Symptom Checklist-90 scores. Neural Regen Res. 2014;9:213–22.

Chiu CC, Liu JP, Su KP. The use of omega-3 fatty acids in treatment of depression: the lights and shadows. Psychiatric Times. 2008;25:76–80.

Choi DC, Lee JY, Moon YJ, Kim SW, Oh TH, Yune TY. Acupuncture-mediated inhibition of inflammation facilitates significant functional recovery after spinal cord injury. Neurobiol Dis. 2010;39:272–82.

Chung KF, Yeung WF, Zhang ZJ, Yung KP, Man SC, Lee CP, Lam SK, Leung TW, Leung KY, Ziea ET, Taam Wong V. Randomized non-invasive sham-controlled pilot trial of electroacupuncture for postpartum depression. J Affect Disord. 2012;142:115–21.

Chung JY, Yoo DY, Im W, Choi JH, Yi SS, Youn HY, Hwang IK, Seong JK, Yoon YS. Electroacupuncture at the Zusanli and Baihui acupoints ameliorates type-2 diabetes-induced reductions in proliferating cells and differentiated neuroblast in the hippocampal dentate gyrus with increasing brain-derived neurotrophic factor levels. J Vet Med Sci. 2014;77(2):167–73.

Consensus N. NIH consensus conference. Acupuncture. JAMA. 1998;280:1518–24.

Danese A, Moffitt TE, Pariante CM, Ambler A, Poulton R, Caspi A. Elevated inflammation levels in depressed adults with a history of childhood maltreatment. Arch Gen Psychiatry. 2008;65:409–15.

Duan DM, Tu Y, Jiao S, Qin W. The relevance between symptoms and magnetic resonance imaging analysis of the hippocampus of depressed patients given electro-acupuncture combined with fluoxetine intervention—a randomized, controlled trial. Chin J Integr Med. 2011;17:190–9.

Duman RS, Charney DS. Cell atrophy and loss in major depression. Biol Psychiatry. 1999;45:1083–4.

Duman RS, Malberg J, Thome J. Neural plasticity to stress and antidepressant treatment. Biol Psychiatry. 1999;46:1181–91.

Gallagher SM, Allen JJ, Hitt SK, Schnyer RN, Manber R. Six-month depression relapse rates among women treated with acupuncture. Complement Ther Med. 2001;9:216–8.

Gao J, Wang S, Wang X, Zhu C. Electroacupuncture enhances cell proliferation and neuronal differentiation in young rat brains. Neurol Sci. 2011;32:369–74.

Gaynes BN, Rush AJ, Trivedi MH, Wisniewski SR, Spencer D, Fava M. The STAR*D study: treating depression in the real world. Cleve Clin J Med. 2008;75:57–66.

Gibertini M, Nations KR, Whitaker JA. Obtained effect size as a function of sample size in approved antidepressants: a real-world illustration in support of better trial design. Int Clin Psychopharmacol. 2012;27:100–6.

Gozzelino R, Jeney V, Soares MP. Mechanisms of cell protection by heme oxygenase-1. Annu Rev Pharmacol Toxicol. 2010;50:323–54.

Han JS. Electroacupuncture: an alternative to antidepressants for treating affective diseases? Int J Neurosci. 1986;29:79–92.

He Q, Zhang J, Tang Y. A controlled study on treatment of mental depression by acupuncture plus TCM medication. J Tradit Chin Med. 2007;27:166–9.

Hochstrasser T, Ullrich C, Sperner-Unterweger B, Humpel C. Inflammatory stimuli reduce survival of serotonergic neurons and induce neuronal expression of indoleamine 2,3-dioxygenase in rat dorsal raphe nucleus organotypic brain slices. Neuroscience. 2011;184:128–38.

Hwang IK, Chung JY, Yoo DY, Yi SS, Youn HY, Seong JK, Yoon YS. Comparing the effects of acupuncture and electroacupuncture at Zusanli and Baihui on cell proliferation and neuroblast differentiation in the rat hippocampus. J Vet Med Sci. 2010;72:279–84.

Krishnan V, Nestler EJ. The molecular neurobiology of depression. Nature. 2008;455:894–902.

Kwon S, Kim D, Park H, Yoo D, Park HJ, Hahm DH, Lee H, Kim ST. Prefrontal-limbic change in dopamine turnover by acupuncture in maternally separated rat pups. Neurochem Res. 2012a;37:2092–8.

Kwon S, Lee B, Yeom M, Sur BJ, Kim M, Kim ST, Park HJ, Lee H, Hahm DH. Modulatory effects of acupuncture on murine depression-like behavior following chronic systemic inflammation. Brain Res. 2012b;1472:149–60.

Lao L, Zhang G, Wei F, Berman BM, Ren K. Electro-acupuncture attenuates behavioral hyperalgesia and selectively reduces spinal Fos protein expression in rats with persistent inflammation. J Pain. 2001;2:111–7.

Lewith GT, White PJ, Kaptchuk TJ. Developing a research strategy for acupuncture. Clin J Pain. 2006;22:632–8.

Lin PY, Huang SY, Su KP. A meta-analytic review of polyunsaturated fatty acid compositions in patients with depression. Biol Psychiatry. 2010;68:140–7.

Lin PY, Mischoulon D, Freeman MP, Matsuoka Y, Hibbeln J, Belmaker RH, Su KP. Are omega-3 fatty acids antidepressants or just mood-improving agents? The effect depends upon diagnosis, supplement preparation, and severity of depression. Mol Psychiatry. 2012;17: 1161–3.

Liu XY, Zhou HF, Pan YL, Liang XB, Niu DB, Xue B, Li FQ, He QH, Wang XH, Wang XM. Electro-acupuncture stimulation protects dopaminergic neurons from inflammation-mediated damage in medial forebrain bundle-transected rats. Exp Neurol. 2004;189:189–96.

Lu DY, Tsao YY, Leung YM, Su KP. Docosahexaenoic acid suppresses neuroinflammatory responses and induces heme oxygenase-1 expression in BV-2 microglia: implications of anti-depressant effects for omega-3 fatty acids. Neuropsychopharmacology. 2010;35:2238–48.

Lu DY, Leung YM, Su KP. Interferon-alpha induces nitric oxide synthase expression and haem oxygenase-1 down-regulation in microglia: implications of cellular mechanism of IFN-alpha-induced depression. Int J Neuropsychopharmacol. 2013;16:433–44.

Luo H, Meng F, Jia Y, Zhao X. Clinical research on the therapeutic effect of the electro-acupuncture treatment in patients with depression. Psychiatry Clin Neurosci. 1998;52(Suppl):S338–40.

Luo D, Fan X, Ma C, Fan T, Wang X, Chang N, Li L, Zhang Y, Meng Z, Wang S, Shi X. A study on the effect of neurogenesis and regulation of GSK3beta/PP2A expression in acupuncture treatment of neural functional damage caused by focal ischemia in MCAO rats. Evid Based Complement Alternat Med. 2014;2014:962343.

Maciocia G. The practice of Chinese medicine: the treatment of diseases with acupuncture and Chinese herbal medicine. Edinburgh: Churchill Livingstone; 1994.

MacPherson H. Acupuncture for depression: state of the evidence. Acupunct Med. 2014;32:304–5.

MacPherson H, Altman DG, Hammerschlag R, Youping L, Taixiang W, White A, Moher D, STRICTA Revision Group. Revised STandards for Reporting Interventions in Clinical Trials of Acupuncture (STRICTA): extending the CONSORT statement. J Altern Complement Med. 2010;16:ST1–14.

MacPherson H, Richmond S, Bland M, Brealey S, Gabe R, Hopton A, Keding A, Lansdown H, Perren S, Sculpher M, et al. Acupuncture and counselling for depression in primary care: a randomised controlled trial. PLoS Med. 2013;10:e1001518.

Maes M, Leonard B, Fernandez A, Kubera M, Nowak G, Veerhuis R, Gardner A, Ruckoanich P, Geffard M, Altamura C, et al. (Neuro)inflammation and neuroprogression as new pathways and drug targets in depression: from antioxidants to kinase inhibitors. Prog Neuropsychopharmacol Biol Psychiatry. 2011;35:659–63.

Man SC, Hung BH, Ng RM, Yu XC, Cheung H, Fung MP, Li LS, Leung KP, Leung KP, Tsang KW, et al. A pilot controlled trial of a combination of dense cranial electroacupuncture stimulation and body acupuncture for post-stroke depression. BMC Complement Altern Med. 2014;14:255.

Manber R, Schnyer RN, Allen JJ, Rush AJ, Blasey CM. Acupuncture: a promising treatment for depression during pregnancy. J Affect Disord. 2004;83:89–95.

Manber R, Schnyer RN, Lyell D, Chambers AS, Caughey AB, Druzin M, Carlyle E, Celio C, Gress JL, Huang MI, et al. Acupuncture for depression during pregnancy: a randomized controlled trial. Obstet Gynecol. 2010;115:511–20.

Mischoulon D, Brill CD, Ameral VE, Fava M, Yeung AS. A pilot study of acupuncture mono-therapy in patients with major depressive disorder. J Affect Disord. 2012;141:469–73.

Murray CJ, Lopez AD. Global mortality, disability, and the contribution of risk factors: Global Burden of Disease Study. Lancet. 1997;349:1436–42.

Nam MH, Ahn KS, Choi SH. Acupuncture stimulation induces neurogenesis in adult brain. Int Rev Neurobiol. 2013;111:67–90.

Norheim AJ. Adverse effects of acupuncture: a study of the literature for the years 1981-1994. J Altern Complement Med. 1996;2:291–7.

Pariante CM, Miller AH. Glucocorticoid receptors in major depression: relevance to pathophysiology and treatment. Biol Psychiatry. 2001;49:391–404.

Park H, Yoo D, Kwon S, Yoo TW, Park HJ, Hahm DH, Lee H, Kim ST. Acupuncture stimulation at HT7 alleviates depression-induced behavioral changes via regulation of the serotonin system in the prefrontal cortex of maternally-separated rat pups. J Physiol Sci. 2012;62:351–7.

Pezawas L, Meyer-Lindenberg A, Drabant EM, Verchinski BA, Munoz KE, Kolachana BS, Egan MF, Mattay VS, Hariri AR, Weinberger DR. 5-HTTLPR polymorphism impacts human cingulate-amygdala interactions: a genetic susceptibility mechanism for depression. Nat Neurosci. 2005;8:828–34.

Popoli M, Yan Z, McEwen BS, Sanacora G. The stressed synapse: the impact of stress and gluco-corticoids on glutamate transmission. Nat Rev Neurosci. 2012;13:22–37.

Qu SS, Huang Y, Zhang ZJ, Chen JQ, Lin RY, Wang CQ, Li GL, Wong HK, Zhao CH, Pan JY, et al. A 6-week randomized controlled trial with 4-week follow-up of acupuncture combined with paroxetine in patients with major depressive disorder. J Psychiatr Res. 2013;47:726–32.

Quah-Smith JI, Tang WM, Russell J. Laser acupuncture for mild to moderate depression in a pri-mary care setting—a randomised controlled trial. Acupunct Med. 2005;23:103–11.

Quah-Smith I, Smith C, Crawford JD, Russell J. Laser acupuncture for depression: a ran-domised double blind controlled trial using low intensity laser intervention. J Affect Disord. 2013a;148:179–87.

Quah-Smith I, Suo C, Williams MA, Sachdev PS. The antidepressant effect of laser acupuncture: a comparison of the resting brain's default mode network in healthy and depressed subjects dur-ing functional magnetic resonance imaging. Med Acupunct. 2013b;25:124–33.

Raison CL, Capuron L, Miller AH. Cytokines sing the blues: inflammation and the pathogenesis of depression. Trends Immunol. 2006;27:24–31.

Raison CL, Borisov AS, Majer M, Drake DF, Pagnoni G, Woolwine BJ, Vogt GJ, Massung B, Miller AH. Activation of central nervous system inflammatory pathways by interferon-alpha: relationship to monoamines and depression. Biol Psychiatry. 2009;65:296–303.

Röschke J, Wolf C, Muller MJ, Wagner P, Mann K, Grozinger M, Bech S. The benefit from whole body acupuncture in major depression. J Affect Disord. 2000;57:73–81.

Rush AJ. STAR*D: what have we learned? Am J Psychiatry. 2007;164:201–4.

Santarelli L, Saxe M, Gross C, Surget A, Battaglia F, Dulawa S, Weisstaub N, Lee J, Duman R, Arancio O, et al. Requirement of hippocampal neurogenesis for the behavioral effects of anti-depressants. Science. 2003;301:805–9.

Santen G, van Zwet E, Bettica P, Gomeni RA, Danhof M, Della Pasqua O. From trial and error to trial simulation III: a framework for interim analysis in efficacy trials with antidepressant drugs. Clin Pharmacol Ther. 2011;89:602–7.

Sapolsky RM. Glucocorticoids and hippocampal atrophy in neuropsychiatric disorders. [Review] [83 refs]. Arch Gen Psychiatry. 2000;57:925–35.

Schnyer RN, Iuliano D, Kay J, Shields M, Wayne P. Development of protocols for random-ized sham-controlled trials of complex treatment interventions: Japanese acupuncture for endometriosis-related pelvic pain. J Altern Complement Med. 2008;14:515–22.

Shiue HS, Lee YS, Tsai CN, Hsueh YM, Sheu JR, Chang HH. DNA microarray analysis of the effect on inflammation in patients treated with acupuncture for allergic rhinitis. J Altern Complement Med. 2008;14:689–98.

Sinyor M, Schaffer A, Levitt A. The sequenced treatment alternatives to relieve depression (STAR*D) trial: a review. Can J Psychiatry. 2010;55:126–35.

Song C, Wang H. Cytokines mediated inflammation and decreased neurogenesis in animal models of depression. Prog Neuro-Psychopharmacol Biol Psychiatry. 2011;35:760–8.

Song Y, Zhou D, Fan J, Luo H, Halbreich U. Effects of electroacupuncture and fluoxetine on the density of GTP-binding-proteins in platelet membrane in patients with major depressive disor-der. J Affect Disord. 2007;98:253–7.

Song C, Halbreich U, Han C, Leonard BE, Luo H. Imbalance between pro- and anti-inflammatory cytokines, and between Th1 and Th2 cytokines in depressed patients: the effect of electroacu-puncture or fluoxetine treatment. Pharmacopsychiatry. 2009;42:182–8.

Song Q, Hu S, Wang H, Lv Y, Shi X, Sheng Z, Sheng W. Electroacupuncturing at Zusanli point (ST36) attenuates pro-inflammatory cytokine release and organ dysfunction by activating cholinergic anti-inflammatory pathway in rat with endotoxin challenge. Afr J Tradit Complement Altern Med. 2014;11:469–74.

Stahl S, Briley M. Understanding pain in depression. Hum Psychopharmacol. 2004;19(Suppl 1):S9–S13.

Su KP. Mind-body interface: the role of n-3 fatty acids in psychoneuroimmunology, somatic presentation, and medical illness comorbidity of depression. Asia Pac J Clin Nutr. 2008; 17(Suppl 1):151–7.

Su KP. Biological mechanism of antidepressant effect of omega-3 fatty acids: how does fish oil act as a 'Mind-Body Interface'. Neurosignals. 2009;17:144–52.

Su KP. Inflammation in psychopathology of depression: clinical, biological, and therapeutic implications. Biomedicine. 2012;2:68–74.

Su KP, Balanzá-Martínez V. Role of omega-3 fatty acids in mood disorders. In: McNamara RK, editor. The omega-3 fatty acid deficiency syndrome: opportunities for disease prevention. New York: Nova Science; 2013. p. 315–36.

Su KP, Huang SY, Chiu TH, Huang KC, Huang CL, Chang HC, Pariante CM. Omega-3 fatty acids for major depressive disorder during pregnancy: results from a randomized, double-blind, placebo-controlled trial. J Clin Psychiatry. 2008;69:644–51.

Su KP, Huang SY, Peng CY, Lai HC, Huang CL, Chen YC, Aitchison KJ, Pariante CM. Phospholipase A2 and cyclooxygenase 2 genes influence the risk of interferon-alpha-induced depression by regulating polyunsaturated fatty acids levels. Biol Psychiatry. 2010;67:550–7.

Su KP, Wang SM, Pae CU. Omega-3 polyunsaturated fatty acids for major depressive disorder. Expert Opin Investig Drugs. 2013;22:1519–34.

Su KP, Lai HC, Yang HT, Su WP, Peng CY, Chang JP, Chang HC, Pariante CM. Omega-3 fatty acids in the prevention of interferon-alpha-induced depression: results from a randomized, controlled trial. Biol Psychiatry. 2014;76:559–66.

Sun H, Zhao H, Ma C, Bao F, Zhang J, Wang DH, Zhang YX, He W. Effects of electroacupuncture on depression and the production of glial cell line-derived neurotrophic factor compared with fluoxetine: a randomized controlled pilot study. J Altern Complement Med. 2013;19:733–9.

Talarowska M, Bobinska K, Zajaczkowska M, Su KP, Maes M, Galecki P. Impact of oxidative/nitrosative stress and inflammation on cognitive functions in patients with recurrent depressive disorders. Med Sci Monit. 2014a;20:110–5.

Talarowska M, Orzechowska A, Szemraj J, Su KP, Maes M, Galecki P. Manganese superoxide dismutase gene expression and cognitive functions in recurrent depressive disorder. Neuropsychobiology. 2014b;70:23–8.

Trivedi MH, Rush AJ, Wisniewski SR, Nierenberg AA, Warden D, Ritz L, Norquist G, Howland RH, Lebowitz B, McGrath PJ, et al. Evaluation of outcomes with citalopram for depression using measurement-based care in STAR*D: implications for clinical practice. Am J Psychiatry. 2006;163:28–40.

Wang W, Wu SX. JAMA patient page. Treating pain with acupuncture. JAMA. 2014;312:1365.

Whiting M, Leavey G, Scammell A, Au S, King M. Using acupuncture to treat depression: a feasibility study. Complement Ther Med. 2008;16:87–91.

WHO. International classification of diseases. 10th ed. New York: World Health Organization Publications Center; 1999.

WHO. WHO International Standard Terminologies on traditional medicine in the Western Pacific Region. Western Pacific Region: World Health Organization; 2007.

WHO. Media Center. Fact sheet. Depression. 2016. Page last reviewed April 2016. http://www.who.int/mediacentre/factsheets/fs369/en/.

Wittchen HU. The burden of mood disorders. Science. 2012;338:15.

Witzel T, Napadow V, Kettner NW, Vangel MG, Hamalainen MS, Dhond RP. Differences in cortical response to acupressure and electroacupuncture stimuli. BMC Neurosci. 2011;12:73.

Yeung AS, Ameral VE, Chuzi SE, Fava M, Mischoulon D. A pilot study of acupuncture augmentation therapy in antidepressant partial and non-responders with major depressive disorder. J Affect Disord. 2011;130:285–9.

Yeung WF, Chung KF, Ng KY, et al. Prescription of Chinese herbal medicine in pattern-based traditional Chinese medicine treatment for depression: a systematic review. Evid Based Complement Alternat Med. 2015;2015:160189. https://doi.org/10.1155/2015/160189.

Yu JS, Zeng BY, Hsieh CL. Acupuncture stimulation and neuroendocrine regulation. Int Rev Neurobiol. 2013;111:125–40.

Zhang C. The brain-resuscitation acupuncture method for treatment of post wind-stroke mental depression—a report of 45 cases. J Tradit Chin Med. 2005;25:243–6.

Zhang GJ, Shi ZY, Liu S, Gong SH, Liu JQ, Liu JS. Clinical observation on treatment of depression by electro-acupuncture combined with Paroxetine. Chin J Integr Med. 2007;13(3):228–30.

Zhang WJ, Yang XB, Zhong BL. Combination of acupuncture and fluoxetine for depression: a randomized, double-blind, sham-controlled trial. J Altern Complement Med. 2009;15:837–44.

Zhang F, Zhou H, Wilson BC, Shi JS, Hong JS, Gao HM. Fluoxetine protects neurons against microglial activation-mediated neurotoxicity. Parkinsonism Relat Disord. 2012a;18(Suppl 1):S213–7.

Zhang GC, Fu WB, Xu NG, Liu JH, Zhu XP, Liang ZH, Huang YF, Chen YF. Meta analysis of the curative effect of acupuncture on post-stroke depression. J Tradit Chin Med. 2012b;32:6–11.

Zhang ZJ, Ng R, Man SC, Li JT, Wong W, Wong HK, Wang D, Wong MT, Tsang AW, Yip KC, Sze SC. Use of electroacupuncture to accelerate the antidepressant action of selective serotonin reuptake inhibitors: a single-blind, randomised, controlled study. Hong Kong Med J. 2013;19(Suppl 9):12–6.

Acupuncture and Itch: Basic Research Aspects

5

Yi-Hung Chen and Jaung-Geng Lin

Abstract

Acupuncture has been used in traditional Chinese medicine for over 2500 years. Clinical evidence supports the efficacy of acupuncture in the treatment of itch. In particular, acupuncture can relieve histamine-induced itch, refractory uremic pruritus and neurogenic pruritus. However, very little clinical evidence is available as to how acupuncture can assist in itch. Preclinical investigations into itch typically use rodents, in which scratching behavior reliably serves as a behavioral readout of itch. Typically, researchers count the numbers of hindlimb scratch bouts at the site of an injected pruritogen in the nape of the neck. Using murine models of itch, we have demonstrated that EA at Hegu (LI4) and Quchi (LI11) or cold stimulation at LI11 significantly attenuates pruritogen-induced scratching behavior. This chapter discusses evidence suggesting that this effect is mediated by the inhibition of microglial activation in the spinal cord.

Keywords

Itch · Pruritogen · Mouse · Acupuncture · Microglia

Y.-H. Chen
Graduate Institute of Acupuncture Science, College of Chinese Medicine, China Medical University, Taichung, Taiwan

J.-G. Lin (✉)
School of Chinese Medicine, College of Chinese Medicine, China Medical University, Taichung, Taiwan
e-mail: jglin@mail.cmu.edu.tw

5.1   Introduction

5.1.1   Definition of Itch

Itch has long been recognized as an "unpleasant sensation that elicits the desire to scratch" (Bergasa 2008; Carlsson and Wallengren 2010). Modern definitions describe itch as "a common symptom that may be associated with a specific dermatologic condition or systemic disease. The cause of itch can be multifactorial or due to a single underlying disorder" (Fazio and Yosipovitch 2018).

5.1.2   Pathology of Itch

Itch may be widespread or localized, without any obvious cause. Besides the skin, itch may occur in the epithelium of the conjunctivae, mouth, nose, pharynx, anogenital area, and trachea (Twycross et al. 2003).

No unique peripheral receptors for pruritus have been identified. However, the specificity of the itch stimulus is related to connections at the spinal level, where a specific class of dorsal horn neurons is located (see Fig. 5.1). From the spinal cord, the stimulus transmits via the lateral spinothalamic tract to the thalamus and on to the cerebral cortex to cause the sensation of itch. The sensation of pruritus is transmitted by unmyelinated C-fibers with a slow conduction velocity and extensive terminal branching (Schmelz et al. 1997). These fibers are distinct from those that

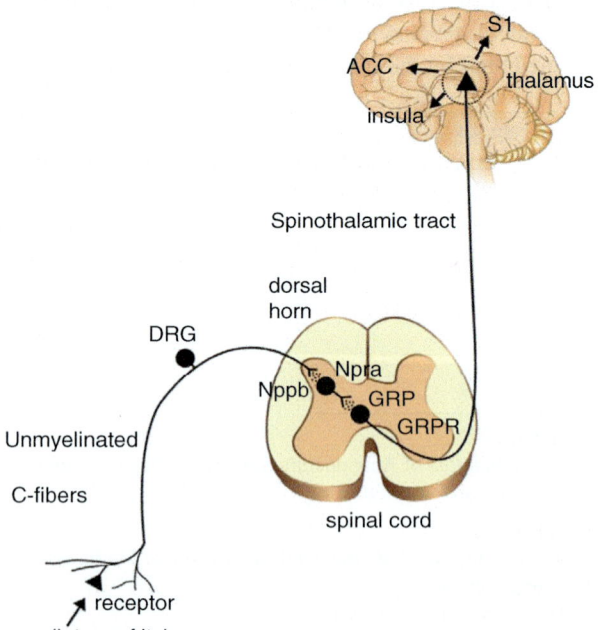

Fig. 5.1 Itch-specific neural pathway (adapted from Ikoma 2006). *DRG* dorsal root ganglion, *ACC* anterior cingulated cortex, *S1* primary somatosensory cortex, *GRP* gastrin-releasing peptide, *NPPB* natriuretic precursor peptide B

transmit pain: it is now recognized that separate sets of neurons mediate itch and pain input from the peripheral nerve (Galatian et al. 2009).

Gastrin-releasing peptide (GRP) has been recognized as a key neurotransmitter in the itch sensation. GRP receptors (GRPRs) are expressed in the superficial dorsal horn, and pharmacological inhibition and genetic deletion of GRP signaling pathways can reduce itch responses (Sun and Chen 2007; Sun et al. 2009). Recently, another neuropeptide, natriuretic precursor peptide B (NPPB), has been indicated as a neurotransmitter in spinal cord that provokes scratching behavior in mice (Mishra and Hoon 2013).

5.2   Itch Classification

Although the pathophysiology of most clinical itch conditions is not completely understood, operational classifications are needed for clinical use. The following definitions are taken from a review of itch published in 2003 by the *Lancet* (Yosipovitch et al. 2003):

> "Pruritoceptive itch
>
> Itch originating in the skin, due to inflammation, dryness, or other skin damage, is termed pruritoceptive and is transmitted by C nerve fibres. Examples are itch due to scabies, urticaria, and reactions to insect bite.
>
> Neuropathic itch
>
> Itch that arises because of disease located at any point along the afferent pathway is called neuropathic itch. Five Post-herpes zoster neuropathy and the itch occasionally associated with multiple sclerosis and brain tumours are in this category.
>
> Neurogenic itch
>
> Neurogenic itch is defined as that which originates centrally but without evidence of neural pathology, such as the itch of cholestasis, which is due to the action of opioid neuropeptides on μ-opioid receptors.
>
> Psychogenic itch
>
> The fourth type of itch is psychogenic, as in the delusional state of parasitophobia. This classification is both clinically relevant and informative as to the pathomechanisms of pruritus."

5.3   Modulators for Itch and Pain

Evidence has revealed that the peripheral mediators and/or receptors responsible for itch and pain broadly overlap (Ikoma et al. 2006). Some of them are described as follows:

5.3.1   Histamine

Histamine is the best-known pruritogen. Activation of H_1 receptors can increase vasodilation of vascular endothelium. In general, histamine-induced itch and wheal and flare in the skin can be suppressed by H_1 antagonists (Morita et al. 2005).

However, H_1 antagonists are ineffective in many pruritic diseases, such as atopic dermatitis (Klein and Clark 1999). Other histamine receptors such as H_4 receptors have been indicated as playing an independent role in pruritus (Bell et al. 2004).

5.3.2 Interleukins (ILs)

Specific neuronal pathways for itch have only recently been discovered. IL-6 has been proposed to play a role in the pathophysiology of some types of itch (Ikoma et al. 2006). IL-31 has been found to induce pruritic dermatitis in mice (Dillon et al. 2004; Sun et al. 2004), which indicates a special role for IL-31 in pruritus.

5.3.3 Protease-Activated Receptors

Microbes and plants, as well as inflammatory cells, can induce the production of proteases, which in turn activate protease-activated receptors (PARs). Recently, PAR-2 has been implicated in pain (Cottrell et al. 2003) and itch (Steinhoff et al. 2003). Intradermal (i.d.) injection of PAR-2 agonists induced scratching in mice (Shimada et al. 2006; Tsujii et al. 2008; Ui et al. 2006). The scratching behavior induced by PAR-2 is histamine-independent and PAR-2 is considered to be a non-histaminergic mechanism for itch.

5.3.4 Mas-Related G Protein-Coupled Receptors (Mrgprs)

The mouse genome contains approximately 50 identified Mas-related G protein-coupled receptor (Mrgpr) genes, grouped by their sequence homology into the MrgprA, MrgprB, MrgprC and MrgprD subfamilies, located only in the small-diameter sensory neurons in the dorsal root ganglia (DRG) and trigeminal ganglia (Dong et al. 2001; Zylka et al. 2003). MrgprA3 and MrgprC11, which belong to the sensory neuron-specific Mrgpr family, play key roles in histamine-independent pruritus. Activation of MrgprA3 by the antimalarial chloroquine leads to acute itch in rodents and intolerable itch in some patients (Wilson et al. 2011), while mast cell pruritogens released during allergic inflammation target MrgprC11 (Lee et al. 2008).

5.3.5 Peripheral μ- and κ-Opioid Receptors

Pruritus is a well-known side effect of treatment of opioids administered for pain relief (Friedman and Dello Buono 2001). There is growing evidence, however, that opioid receptors and endogenous opioid agonists are also functional in the skin, and they have been found on peripheral nerve fibers, keratinocytes, and immune cells (Bigliardi et al. 2009). Recent evidence indicates that the μ-opioid receptors mediate itch, whereas the κ-opioid receptors suppress itch. Stimulation of the κ-opioid receptor was found to inhibit μ-opioid receptor effects both centrally and peripherally (Inan et al. 2009; Pan 1998; Umeuchi et al. 2003).

Since μ-opioid receptors may mediate itch, μ-opioid receptor antagonists, such as naltrexone and naloxone, have been used to treat chronic pruritus (Metze et al. 1999; Terra and Tsunoda 1998; Zylicz et al. 2005). Several double-blind, placebo-controlled studies have proven the efficacy of systemically applied naltrexone and naloxone in hepatogenic pruritus (Bergasa et al. 1995; Terg et al. 2002; Wolfhagen et al. 1997). On the other hand, a κ-opioid receptor agonist has been used to treat uremic pruritus (Nakao and Mochizuki 2009).

5.4   Itch Is Frequently Poorly Controlled by Antihistamines and Other Treatments

Antihistamines are used to relieve itching caused by various allergies, but they fail to lessen itch in skin, liver, or kidney diseases. Gabapentin (a GABA analog) and cholestyramine (an anion exchange resin) have been clinically tested, but an efficacious treatment against itch remains to be identified (Bergasa 2008; Patel et al. 2007). Pruritus may be a debilitating condition in some patients, and treatment is often ineffective (Fazio and Yosipovitch 2018).

5.5   Acupuncture

Acupuncture has been used in traditional Chinese medicine for over 2500 years (Wu 1996). Its practice is becoming more widespread worldwide (Conference 1998). In 1998, the US National Institutes of Health stated that acupuncture is useful for treating particular conditions and that it has fewer side effects than other medical procedures, such as surgery or pharmaceuticals (NIH 1998).

5.6   Acupuncture and Pruritus: Acupuncture Treatment Is Effective for Itch in Clinical Studies

Several small, placebo-controlled studies have evaluated the effect of acupuncture on histamine-induced itch and other pruritus conditions. Hegu (LI4; 合谷) and Quchi (LI11; 曲池) are commonly used acupoints.

5.6.1   Acupuncture Decreases the Histamine-Induced Itch Response

In experimentally-induced itch in healthy volunteers, acupuncture at Quchi (LI11) reduced histamine-induced flares, duration and intensity of itch, but had little or no effect on the itch onset time or maximal itch intensity (Belgrade et al. 1984). Another study has examined whether acupuncture can prevent histamine-induced itch (Lundeberg et al. 1987). In that study, itching was induced by intradermally-injected histamine in ten healthy volunteers who then underwent 'placebo-acupuncture' (superficial insertion of needles), manual acupuncture (MA), and electroacupuncture (EA) (2 and 80 Hz) sessions, in a crossover fashion. When applied intrasegmentally (proximal to the injection site) prior to the induction of itch on the arm, MA and EA significantly reduced subjective itch intensity. In more recent research, acupuncture at Quchi (LI11) prevented skin prick test histamine-induced itch in healthy volunteers (Pfab et al. 2005).

5.6.2 Acupuncture Decreases Pruritus Scores in Patients with Refractory Uremic Pruritus

Che-Yi et al. tested the effects of acupuncture on pruritus scores in patients with refractory uremic pruritus. The acupuncture group received acupuncture at the LI11 acupoint 3 times weekly for 1 month, while the control group received acupuncture at a non-acupoint 2 cm laterally from the elbow, for the same number of treatment sessions. In the acupuncture group, pruritus scores were reduced from baseline by about 50% after acupuncture and at the 3-month follow-up visit; the controls experienced no such change (Che-Yi et al. 2005).

5.6.3 Acupuncture Alleviates Itching in Patients with Neurogenic Pruritus

Another study retrospectively examined the symptomatic relief of acupuncture in 16 patients with neurogenic pruritus. The majority (75%) of patients experienced total resolution of symptoms, as evidenced by VAS scores (Stellon 2002).

5.7 Basic Research on the Acupuncture Treatment of Itch Is Limited

Many studies have examined the effect of acupuncture and EA on pain, but few studies have examined their effect on pruritus; the antipruritic mechanism of EA remains unclear.

5.8 Animal Models of Pruritogen-Induced Scratching Behavior

Animal models of itch can be performed in rodents. As itch is always accompanied by a desire to scratch, scratching behavior is used as an indicator of itching intensity. This can be measured by counting numbers of hindlimb scratch bouts directed to the site of subcutaneous (s.c.) injection or i.d. microinjection of a pruritogen to the nape of the neck (Akiyama et al. 2009; Kuraishi et al. 1995; Nojima and Carstens 2003).

5.8.1 GNTI-Induced Scratching

5′-Guanidinonaltrindole (GNTI) is a selective κ-opioid receptor antagonist (Jones and Portoghese 2000) that elicits immediate and excessive scratching in mice (Cowan and Inan 2009; Kuraishi et al. 1995). The scratching behavior induced by s.c. injection of GNTI to the neck is abolished by the κ-opioid agonist, nalfurafine (Cowan and Inan 2009).

5.8.2 Compound 48/80-Induced Scratching

Compound 48/80 induces a rapid release of inflammatory mediators such as histamine from mast cells in the connective tissue and skin (Enerback 1966; Koibuchi et al. 1985). S.c. injection or i.d. microinjection of compound 48/80 to the nape of the neck induced scratching behavior in mice, which was effectively suppressed by various H_1 antagonists (Inagaki et al. 2002).

5.8.3 5-HT-Induced Scratching

5-HT (5-hydroxytryptamine or serotonin) is a common neurotransmitter located in the gastrointestinal tract and nervous system that exerts excitatory and inhibitory effects by activating 5-HT receptors. 5-HT is also considered to be a pruritogen (Yamaguchi et al. 1999). Although only weak pruritus is elicited in human skin, i.d. application of 5-HT induces significant scratching behavior in rodents, which is most probably mediated by peripheral 5-HT2 receptors.

5.9 Itch-Related Scratching Behavior Is Associated with c-Fos Expression in the Superficial Dorsal Horn of the Spinal Cord

5.9.1 A Tool to Visualize the Pathway Involved in the Integration of Noxious Inputs

C-Fos is an immediate early gene. Its activation generates the immunologically detectable nuclear protein Fos (Curran and Morgan 1995; Morgan and Curran 1991), which is widely used to indicate neuronal activation pathways involved in noxious inputs. The dorsal horn neuron is at the origin of nociceptive integration, where strong Fos expression follows nociceptive stimuli. Fos or c-Fos expression indicates populations of neurons that are activated or excited by nociceptive input (Buritova et al. 1997; Munglani et al. 1996).

5.9.2   Pruritogen-Induced c-Fos Expression

Nojima and Carstens (2003) reported spontaneous itch-related scratching behavior and associated c-Fos expression in the superficial dorsal horn of the spinal cord in a rat model of dry skin. Subsequent studies reported that GNTI and compound 48/80 provoked c-Fos expression in different neurons at the lateral side of the dorsal horn (Inan et al. 2009).

The expression of Fos in the dorsal horn provides the single best technique for visualizing the individual neurons activated by noxious inputs in awake and mobile animals (Buritova et al. 1997; Coggeshall 2005; Hunt et al. 1987; Nojima et al. 2003, 2004).

5.10   Recent Results

Han et al. (2008) reported an antipruritic effect of acupuncture in a rat model of hindlimb scratching. Their results suggest that acupuncture and EA stimulation are effective treatments for scratching induced by i.d. injection of 2% 5-HT (20 μL) into the rostral back in rats. We have performed a series of studies to characterize the protective profile of EA on pruritogen-induced itch.

5.10.1 EA at LI4 and LI11 Attenuates Scratching Behavior and c-Fos Expression Induced by GNTI

Our recent study revealed that EA at LI4 and LI11 attenuates scratching behavior and c-Fos expression induced by GNTI in anesthetized mice (Chen et al. 2013). Figure 5.2 shows the positioning of the acupuncture needles and the electric stimulator used in the study. Two needles were inserted into the LI4 and LI11 acupoints. To test the effects of EA at different frequencies on pruritogen-induced scratching behavior, the mice were divided into three groups in each pruritogen test: (1) control, (2) 2 Hz EA, and (3) 100 Hz EA. Mice started scratching at 2–3 min after GNTI (a κ-opioid receptor antagonist; 0.3 mg/kg; s.c. behind the neck). Strong, stereotypic behavior continued throughout the 40-min observation period.

As shown in Table 5.1, the application of EA 2 Hz to the LI4 and LI11 acupoints attenuated GNTI-induced scratching; no such effect was seen with EA 100 Hz.

This study also determined the effects on GNTI-induced scratching behavior of EA 2 Hz applied to bilateral ST36 acupoints. As shown in Table 5.2, application of EA at 2 Hz to bilateral ST36 did not affect GNTI (0.3 mg/kg)-evoked scratching.

As reported by Inan et al. in 2009, GNTI significantly increased the number of c-Fos-positive nuclei on the lateral side of the superficial layers of the dorsal horn in

Fig. 5.2 Photograph of a mouse under isoflurane anesthesia with acupuncture needles administering EA at the Hegu (LI4) and Quchi (LI11) acupoints

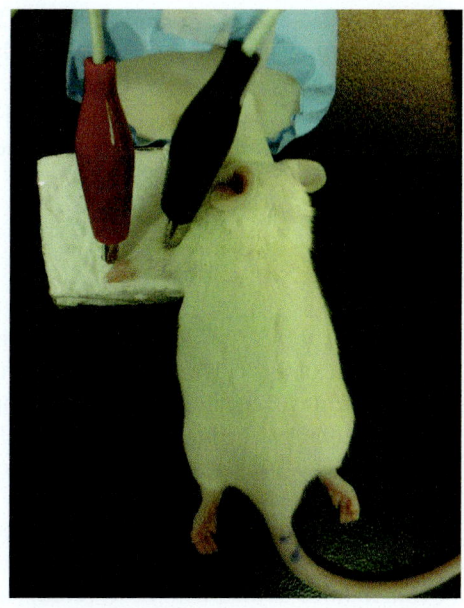

Table 5.1 EA 2 Hz administered to the LI4 and LI11 acupoints attenuated GNTI-induced scratching, whereas EA 100 Hz had no such effect

	Control	EA 2 Hz	EA 100 Hz
Number of scratches mean ± S.E.M.	477.7 ± 48 (n = 20)	290.6 ± 36.1 (n = 14)[a]	398.3 ± 53.7 (n = 14)

[a]p < 0.05 compared with control

Table 5.2 EA to the bilateral ST36 acupoints at 2 Hz did not affect GNTI-induced scratching

	Control	EA 2 Hz
Number of scratches mean ± S.E.M.	438.1 ± 41.1 (n = 8)	427.2 ± 55.4 (n = 6)

cervical spinal cord sections compared to the saline control group. While EA 2 Hz by itself had no significant effect on c-Fos expression, pretreatment with EA 2 Hz significantly reduced the number of c-Fos-positive cells induced by GNTI (Chen et al. 2013).

5.10.2 EA at LI4 and LI11 Attenuates GNTI-Induced Spinal Microglial Activation

Microglia are glial cells that are responsible for immune function in the CNS. It has been indicated that microglia participate in the initiation and progression of neurological disorders. Recent research revealed that scratching behavior induced by GNTI and compound 48/80 is accompanied by an acute activation of microglial cells in the spinal cord of mice (Zhang et al. 2015). We therefore tested whether EA suppresses pruritogen-induced microglial activation. The results found that EA (2 Hz) at LI4 and LI11 effectively reduced the scratching response and activation of microglia in the spinal cord induced by GNTI (Lin et al. 2016). This suggests that EA may be a useful treatment for itch and also for disorders involving microglial dysregulation.

5.10.3 Cold Stimulation

The effects of cold stimulation on acupoints have not previously been addressed. Our group examined the effects of different thermal stimulations at murine LI11 upon scratching behavior elicited by compound 48/80 (Tsai et al. 2014). We also assessed whether ruthenium red (a non-selective transient receptor potential [TRP] channel blocker) pretreatment at LI11 modifies the antipruritic effects of thermal stimulation.

The number of scratches in mice injected with compound 48/80 was 290.1 ± 20.9 bouts/30 min. Itch behavior was significantly reduced to 139.8 ± 31.9 bouts per 30 min in mice treated with 20°C (cold) stimulation at LI11, whereas stimulation at 5, 15, 25, 35, or 45°C had no such effects, suggesting that 20°C is an optimal temperature for cold stimulation at LI11 for attenuating pruritogen-induced scratching. Interestingly, 20°C stimulation at the sham acupoints (located at the midpoint of the acromial part of the deltoid muscle) had no effect on scratching induced by compound 48/80. Similarly to the previous study (Chen et al. 2013), cold stimulation at LI11 attenuated increases in c-Fos expression induced by compound 48/80 in the cervical spinal cord. Interestingly, injecting mice subcutaneously with ruthenium red (0.5 μmoL/site) at LI11 5 min before 20°C stimulation lowered the antipruritic effect of cold stimulation. These results demonstrated that cold stimulation at LI11 appears to attenuate pruritogen-induced scratching behavior via a TRP-related pathway.

Conclusions

The sensations of pain and itch share many interactions in acute transmission and sensitization processes, but they have many differences as well. Pain sensation evokes withdrawal behavior, while itch evokes scratching as a reflex or conscious mechanical stimulation to relieve the hazardous stimulant and act as a helpful warning of potential hazards (Ikoma et al. 2006). Separate sets of neurons mediate itch and pain input from the peripheral nerve. Primary afferents for pain sensation are mechano-sensitive and mechano-insensitive Aδ- and polymodal C-fibers (Andrew and Craig 2001; Schmidt et al. 2000), whereas primary afferents for itch sensation are histamine-activated mechano-insensitive C-fibers (Schmelz et al. 1997) and cowhage-activated mechano-sensitive fibers (Namer et al. 2008). Histamine stimulates neurons that project to the posterior part of the ventromedial nucleus of the thalamus (Andrew and Craig 2001), whereas pain stimulates neurons that project to the ventroposterior lateral nucleus of the thala-

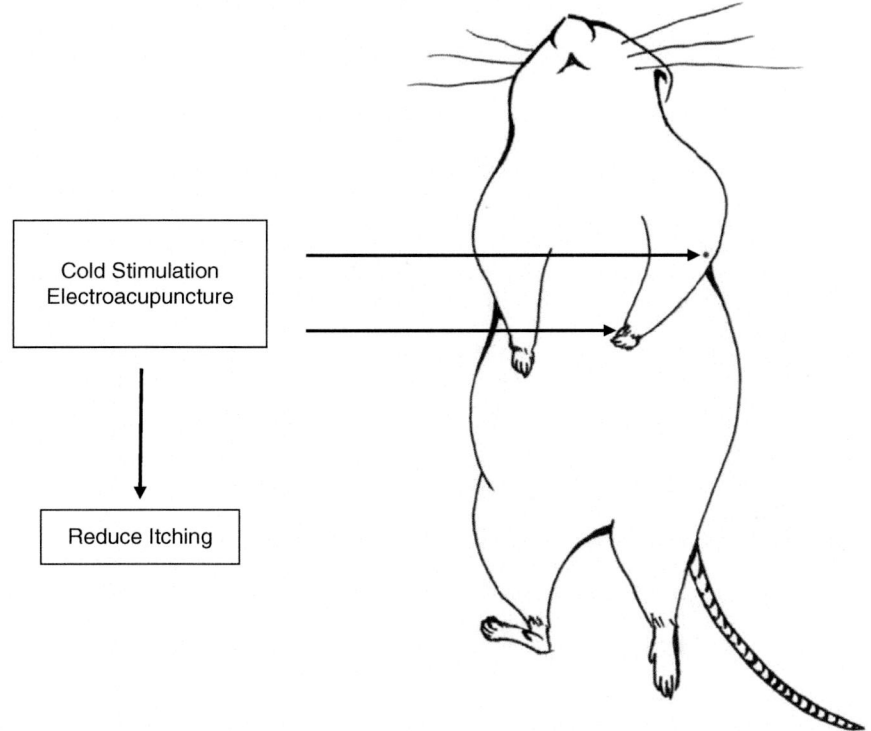

Fig. 5.3 EA at LI4 and LI11 or cold stimulation at LI11 significantly attenuates pruritogen-induced scratching behavior in mice

mus (Craig 2002). Much clinical and basic research evidence has proven the efficacy of acupuncture in pain relief. However, scant evidence exists as to the efficacy of acupuncture in itch. Our studies have shown that EA at LI4 and LI11 or cold stimulation at LI11 can significantly attenuate pruritogen-induced scratching behavior in mice (Fig. 5.3). Studies into acupuncture for itch treatment are expected to attract more attention and research in the near future, with a growing familiarity of the animal model of itch and greater understanding of the neurotransmission of itch.

References

Akiyama T, Merrill AW, Zanotto K, Carstens MI, Carstens E. Scratching behavior and Fos expression in superficial dorsal horn elicited by protease-activated receptor agonists and other itch mediators in mice. J Pharmacol Exp Ther. 2009;329:945–51.
Andrew D, Craig AD. Spinothalamic lamina I neurons selectively sensitive to histamine: a central neural pathway for itch. Nat Neurosci. 2001;4:72–7.
Belgrade MJ, Solomon LM, Lichter EA. Effect of acupuncture on experimentally induced itch. Acta Derm Venereol. 1984;64:129–33.

Bell JK, McQueen DS, Rees JL. Involvement of histamine H4 and H1 receptors in scratching induced by histamine receptor agonists in Balb C mice. Br J Pharmacol. 2004;142:374–80.

Bergasa NV. Update on the treatment of the pruritus of cholestasis. Clin Liver Dis. 2008;12:219–34, x.

Bergasa NV, Alling DW, Talbot TL, Swain MG, Yurdaydin C, Turner ML, Schmitt JM, Walker EC, Jones EA. Effects of naloxone infusions in patients with the pruritus of cholestasis. A double-blind, randomized, controlled trial. Ann Intern Med. 1995;123:161–7.

Bigliardi PL, Tobin DJ, Gaveriaux-Ruff C, Bigliardi-Qi M. Opioids and the skin—where do we stand? Exp Dermatol. 2009;18:424–30.

Buritova J, Chapman V, Honore P, Besson JM. The contribution of peripheral bradykinin B2 receptors to carrageenan-evoked oedema and spinal c-Fos expression in rats. Eur J Pharmacol. 1997;320:73–80.

Carlsson CP, Wallengren J. Therapeutic and experimental therapeutic studies on acupuncture and itch: review of the literature. J Eur Acad Dermatol Venereol. 2010;24(9):1013–6.

Chen YH, Yang HY, Lin CH, Dun NJ, Lin JG. Electroacupuncture attenuates 5'-Guanidinonaltrindole-evoked scratching and spinal c-Fos expression in the mouse. Evid Based Complement Alternat Med. 2013;2013:319124.

Che-Yi C, Yu Wen C, Min-Tsung K, Chiu-Ching H. Acupuncture in haemodialysis patients at the Quchi (LI11) acupoint for refractory uraemic pruritus. Nephrol Dial Transplant. 2005;20(9):1912–5.

Coggeshall RE. Fos, nociception and the dorsal horn. Prog Neurobiol. 2005;77:299–352.

Conference NC. NIH consensus conference, acupuncture. JAMA. 1998;280(17):1518–24.

Cottrell GS, Amadesi S, Schmidlin F, Bunnett N. Protease-activated receptor 2: activation, signalling and function. Biochem Soc Trans. 2003;31:1191–7.

Cowan A, Inan S. Kappa-opioid antagonists as pruritogenic agents. New York: Humana Press; 2009. p. 541–9.

Craig AD. How do you feel? Interoception: the sense of the physiological condition of the body. Nat Rev Neurosci. 2002;3:655–66.

Curran T, Morgan JI. Fos: an immediate-early transcription factor in neurons. J Neurobiol. 1995;26:403–12.

Dillon SR, Sprecher C, Hammond A, Bilsborough J, Rosenfeld-Franklin M, Presnell SR, Haugen HS, Maurer M, Harder B, Johnston J, et al. Interleukin 31, a cytokine produced by activated T cells, induces dermatitis in mice. Nat Immunol. 2004;5:752–60.

Dong X, Han S, Zylka MJ, Simon MI, Anderson DJ. A diverse family of GPCRs expressed in specific subsets of nociceptive sensory neurons. Cell. 2001;106:619–32.

Enerback L. Mast cells in rat gastrointestinal mucosa. 3. Reactivity towards compound 48/80. Acta Pathol Microbiol Scand. 1966;66:313–22.

Fazio SB, Yosipovitch G. Pruritus: overview of management. UpToDate Topic 5576 Version 25.0; 2018.

Friedman JD, Dello Buono FA. Opioid antagonists in the treatment of opioid-induced constipation and pruritus. Ann Pharmacother. 2001;35:85–91.

Galatian A, Stearns G, Grau R. Pruritus in connective tissue and other common systemic disease states. Cutis. 2009;84:207–14.

Han J-B, Kim CW, Sun B, Kim SK, Lee MG, Park DS, Min B. The antipruritic effect of acupuncture on serotonin-evoked itch in rats. Acupunct Electrother Res. 2008;33(3):145–56.

Hunt SP, Pini A, Evan G. Induction of c-fos-like protein in spinal cord neurons following sensory stimulation. Nature. 1987;328:632–4.

Ikoma A, Steinhoff M, Stander S, Yosipovitch G, Schmelz M. The neurobiology of itch. Nat Rev Neurosci. 2006;7:535–47.

Inagaki N, Igeta K, Kim JF, Nagao M, Shiraishi N, Nakamura N, Nagai H. Involvement of unique mechanisms in the induction of scratching behavior in BALB/c mice by compound 48/80. Eur J Pharmacol. 2002;448:175–83.

Inan S, Dun NJ, Cowan A. Nalfurafine prevents 5'-guanidinonaltrindole- and compound 48/80-induced spinal c-fos expression and attenuates 5'-guanidinonaltrindole-elicited scratching behavior in mice. Neuroscience. 2009;163:23–33.

Jones RM, Portoghese PS. 5′-Guanidinonaltrindole, a highly selective and potent kappa-opioid receptor antagonist. Eur J Pharmacol. 2000;396:49–52.

Klein PA, Clark RA. An evidence-based review of the efficacy of antihistamines in relieving pruritus in atopic dermatitis. Arch Dermatol. 1999;135:1522–5.

Koibuchi Y, Ichikawa A, Nakagawa M, Tomita K. Histamine release induced from mast cells by active components of compound 48/80. Eur J Pharmacol. 1985;115:163–70.

Kuraishi Y, Nagasawa T, Hayashi K, Satoh M. Scratching behavior induced by pruritogenic but not algesiogenic agents in mice. Eur J Pharmacol. 1995;275:229–33.

Lee MG, Dong X, Liu Q, Patel KN, Choi OH, Vonakis B, Undem BJ. Agonists of the MAS-related gene (Mrgs) orphan receptors as novel mediators of mast cell-sensory nerve interactions. J Immunol. 2008;180:2251–5.

Lin JG, Lee YC, Tseng CH, Chen DY, Shih CY, MacDonald I, Hung SY, Chen YH. Electroacupuncture inhibits pruritogen-induced spinal microglial activation in mice. Brain Res. 2016;1649:23–9.

Lundeberg T, Bondesson L, Thomas M. Effect of acupuncture on experimentally induced itch. Br J Dermatol. 1987;117:771–7.

Metze D, Reimann S, Beissert S, Luger T. Efficacy and safety of naltrexone, an oral opiate receptor antagonist, in the treatment of pruritus in internal and dermatological diseases. J Am Acad Dermatol. 1999;41:533–9.

Mishra SK, Hoon MA. The cells and circuitry for itch responses in mice. Science. 2013;340:968–71.

Morgan JI, Curran T. Stimulus-transcription coupling in the nervous system: involvement of the inducible proto-oncogenes fos and jun. Annu Rev Neurosci. 1991;14:421–51.

Morita E, Matsuo H, Zhang Y. Double-blind, crossover comparison of olopatadine and cetirizine versus placebo: suppressive effects on skin response to histamine iontophoresis. J Dermatol. 2005;32:58–61.

Munglani R, Fleming BG, Hunt SP. Remembrance of times past: the significance of c-fos in pain. Br J Anaesth. 1996;76:1–4.

Nakao K, Mochizuki H. Nalfurafine hydrochloride: a new drug for the treatment of uremic pruritus in hemodialysis patients. Drugs Today (Barc). 2009;45:323–9.

Namer B, Carr R, Johanek LM, Schmelz M, Handwerker HO, Ringkamp M. Separate peripheral pathways for pruritus in man. J Neurophysiol. 2008;100:2062–9.

NIH. NIH consensus development conference on acupuncture. JAMA. 1998;280(17):1518–24.

Nojima H, Carstens E. 5-Hydroxytryptamine (5-HT)2 receptor involvement in acute 5-HT-evoked scratching but not in allergic pruritus induced by dinitrofluorobenzene in rats. J Pharmacol Exp Ther. 2003;306:245–52.

Nojima H, Simons CT, Cuellar JM, Carstens MI, Moore JA, Carstens E. Opioid modulation of scratching and spinal c-fos expression evoked by intradermal serotonin. J Neurosci. 2003;23:10784–90.

Nojima H, Cuellar JM, Simons CT, Carstens MI, Carstens E. Spinal c-fos expression associated with spontaneous biting in a mouse model of dry skin pruritus. Neurosci Lett. 2004;361:79–82.

Pan ZZ. mu-Opposing actions of the kappa-opioid receptor. Trends Pharmacol Sci. 1998;19:94–8.

Patel TS, Freedman BI, Yosipovitch G. An update on pruritus associated with CKD. Am J Kidney Dis. 2007;50:11–20.

Pfab F, Hammes M, Backer M, Huss-Marp J, Athanasiadis GI, Tolle TR, Behrendt H, Ring J, Darsow U. Preventive effect of acupuncture on histamine-induced itch: a blinded, randomized, placebo-controlled, crossover trial. J Allergy Clin Immunol. 2005;116:1386–8.

Schmelz M, Schmidt R, Bickel A, Handwerker HO, Torebjörk HE. Specific C-receptors for itch in human skin. J Neurosci. 1997;17:8003–8.

Schmidt R, Schmelz M, Torebjork HE, Handwerker HO. Mechano-insensitive nociceptors encode pain evoked by tonic pressure to human skin. Neuroscience. 2000;98:793–800.

Shimada SG, Shimada KA, Collins JG. Scratching behavior in mice induced by the proteinase-activated receptor-2 agonist, SLIGRL-NH2. Eur J Pharmacol. 2006;530:281–3.

Steinhoff M, Neisius U, Ikoma A, Fartasch M, Heyer G, Skov PS, Luger TA, Schmelz M. Proteinase-activated receptor-2 mediates itch: a novel pathway for pruritus in human skin. J Neurosci. 2003;23:6176–80.

Stellon A. Neurogenic pruritus: an unrecognised problem? A retrospective case series of treatment by acupuncture. Acupunct Med. 2002;20:186–90.

Sun YG, Chen ZF. A gastrin-releasing peptide receptor mediates the itch sensation in the spinal cord. Nature. 2007;448:700–3.

Sun RQ, Tu YJ, Lawand NB, Yan JY, Lin Q, Willis WD. Calcitonin gene-related peptide receptor activation produces PKA- and PKC-dependent mechanical hyperalgesia and central sensitization. J Neurophysiol. 2004;92:2859–66.

Sun YG, Zhao ZQ, Meng XL, Yin J, Liu XY, Chen ZF. Cellular basis of itch sensation. Science. 2009;325:1531–4.

Terg R, Coronel E, Sorda J, Munoz AE, Findor J. Efficacy and safety of oral naltrexone treatment for pruritus of cholestasis, a crossover, double blind, placebo-controlled study. J Hepatol. 2002;37:717–22.

Terra SG, Tsunoda SM. Opioid antagonists in the treatment of pruritus from cholestatic liver disease. Ann Pharmacother. 1998;32:1228–30.

Tsai KS, Chen YH, Chen HY, Shen EY, Lee YC, Shen JL, Wu SY, Lin JG, Chen YH, Chen WC. Antipruritic effect of cold stimulation at the Quchi acupoint (LI11) in mice. BMC Complement Altern Med. 2014;14:341.

Tsujii K, Andoh T, Lee JB, Kuraishi Y. Activation of proteinase-activated receptors induces itch-associated response through histamine-dependent and -independent pathways in mice. J Pharmacol Sci. 2008;108:385–8.

Twycross R, Greaves MW, Handwerker H, Jones EA, Libretto SE, Szepietowski JC, Zylicz Z. Itch: scratching more than the surface. QJM. 2003;96:7–26.

Ui H, Andoh T, Lee JB, Nojima H, Kuraishi Y. Potent pruritogenic action of tryptase mediated by PAR-2 receptor and its involvement in anti-pruritic effect of nafamostat mesilate in mice. Eur J Pharmacol. 2006;530:172–8.

Umeuchi H, Togashi Y, Honda T, Nakao K, Okano K, Tanaka T, Nagase H. Involvement of central mu-opioid system in the scratching behavior in mice, and the suppression of it by the activation of kappa-opioid system. Eur J Pharmacol. 2003;477:29–35.

Wilson SR, Gerhold KA, Bifolck-Fisher A, Liu Q, Patel KN, Dong X, Bautista DM. TRPA1 is required for histamine-independent, Mas-related G protein-coupled receptor-mediated itch. Nat Neurosci. 2011;14:595–602.

Wolfhagen FH, Sternieri E, Hop WC, Vitale G, Bertolotti M, Van Buuren HR. Oral naltrexone treatment for cholestatic pruritus: a double-blind, placebo-controlled study. Gastroenterology. 1997;113:1264–9.

Wu JN. A short history of acupuncture. J Altern Complement Med. 1996;2:19–21.

Yamaguchi T, Nagasawa T, Satoh M, Kuraishi Y. Itch-associated response induced by intradermal serotonin through 5-HT2 receptors in mice. Neurosci Res. 1999;35:77–83.

Yosipovitch G, Greaves MW, Schmelz M. Itch. Lancet. 2003;361:690–4.

Zhang Y, Dun SL, Chen YH, Luo JJ, Cowan A, Dun NJ. Scratching activates microglia in the mouse spinal cord. J Neurosci Res. 2015;93:466–74.

Zylicz Z, Stork N, Krajnik M. Severe pruritus of cholestasis in disseminated cancer: developing a rational treatment strategy. A case report. J Pain Symptom Manag. 2005;29:100–3.

Zylka MJ, Dong X, Southwell AL, Anderson DJ. Atypical expansion in mice of the sensory neuron-specific Mrg G protein-coupled receptor family. Proc Natl Acad Sci U S A. 2003;100:10043–8.

Effects of Acupuncture on Peripheral Nerve Regeneration

6

Yueh-Sheng Chen, Cherng-Jyh Ke, Ching-Yun Chen, and Jaung-Geng Lin

Abstract

While Western medicine focuses on the use of surgery or drug treatment in the repair of peripheral nerve injury, the use of non-surgical physical stimulation in nerve repair is attracting increasing attention. As a part of traditional Chinese medicine, the practice of acupuncture has spread worldwide and is used to treat various diseases and symptoms. A search of the keywords "acupuncture" and "peripheral nerve regeneration" in the online bibliographic databases covering

Y.-S. Chen
Lab of Biomaterials, School of Chinese Medicine, China Medical University, Taichung, Taiwan

Department of Biomedical Imaging and Radiological Science, China Medical University, Taichung, Taiwan

Department of Biomaterials Translational Research Center, China Medical University Hospital, Taichung, Taiwan

C.-J. Ke
Department of Biological Science and Technology, College of Biopharmaceutical and Food Sciences, China Medical University, Taichung, Taiwan

Department of Biomaterials Translational Research Center, China Medical University Hospital, Taichung, Taiwan

C.-Y. Chen
Institute of Biomedical Engineering, College of Medicine and College of Engineering, National Taiwan University, Taipei, Taiwan

Institute of Biomedical Engineering and Nanomedicine, National Health Research Institutes, Miaoli, Taiwan

J.-G. Lin (✉)
School of Chinese Medicine, College of Chinese Medicine, China Medical University, Taichung, Taiwan
e-mail: jglin@mail.cmu.edu.tw

© Springer Nature Singapore Pte Ltd. 2018
J.-G. Lin (ed.), *Experimental Acupuncturology*,
https://doi.org/10.1007/978-981-13-0971-7_6

the clinical medicine literature, including MedLine and PubMed, reveals a wealth of related literature, including experimental animal models, in vitro testing and clinical studies, suggesting that acupuncture improves the symptoms of nerve damage. This chapter reviews the effects of different types of stimulation (traditional acupuncture, electro-acupuncture, or stem cell transplantation as an adjuvant therapy) on promoting repair following peripheral nerve damage caused by various conditions (including traumatic injury, degenerative diseases, or side effects of chemotherapy). We propose future directions for research into the use of acupuncture in nerve regeneration.

Keywords

Acupuncture · Nerve regeneration · Neurotrophin · Diabetic peripheral neuropathy · Chemotherapy-induced peripheral neuropathy

6.1   Introduction

Peripheral nerve injury and degeneration, whether caused by traumatic injury, diseases (such as Alzheimer's disease, diabetes, and stroke) (Ho et al. 2014a; Zhang et al. 2014; Lin et al. 2014) or cancer treatments, reduce patients' quality of life and impose a heavy burden on their families. Many researchers have focused on the effective treatment or repair of the damaged nerve. However, nerve repair is difficult. For damage over short lengths, such as stab and scratch wounds, nerves can be repaired with wound healing and the severed nerve fiber can self-regenerate. However, in cases of massive damage, such as that involving broken limbs (Yoo et al. 2003), disease-induced damage (Schröder et al. 2007) or nerve degeneration caused by chemotherapy drugs (Wong and Sagar 2006; Franconi et al. 2013), the lengths are beyond self-regeneration capacity and the nerve damage may become permanent (Lundborg et al. 1982). This difference in regeneration capacity may be explained by the structure of the nerve. In general, the nerve structure includes the cell body (soma), dendrites, axon, and the surrounding myelin sheath. The electrical signals are received by dendrites, sent to the cell body, then transmitted by axons out of the cell body. In the peripheral nervous system, the surrounding Schwann cells form myelin sheaths to support and insulate axons, increase the speed of signal transmission and conduct action potentials (Kagitani et al. 2010).

If the nerve is transected, a temporary loss of nerve function may occur. The distal end of the nerve may degenerate and die, while the proximal end near the cell body can grow towards the distal end at the speed of about 1–2 mm/day (Detrait et al. 2000). Meanwhile, the demyelinated Schwann cells and the surrounding endoneurial tubes formed by the basal lamina, release neurotrophic substances and function as scaffolds to support axonal growth toward the distal end. If the distance is too great, the distal nerve is unable to receive a steady, prolonged supply of nutrients, leading to progressive degeneration and death of the nerve fibers, as well as the formation of neurofibromatosis. Alternatively, the lack of formation of long endoneurial tubes prevents the axon from growing to the distal end, leading to the failure of nerve regeneration (Yoo et al. 2003; Wang et al. 2011b; Chang et al. 2011; Chen et al. 2004, 2005b, 2008).

In nerve damage caused by disease, problems with regeneration are usually due to inadequate blood flow. For example, in patients with diabetes, long-term hyperglycemia, abnormal blood lipid level, and an elevated inflammatory response lead to abnormal thickening of blood vessel walls, inadequate nutrient supply, and reduced blood permeability. In other scenarios, a reduced blood oxygen level and higher inflammation index may lead to an environment with higher chemical factors or lower neurotrophic factors, leading to nerve damage (Lin et al. 2014; Piao and Liang 2012; Yao et al. 2012; Kao et al. 2013; Kennedy and Zochodne 2005, 2000). About 20–30% of patients with diabetes exhibit various types of nerve damage; the prevalence is as high as 50% in patients aged over 60 years. Symptoms include a sensation of numbness, tingling or burning in extremities, an occasional sense of imbalance, or complete loss of sensory functions (such as touch, pressure, cold, heat, and pain) in the extremities (Young et al. 1993).

Chemotherapy drugs invariably damage normal cells (Windebank and Grisold 2008). Chemotherapy-induced peripheral neuropathy (CIPN) is a common treatment-related adverse effect of several commonly used cancer treatments, including docetaxel and cisplatin. Although the symptoms of discomfort can be reduced by limiting or decreasing the drug dosage, the sensory or motor nerves may still be affected (Wolf et al. 2008). The neurotoxic mechanism can cause mitochondrial damage, axonal atrophy and myelin degeneration, thereby depriving the dorsal root ganglia (DRG) neurons of their barriers, and resulting in symptoms of peripheral pain, numbness, or neuropathic pain (Podratz et al. 2011).

In certain injuries, the damage results in nerve fiber degeneration or a neuroma developing at the nerve stump, preventing functional recovery. Currently, surgical treatments, including direct suture repair, nerve grafting and the use of nerve conduits, are commonly used to repair the damaged nerve. Nerve endings, as well as the related nerve membrane and blood vessels, are sutured under a microscope of high magnification. Successful operations depend on the length of nerve damage. For damage extending over a significant length, nerve grafting is commonly used. Autografts can avoid immune rejection and have a good postoperative recovery rate in clinical practice; however, they have limited availability and may cause donor site damage. In contrast, allografts or xenografts induce immune rejection and have poor physical properties (Ide 1996; Fowler et al. 2015; Fawcett and Keynes 1990). Use of nerve conduits to bridge nerve gaps shows enormous potential, providing a scaffold for attached migration of the regenerating nerves, and avoiding a second surgery and pressure on the nerve, due to the use of biodegradable materials used in nerve conduits (gelatin, chitosan, polyester materials polylactic acid [PLA], polyglycolic acid [PGA], and poly lactic-co-glycolic acid [PLGA]). Although many successful cases have been reported (Lin et al. 2014; Wang et al. 2011a, b; Chen et al. 2005a, b, 2008, 2013; Chang et al. 2007; Lu et al. 2007; Hsiang et al. 2011a, b; Huang et al. 2011), nerve conduits are ineffective for degenerative neuropathy and damage in areas where surgical treatment is impossible.

6.2   Application of Acupuncture in Nerve Repair

Traditional Chinese acupuncture techniques have become a valuable alternative tool or form of complementary medicine used increasingly by Western medical practitioners (Mayer 2000). In 2007, Schröder et al. reported the use of acupuncture stimulation in restoring the conducting capability of lesioned nerves. At 1 year after treatment, nerve conduction studies revealed symptomatic and objective improvement in 76% of the patients in the experimental group, as compared with only 15% of the control group. Investigations using functional magnetic resonance imaging (fMRI) to examine the effect of acupuncture on the brain reveal that acupuncture stimulation at specific acupoints induces activity in the corresponding brain areas (Bai and Lao 2013). Western clinical literature provides evidence showing that acupuncture exerts beneficial stimulation to nerves (Mayer 2000).

6.2.1   Nerve Transection Injury

Peripheral nerve transection injury is usually repaired by surgery (Nawabi et al. 2006). The use of complementary acupuncture or electro-acupuncture on animal models has recently advanced and has become the mainstream approach in complementary medicine (Ide 1996; Chen et al. 2001; Inoue et al. 2003; de Albornoz et al. 2011). In 2001, Chen et al. (2001) used a silicon rubber tube as a nerve conduit to bridge a 1-cm long gap in a rat model of sciatic nerve injury and then applied acupuncture stimulation. Six weeks after implantation of the conduits, animals that received acupuncture in the experimental group exhibited a more developed and complete nerve structure. In further examinations into the difference between traditional acupuncture and electroneedling stimulation (Ho et al. 2013), low-frequency electro-acupuncture was found to potentiate the nerve-growth promoting effect. The animal behavior study also found that rats with sciatic nerve injury exhibited signs of sensory and motor function recovery after 6 weeks of treatment with electro-acupuncture at acupoints GB30 and GB34. In particular, gait analysis indicated that electro-acupuncture significantly improved motor function recovery (Hoang et al. 2012).

Clinically, many case studies have indicated that acupuncture may promote nerve repair. In an analysis of 100 patients with acute spinal cord injury, neurological recovery was better amongst patients in the experimental group treated with electro-acupuncture at points S13, BL62, and others (Wong et al. 2003). In 2010, a study using intermittent direct current (DC, 100 Hz, 20 min) to stimulate patients with injured peripheral nerves (including functional nerve palsy, axonal truncation, and truncated nerve) showed that in most patients (except those with axonal truncation), motor function was restored (Inoue et al. 2011), indicating that it is feasible to use acupuncture to aid nerve repair in clinical practice.

6.2.2 Disease-Related Nerve Damage

Diabetic peripheral neuropathy (DPN) is a common complication of diabetes (Harati 1987; Younger 1998; Pinzur 2011). Stroke is also likely to cause hypoxic neuronal necrosis (Palumbo et al. 1978). For disease-related nerve damage, which affects broader areas and cannot be easily treated by surgery, acupuncture is an attractive alternative treatment.

A review published in 1976 (Becker et al. 1976) described how DC electrical stimulation with acupuncture needles could affect nerve repair by promoting the proliferation of Schwann cells. A 1989 study by Cameron et al. (1989) showed that using continuous electro-acupuncture stimulation (10 Hz, 8 h or more each day) to treat streptozotocin (STZ)-induced diabetic rats restored the conduction velocity (CV) of the anterior tibial nerve to a level (no significant difference) comparable to that in control rats. This research group published another paper in 1993, using the same animal model and stimulation condition to explore the effects upon the peroneal sciatic nerve (Cameron et al. 1993). In this study, acupuncture stimulation increased the CV by 60%. The group also proposed that the increased blood flow and metabolism induced by the electrical stimulation led to the effective repair of the damaged nerve.

In 2012, Chen et al. constructed a rat model of diabetes, using a silicon rubber tube as the nerve conduit, and applied continuous electro-acupuncture stimulation (1 mA, 2 Hz, 15 min each day) for 3 weeks. They found that after electrical stimulation, in animals with or without diabetes, the propagation delay time was shortened, the CV was increased, and the proportion of macrophages in the regenerated tissue increased. Tissue section analysis also revealed that the electrical stimulation effectively increased the density of axons and the endoneurium area. Moreover, the index values of the diabetic rats were restored to levels similar to those in control rats (normal animals) (Yao et al. 2012). In 2013 (Kao et al. 2013) and 2014 (Lin et al. 2014), the same group examined the effects of different frequencies (0, 2, 20, and 200 Hz) and currents (1, 10, and 20 mA) on neural conduit-mediated repair of the sciatic nerve in a rat model of diabetes. Under conditions of the same current level (1 mA) and different frequencies, a higher frequency (200 Hz) had better effect on nerve regeneration in diabetic rats. In the experiments with different current levels, complete nerve regeneration was found in the 10-mA group.

Many clinical reports have also confirmed the treatment effect of acupuncture on DPN. In 1998, Abuaisha et al. published the results of a clinical trial, in which 64 patients with DPN, 29 of whom had already received general pain treatment, received acupuncture treatment. Ten weeks after treatment with acupuncture, 77% of patients who completed the course felt a significant improvement in pain. Another treatment cycle of 18–25 weeks led to a reduced dosage of pain medications in 67% of the patients. Among them, 21% became pain-free and stopped the medications. None of the patients showed side effects after acupuncture treatment.

In 2014, a randomized controlled trial (RCT) explored the role of acupuncture on the management of DPN. The experimental group received a 10-week course of acupuncture stimulation at acupoints LV3, K13, SP6, SP10, ST36, and others. Compared with the control group given placebo treatment, patients in the experimental group exhibited significant improvement when assessed with the Leeds Assessment of Neuropathic Symptoms and Signs (LANSS), LANSS scale the Sleep Problem Scale (SPS), the lower limb pain Visual Analogue Scale (VAS), the Measure Yourself Medical Outcome Profile (MYMOP), and blood pressure measurements (Richardson and Vincent 1986). In addition, diabetes-related discomfort was reduced.

Nerve damage caused by disease often results from a lack of nutrients or insufficient blood supply. Acupuncture can increase blood flow and metabolism, and increase the proportion of macrophages in the damaged areas. Macrophages secrete high levels of growth factors and accelerate the clearance of necrotic tissue, thereby effectively improving nerve regeneration in rat models of diabetes. Clinical trials have also shown that acupuncture reduces discomfort in patients with DPN and enables them to return to a normal lifestyle without pain medications.

6.2.3   Nerve Damage Caused by Chemotherapy Drugs

Chemotherapy-induced peripheral neuropathy (CIPN) is one of the major side effects of cancer therapy, with an incidence of about 30–40% (Windebank and Grisold 2008; Fernandez et al. 2014). Currently, chemotherapy drugs including platinum drugs, taxanes, and interferon alpha are associated with the well-known side effect of degenerative nerve damage (Wong and Sagar 2006; Franconi et al. 2013; Wolf et al. 2008; Windebank and Grisold 2008; Fernandez et al. 2014; Quasthoff and Hartung 2002; Visovsky et al. 2007). Vitamin E (Pace et al. 2003; Argyriou et al. 2005), calcium/magnesium infusion (Gamelin et al. 2008), glutamine (Gwag et al. 1997; Wang et al. 2007a), glutathione (Cascinu et al. 1995; Smyth et al. 1997), and other preparations have been used to prevent peripheral neuropathy, but the mechanisms that improve nerve regeneration are not yet established (Pachman et al. 2011).

Many studies have explored the protective effect of acupuncture on CIPN (Dorsher 2011; Dyson-Hudson et al. 2007; Trinh et al. 2004; Lee et al. 2005; Richardson and Vincent 1986; Pomeranz 1989; Inoue et al. 2008; Madsen et al. 2009; Gavronsky et al. 2012). In 2006, Wong and Sagar (2006) reported that acupuncture stimulation at acupoints CV6, ST36, LI11, EX-LE10, EX-UE9, etc. led to a significant improvement in pain in 80% of patients with CIPN, with no side effects. A case report by Bao et al. (2011) described how a 48-year-old male patient with myeloma, who had severe pain and paralysis of the leg after bortezomib treatment, received acupuncture at acupoints L14, SJ5, LI11, ST40, EX-LE10, etc. Initially, the pain was relieved for only a few hours. Subsequently, the patient gradually became pain-free and the dosage of pain medication was reduced. After 14 acupuncture treatments, the patient stopped his pain medication and was able to return to a normal work schedule.

In 2011, a report by Donald et al. described the effects of acupuncture upon CIPN. Eighteen patients received acupuncture treatment on the same day of chemotherapy; this continued for six cycles of chemotherapy (cycles were repeated every 6 weeks). The needle remained in situ for 30–45 min each time and the acupoints were selected based on the areas of discomfort that the patients complained about. The results showed that 80% of the patients reported an improvement in symptoms following their course of acupuncture, a reduction in analgesic use, and an improved sleeping pattern. The results also indicated that the more effective acupoints were SP6, ST36 and LV3 in 14 patients.

In 2013, Ogawa et al. observed that acupuncture was effective in treating taxane- and oxaliplatin-induced nerve degeneration. Six patients who had undergone chemotherapy were treated with acupuncture. For each treatment, the needle remained in situ for 30 s to 1 min, and the patients received 4–6 treatments in 3 months. Acupoints CV12, CV4, ST25 and K12 were used in all patients. In addition, based on different conditions, the following points were used: LR8, LR14, SP3, LR13, LU9, LU1, K17, GB25, PC7, CV17, CV6, CV4, ST36, BL20, BL13, BL18, and BL23. All patients showed improvement in pain and some had no pain after the treatment. Two of the cases showed apparent improvement after only 1–2 treatments.

CIPN not only causes pain and discomfort, but also lowers quality of life. Current studies indicate that acupuncture does reduce the pain and related side effects, and is a safe and effective method.

6.3   Influence of Acupuncture on Neurotrophins

The neurotrophin (NT) family regulates neuronal growth and differentiation, and maintains the survival of neurons (Gordon 2009; Ernfors 2001; Kaplan and Miller 2000). Upon peripheral nerve damage, a large amount of endogenous NTs is secreted to promote the repair or regeneration of the damaged nerve. When the concentration of NTs is insufficient in the body, axon regeneration is disrupted and the activity of Schwan cells is reduced, resulting in neurological dysfunction (Manni et al. 2010). Increasing the concentration of NTs in vivo is an important way to promote nerve regeneration or repair.

The literature shows that acupuncture is very effective for pain and numbness caused by peripheral nerve damage, and encourages sensory and motor functional recovery, indicating the ability of acupuncture to stimulate the secretion of NTs and increase the ability of the nerve system to repair and regenerate itself and the speed of regeneration. Acupuncture is therefore a promising complementary medical technique for promoting nerve repair and regeneration.

6.3.1   Nerve Growth Factor (NGF)

NGF is the first identified NT; it plays important roles in the growth, differentiation, and functional maintenance of neurons (Gordon 2009; Allen et al. 2013; Thoenen and Sendtner 2002). NGF also promotes nerve regeneration and functional recovery following nerve damage (Lindsay 1988). Studies have found that in patients with type 1 or type 2 diabetes, NGF levels are reduced, which results in DPN (Pittenger and Vinik 2003).

Many studies have explored the efficacy of acupuncture on DPN. In 2007, Dong et al. used electro-acupuncture stimulation at acupoints BL23 and ST36 in an STZ-induced rat model of DPN and examined NGF levels using immunostaining and polymerase chain reaction (PCR) techniques. Their results indicated that electro-acupuncture not only significantly increases NGF levels and its mRNA expression, but also treats DPN symptoms (Dong et al. 2007). Nori et al. published a study in 2013 showing that electro-acupuncture stimulation at ST36 in an STZ-induced DPN rat model, twice a week for 3 weeks (2 Hz, 180 ms), regulated NGF expression, which in turn affected DPN symptoms caused by damage of the DRG (Nori et al. 2013).

Another study found that in a rat model of inherited retinitis pigmentosa (IRP), daily application of electroneedling stimulation at low frequency for 25 min over 11 days increased the expression of NGF and the NGF binding receptor TrkA, as well as blood flow and thickness of the outer nuclear layer (ONL). Moreover, electroneedling stimulated the secretion of brain-derived growth factor (BDGF), thereby protecting and promoting nerve repair (Pagani et al. 2006).

6.3.2   Other NTs

In addition to NGF, brain-derived neurotrophic factor (BDNF) is an important factor that has often been discussed and used in nerve repair and regeneration. In 2002, Liang et al. studied the use of electro-acupuncture in a rat model of Parkinson's disease (PD). They found that, compared with other low-frequency stimulations, BDNF mRNA levels increased significantly with high-frequency stimulation (100 Hz, 24 times). In addition, the ventral mid-brain dopaminergic neurons were protected from degeneration (Liang et al. 2002). With regard to animal models of spinal cord injury, Xinjia et al. (2002) found that in a rat model, electro-acupuncture increased the expression of BDNF and tyrosine receptor kinase B (TrkB), and promoted nerve regeneration and repair of an injured spinal cord.

Currently, many studies have demonstrated an increase in BDNF levels by acupuncture stimulation and its beneficial effect in treating nerve damage (Isackson 1995; Wang et al. 2005a; Chen et al. 2007; Jeon et al. 2008). Given that BDGF is a brain-derived factor, most studies have used models of brain or spinal cord injury. For the repair of peripheral nerves, more studies have focused on NGF and glial cell line-derived neurotrophic factor (GDNF). GDNF, originally isolated from rat glioma cells, has been shown to have a protective effect on dopaminergic neurons, and therefore is often studied in the treatment of PD (Kaplan and Miller 2000; Allen et al. 2013; Thoenen and Sendtner 2002). In 2003, Liang et al. reported that high-frequency electro-acupuncture stimulation increased GDNF mRNA levels, provided nutrients for dopaminergic neurons, improved repair of the damaged area and accelerated nerve regeneration. In 2005, Wang et al. explored the treatment of DRG damage with acupuncture in a cat model. They found that stimulation at acupoints ST32, ST36, GB39, SP6, etc. improved DRG repair and increased the expression of GDNF and fibroblast growth factor-2 (FGF-2) (Wang et al. 2005a, b).

GDNF can also protect peripheral nerves and provide them with nutrients (Frostick et al. 1998). In an animal model of sciatic nerve injury, the mRNA expression of GDNF receptor á-1 (GFRá-1) in the DRG was elevated, indicating the involvement of GDNF in peripheral nerve repair (Höke et al. 2000). Similarly, in another study, after electro-acupuncture stimulation at GB30 and GB34 (alternating 60 Hz for 1.05 s and 2 Hz for 2.85 s), mRNA levels of GDNF and GFRá-1 in the DRG were increased in a rat model, reducing the pain caused by chronic constriction injury (Dong et al. 2005).

6.3.3 Other growth factors

Insulin-like growth factor 1 (IGF-1) promotes cell growth and proliferation. Current studies also indicate that IGF-1 can promote axon outgrowth (Mizisin et al. 2004; Chen et al. 2006). In 2009, Wang et al. discussed the efficacy of electro-acupuncture on spinal cord injury in a rat model. They found that during the gradual recovery of spinal cord injury, many growth factors, including fibroblast growth factor (FGF-1), IGF-1, and ciliary neurotrophic factor (CNTF) were secreted, indicating beneficial roles in nerve repair and regeneration (Wang et al. 2009). In 2007 and 2009, Wang et al. (2007b) and Liu et al. (2009) reported the involvement of neurotrophin (NT)-3 and -4 in nerve repair and regeneration, respectively, under acupuncture stimulation.

Nerve repair and regeneration result from a series of complex regulatory processes, during which the involved growth factors increase gradually. Although many studies have indicated a prominent effect of acupuncture on nerve repair and regeneration, its association with growth factors and the detailed relationship, including the concept of Yinyang, Qi, and the five elements, still need to be further investigated in order to improve the understanding between traditional Chinese medicine and Western medicine practitioners.

6.4   Future Direction of Acupuncture in Nerve Regeneration

Many studies have confirmed that acupuncture can promote nerve regeneration. In 2001, Chen et al. compared the effect of regular acupuncture with that of electro-acupuncture on peripheral nerve regeneration. They found that the electro-acupuncture group exhibited better results than the traditional acupuncture group in terms of the number of regenerated axons, the number and areas of newly-formed blood vessels, and the maturity of nerve structure (Chen et al. 2001). In 2003, a study by Inoue et al. compared the difference between the distal cathode needle and distal anode needle. They showed that nerve regeneration was better and faster in the distal cathode group, indicating that electro-acupuncture with a distal cathode orientation was superior in nerve regeneration (Inoue et al. 2003). However, for damage involving large areas or long nerve tissue, acupuncture treatment alone is inadequate; a combination with the nerve conduit technique permits the repair length of the damaged nerve to be increased (Lin et al. 2014; Kao et al. 2013; Chen et al. 2013; Ho et al. 2014b). With advances in our understanding of stem cells and stem cell technology, several studies have reported on how acupuncture influences stem cells (Ho et al. 2014a). In 2011, Yan investigated the effect of electro-acupuncture on mesenchymal stem cells (MSCs) and spinal cord regeneration. The data indicated that electro-acupuncture promoted the differentiation of MSCs, nerve fiber growth, and NT-3 secretion, and accelerated nerve repair and regeneration (Yan et al. 2011). A combination of acupuncture with nerve conduit technology and stem cell regeneration and differentiation could possibly surpass the current limitations in nerve regeneration and repair.

Acknowledgments This work was supported by the Department of Biomaterials Translational Research Center, China Medical University Hospital and CMU under the Aim for Top University Plan of the Ministry of Education, Taiwan.

References

Abuaisha B, Costanzi J, Boulton A. Acupuncture for the treatment of chronic painful peripheral diabetic neuropathy: a long-term study. Diabetes Res Clin Pract. 1998;39:115–21.

Allen SJ, Watson JJ, Shoemark DK, Barua NU, Patel NK. GDNF, NGF and BDNF as therapeutic options for neurodegeneration. Pharmacol Ther. 2013;138:155–75.

Argyriou AA, Chroni E, Koutras A, Ellul J, Papapetropoulos S, Katsoulas G, Iconomou G, Kalofonos HP. Vitamin E for prophylaxis against chemotherapy-induced neuropathy: a randomized controlled trial. Neurology. 2005;64:26–31.

Bai L, Lao L. Neurobiological foundations of acupuncture: the relevance and future prospect based on neuroimaging evidence. Evid Based Complement Alternat Med. 2013;2013:812568.

Bao T, Zhang R, Badros A, Lao L. Acupuncture treatment for bortezomib-induced peripheral neuropathy: a case report. Pain Res Treat. 2011;2011:920807.

Becker R, Reichmanis M, Marino A, Spadaro J. Electrophysiological correlates of acupuncture points and meridians. Psychoenergetic Syst. 1976;1:105–12.

Cameron NE, Cotter MA, Robertson S. Chronic low frequency electrical activation for one week corrects nerve conduction velocity deficits in rats with diabetes of three months duration. Diabetologia. 1989;32:759–61.

Cameron NE, Cotter MA, Robertson S, Maxfield EK. Nerve function in experimental diabetes in rats: effects of electrical stimulation. Am J Physiol. 1993;264:E161–6.

Cascinu S, Cordella L, Del Ferro E, Fronzoni M, Catalano G. Neuroprotective effect of reduced glutathione on cisplatin-based chemotherapy in advanced gastric cancer: a randomized double-blind placebo-controlled trial. J Clin Oncol. 1995;13:26–32.

Chang JY, Lin JH, Yao CH, Chen JH, Lai TY, Chen YS. In vivo evaluation of a biodegradable EDC/NHS-cross-linked gelatin peripheral nerve guide conduit material. Macromol Biosci. 2007;7:500–7.

Chang YM, Chi WY, Lai TY, Chen YS, Tsai FJ, Tsai CH, Kuo WW, Cheng YC, Lin CC, Huang CY. Dilong: role in peripheral nerve regeneration. Evid Based Complement Alternat Med. 2011;2011:380809.

Chen YS, Yao CH, Chen TH, Lin JG, Hsieh CL, Lin CC, Lao CJ, Tsai CC. Effect of acupuncture stimulation on peripheral nerve regeneration using silicone rubber chambers. Am J Chin Med. 2001;29:377–85.

Chen YS, Liu CJ, Cheng CY, Yao CH. Effect of bilobalide on peripheral nerve regeneration. Biomaterials. 2004;25:509–14.

Chen YS, Chang JY, Cheng CY, Tsai FJ, Yao CH, Liu BS. An in vivo evaluation of a biodegradable genipin-cross-linked gelatin peripheral nerve guide conduit material. Biomaterials. 2005a;26:3911–8.

Chen YS, Hsu SF, Chiu CW, Lin JG, Chen CT, Yao CH. Effect of low-power pulsed laser on peripheral nerve regeneration in rats. Microsurgery. 2005b;25:83–9.

Chen MH, Chen PR, Chen MH, Hsieh ST, Lin FH. Gelatin–tricalcium phosphate membranes immobilized with NGF, BDNF, or IGF-1 for peripheral nerve repair: an in vitro and in vivo study. J Biomed Mater Res A. 2006;79:846–57.

Chen J, Qi JG, Zhang W, Zhou X, Meng QS, Zhang WM, Wang XY, Wang TH. Electro-acupuncture induced NGF, BDNF and NT-3 expression in spared L6 dorsal root ganglion in cats subjected to removal of adjacent ganglia. Neurosci Res. 2007;59:399–405.

Chen HT, Yao CH, Chao PD, Hou YC, Chiang HM, Hsieh CC, Ke CJ, Chen YS. Effect of serum metabolites of Pueraria lobata in rats on peripheral nerve regeneration: in vitro and in vivo studies. J Biomed Mater Res B Appl Biomater. 2008;84:256–62.

Chen YS, Lin WC, Miller C. The role of complementary and alternative medicine in regenerative medicine. Evid Based Complement Alternat Med. 2013;2013:420458.

de Albornoz PM, Delgado PJ, Forriol F, Maffulli N. Non-surgical therapies for peripheral nerve injury. Br Med Bull. 2011;100:73–100.

Detrait ER, Yoo S, Eddleman CS, Fukuda M, Bittner GD, Fishman HM. Plasmalemmal repair of severed neurites of PC12 cells requires Ca(2+) and synaptotagmin. J Neurosci Res. 2000;62:566–73.

Donald GK, Tobin I, Stringer J. Evaluation of acupuncture in the management of chemotherapy-induced peripheral neuropathy. Acupunct Med. 2011;29:230–3.

Dong ZQ, Ma F, Xie H, Wang YQ, Wu GC. Changes of expression of glial cell line-derived neurotrophic factor and its receptor in dorsal root ganglions and spinal dorsal horn during electroacupuncture treatment in neuropathic pain rats. Neurosci Lett. 2005;376:143–8.

Dong HS, Zhang QJ, Yang Q, Zheng M. Experimental study of nerve growth factor of sciatic nerve of rats with diabetes peripheral neuropathy accommodated by electro-acupuncture. Chin J Rehabil Theory Pract. 2007;13:730–3.

Dorsher PT. Acupuncture for chronic pain. Tech Reg Anesth Pain Manag. 2011;15:55–63.

Dyson-Hudson TA, Kadar P, LaFountaine M, Emmons R, Kirshblum SC, Tulsky D, Komaroff E. Acupuncture for chronic shoulder pain in persons with spinal cord injury: a small-scale clinical trial. Arch Phys Med Rehabil. 2007;88:1276–83.

Ernfors P. Local and target-derived actions of neurotrophins during peripheral nervous system development. Cell Mol Life Sci. 2001;58:1036–44.

Fawcett JW, Keynes RJ. Peripheral nerve regeneration. Annu Rev Neurosci. 1990;13:43–60.

Fernandez C, Mehta Z, Espenlaub A, Ellison N. Chemotherapy-induced peripheral neuropathy #197. J Palliat Med. 2014;17:965–6.

Fowler JR, Lavasani M, Huard J, Goitz RJ. Biologic strategies to improve nerve regeneration after peripheral nerve repair. J Reconstr Microsurg. 2015;31:243–8.

Franconi G, Manni L, Schröder S, Marchetti P, Robinson N. A systematic review of experimental and clinical acupuncture in chemotherapy-induced peripheral neuropathy. Evid Based Complement Alternat Med. 2013;2013:516916.

Frostick SP, Yin Q, Kemp GJ. Schwann cells, neurotrophic factors, and peripheral nerve regeneration. Microsurgery. 1998;18:397–405.

Gamelin L, Boisdron-Celle M, Morel A, Poirier AL, Berger V, Gamelin E, Tournigand C, de Gramont A. Oxaliplatin-related neurotoxicity: interest of calcium-magnesium infusion and no impact on its efficacy. J Clin Oncol. 2008;26:1188–9.

Gavronsky S, Koeniger-Donohue R, Steller J, Hawkins JW. Postoperative pain: acupuncture versus percutaneous electrical nerve stimulation. Pain Manag Nurs. 2012;13:150–6.

Gordon T. The role of neurotrophic factors in nerve regeneration. Neurosurg Focus. 2009;26:E3.

Gwag BJ, Sessler FM, Robine VJ, Springe E. Endogenous glutamate levels regulate nerve growth factor mRNA expression in the rat dentate gyrus. Mol Cell. 1997;7:425–30.

Harati Y. Diabetic peripheral neuropathies. Ann Intern Med. 1987;107:546–59.

Ho CY, Yao CH, Chen WC, Shen WC, Bau DT. Electroacupuncture and acupuncture promote the rat's transected median nerve regeneration. Evid Based Complement Alternat Med. 2013;2013:514610.

Ho TJ, Chan TM, Ho LI, Lai CY, Lin CH, Macdonald I, Harn HJ, Lin JG, Lin SZ, Chen YH. The possible role of stem cells in acupuncture treatment for neurodegenerative diseases: a literature review of basic studies. Cell Transplant. 2014a;23:559–66.

Ho CY, Lin HC, Lee YC, Chou LW, Kuo TW, Chang HW, Chen YS, Lo SF. Clinical effectiveness of acupuncture for carpal tunnel syndrome. Am J Chin Med. 2014b;42:303–14.

Hoang NS, Sar C, Valmier J, Sieso V, Scamps F. Electro-acupuncture on functional peripheral nerve regeneration in mice: a behavioural study. BMC Complement Altern Med. 2012;12:141.

Höke A, Cheng C, Zochodne DW. Expression of glial cell line-derived neurotrophic factor family of growth factors in peripheral nerve injury in rats. Neuroreport. 2000;11:1651–4.

Hsiang SW, Lee HC, Tsai FJ, Tsai CC, Yao CH, Chen YS. Puerarin accelerates peripheral nerve regeneration. Am J Chin Med. 2011a;39:1207–17.

Hsiang SW, Tsai CC, Tsai FJ, Ho TY, Yao CH, Chen YS. Novel use of biodegradable casein conduits for guided peripheral nerve regeneration. J R Soc Interface. 2011b;8:1622–34.

Huang KS, Lin JG, Lee HC, Tsai FJ, Bau DT, Huang CY, Yao CH, Chen YS. Paeoniae alba radix promotes peripheral nerve regeneration. Evid Based Complement Alternat Med. 2011;2011:109809.

Ide C. Peripheral nerve regeneration. Neurosci Res. 1996;25:101–21.

Inoue M, Hojo T, Yano T, Katsumi Y. The effects of electroacupuncture on peripheral nerve regeneration in rats. Acupunct Med. 2003;21:9–17.

Inoue M, Kitakoji H, Yano T, Ishizaki N, Itoi M, Katsumi Y. Acupuncture treatment for low back pain and lower limb symptoms- the relation between acupuncture or electroacupuncture stimulation and sciatic nerve blood flow. Evid Based Complement Altern Med. 2008;5:133–43.

Inoue M, Katsumi Y, Itoi M, Hojo T, Nakajima M, Ohashi S, Oi Y, Kitakoji H. Direct current electrical stimulation of acupuncture needles for peripheral nerve regeneration: an exploratory case series. Acupunct Med. 2011;29:88–93.

Isackson PJ. Trophic factor response to neuronal stimuli or injury. Curr Opin Neurobiol. 1995;5:350–7.

Jeon S, Kim YJ, Kim ST, Moon W, Chae Y, Kang M, Chung MY, Lee H, Hong MS, Chung JH, Joh TH, Lee H, Park HJ. Proteomic analysis of the neuroprotective mechanisms of acupuncture treatment in a Parkinson's disease mouse model. Proteomics. 2008;8:4822–32.

Kagitani F, Uchida S, Hotta H. Afferent nerve fibers and acupuncture. Auton Neurosci. 2010;157:2–8.

Kao CH, Chen JJ, Hsu YM, Bau DT, Yao CH, Chen YS. High-frequency electrical stimulation can be a complementary therapy to promote nerve regeneration in diabetic rats. PLoS One. 2013;8:e79078.

Kaplan DR, Miller FD. Neurotrophin signal transduction in the nervous system. Curr Opin Neurobiol. 2000;10:381–91.

Kennedy JM, Zochodne DW. The regenerative deficit of peripheral nerves in experimental diabetes: its extent, timing and possible mechanisms. Brain. 2000;123:2118–29.

Kennedy JM, Zochodne DW. Impaired peripheral nerve regeneration in diabetes mellitus. J Peripher Nerv Syst. 2005;10:144–57.

Lee H, Schmidt K, Ernst E. Acupuncture for the relief of cancer-related pain—a systematic review. Eur J Pain. 2005;9:437–44.

Liang XB, Liu XY, Li FQ, Luo Y, Lu J, Zhang WM, Wang XM, Han JS. Long-term high-frequency electro-acupuncture stimulation prevents neuronal degeneration and up-regulates BDNF mRNA in the substantia nigra and ventral tegmental area following medial forebrain bundle axotomy. Brain Res Mol Brain Res. 2002;108:51–9.

Liang XB, Luo Y, Liu XY, Lu J, Li FQ, Wang Q, Wang XM, Han JS. Electro-acupuncture improves behavior and upregulates GDNF mRNA in MFB transected rats. Neuroreport. 2003;14:1177–81.

Lin YC, Kao CH, Cheng YK, Chen JJ, Yao CH, Chen YS. Current-modulated electrical stimulation as a treatment for peripheral nerve regeneration in diabetic rats. Restor Neurol Neurosci. 2014;32:437–46.

Lindsay RM. Nerve growth factors (NGF, BDNF) enhance axonal regeneration but are not required for survival of adult sensory neurons. J Neurosci. 1988;8:2394–405.

Liu F, Sun WW, Wang Y, Hu LQ, Dai P, Tian CF, Wang TH. Effects of electro-acupuncture on NT-4 expression in spinal dorsal root ganglion and associated segments of the spinal dorsal horn in cats subjected to adjacent dorsal root ganglionectomy. Neurosci Lett. 2009;450:158–62.

Lu MC, Hsiang SW, Lai TY, Yao CH, Lin LY, Chen YS. Influence of cross-linking degree of a biodegradable genipin-cross-linked gelatin guide on peripheral nerve regeneration. J Biomater Sci Polym Ed. 2007;18:843–63.

Lundborg G, Dahlin LB, Danielsen N, Gelberman RH, Longo FM, Powell HC, Varon S. Nerve regeneration in silicone chambers: influence of gap length and of distal stump components. Exp Neurol. 1982;76:361–75.

Madsen MV, Gøtzsche PC, Hróbjartsson A. Acupuncture treatment for pain: systematic review of randomised clinical trials with acupuncture, placebo acupuncture, and no acupuncture groups. BMJ. 2009;338:a3115.

Manni L, Albanesi M, Guaragna M, Barbaro Paparo S, Aloe L. Neurotrophins and acupuncture. Auton Neurosci. 2010;157:9–17.

Mayer DJ. Acupuncture: an evidence-based review of the clinical literature. Annu Rev Med. 2000;51:49–63.

Mizisin AP, Vu Y, Shuff M, Calcutt NA. Ciliary neurotrophic factor improves nerve conduction and ameliorates regeneration deficits in diabetic rats. Diabetes. 2004;53:1807–12.

Nawabi DH, Jayakumar P, Carlstedt T. Peripheral nerve surgery. Ann R Coll Surg Engl. 2006;88:327–8.

Nori SL, Rocco ML, Florenzano F, Ciotti MT, Aloe L, Manni L. Increased nerve growth factor signaling in sensory neurons of early diabetic rats is corrected by electroacupuncture. Evid Based Complement Alternat Med. 2013;2013:652735.

Ogawa K, Ogawa M, Nishijima K, Tsuda M, Nishimura G. Efficacy of contact needle therapy for chemotherapy-induced peripheral neuropathy. Evid Based Complement Alternat Med. 2013;2013:928129.

Pace A, Savarese A, Picardo M, Maresca V, Pacetti U, Del Monte G, Biroccio A, Leonetti C, Jandolo B, Cognetti F, Bove L. Neuroprotective effect of vitamin E supplementation in patients treated with cisplatin chemotherapy. J Clin Oncol. 2003;21:927–31.

Pachman DR, Barton DL, Watson JC, Loprinzi CL. Chemotherapy-induced peripheral neuropathy: prevention and treatment. Clin Pharmacol Ther. 2011;90:377–87.

Pagani L, Manni L, Aloe L. Effects of electroacupuncture on retinal nerve growth factor and brain-derived neurotrophic factor expression in a rat model of retinitis pigmentosa. Brain Res. 2006;1092:198–206.

Palumbo PJ, Elveback LR, Whisnant JP. Neurologic complications of diabetes mellitus: transient ischemic attack, stroke, and peripheral neuropathy. Adv Neurol. 1978;19:593–601.

Piao Y, Liang X. Chinese medicine in diabetic peripheral neuropathy: experimental research on nerve repair and regeneration. Evid Based Complement Alternat Med. 2012;2012:191632.

Pinzur MS. Diabetic peripheral neuropathy. Foot Ankle Clin. 2011;16:345–59.

Pittenger G, Vinik A. Nerve growth factor and diabetic neuropathy. Exp Diabesity Res. 2003;4:271–85.

Podratz JL, Knight AM, Ta LE, Staff NP, Gass JM, Genelin K, Schlattau A, Lathroum L, Windebank AJ. Cisplatin induced mitochondrial DNA damage in dorsal root ganglion neurons. Neurobiol Dis. 2011;41:661–8.

Pomeranz B. Acupuncture research related to pain, drug addiction and nerve regeneration. In: Stux G, Pomeranz B, editors. Scientific bases of acupuncture. Berlin: Springer; 1989. p. 35–52.

Quasthoff S, Hartung HP. Chemotherapy-induced peripheral neuropathy. J Neurol. 2002;249:9–17.

Richardson PH, Vincent CA. Acupuncture for the treatment of pain: a review of evaluative research. Pain. 1986;24:15–40.

Schröder S, Liepert J, Remppis A, Greten JH. Acupuncture treatment improves nerve conduction in peripheral neuropathy. Eur J Neurol. 2007;14:276–81.

Smyth JF, Bowman A, Perren T, Wilkinson P, Prescott RJ, Quinn KJ, Tedeschi M. Glutathione reduces the toxicity and improves quality of life of women diagnosed with ovarian cancer treated with cisplatin: results of a double-blind, randomised trial. Ann Oncol. 1997;8:569–73.

Thoenen H, Sendtner M. Neurotrophins: from enthusiastic expectations through sobering experiences to rational therapeutic approaches. Nat Neurosci. 2002;5:1046–50.

Trinh KV, Phillips SD, Ho E, Damsma K. Acupuncture for the alleviation of lateral epicondyle pain: a systematic review. Rheumatology. 2004;43:1085–90.

Visovsky C, Collins M, Abbott L, Aschenbrenner J, Hart C. Putting evidence into practice: evidence-based interventions for chemotherapy-induced peripheral neuropathy. Clin J Oncol Nurs. 2007;11:901–13.

Wang TW, Wang TH, Zhou X, Zhang LS, Xu XY. Effect of partial ganglionectomy and acupuncture on culturing spared DRG in vitro. Sichuan Da Xue Xue Bao Yi Xue Ban. 2005a;36:630–3.

Wang TT, Yuan Y, Kang Y, Yuan WL, Zhang HT, Wu LY, Feng ZT. Effects of acupuncture on the expression of glial cell line-derived neurotrophic factor (GDNF) and basic fibroblast growth factor (FGF-2/bFGF) in the left sixth lumbar dorsal root ganglion following removal of adjacent dorsal root ganglia. Neurosci Lett. 2005b;382:236–41.

Wang WS, Lin JK, Lin TC, Chen WS, Jiang JK, Wang HS, Chiou TJ, Liu JH, Yen CC, Chen PM. Oral glutamine is effective for preventing oxaliplatin-induced neuropathy in colorectal cancer patients. Oncol. 2007a;12:312–9.

Wang TH, Wang XY, Li XL, Chen HM, Wu LF. Effect of electroacupuncture on neurotrophin expression in cat spinal cord after partial dorsal rhizotomy. Neurochem Res. 2007b;32:1415–22.

Wang XY, Li XL, Hong SQ, Xi-Yang YB, Wang TH. Electroacupuncture induced spinal plasticity is linked to multiple gene expressions in dorsal root deafferented rats. J Mol Neurosci. 2009;37:97–110.

Wang W, Huang CY, Tsai FJ, Tsai CC, Yao CH, Chen YS. Growth-promoting effects of quercetin on peripheral nerves in rats. Int J Artif Organs. 2011a;34:1095–105.

Wang W, Lin JH, Tsai CC, Chuang HC, Ho CY, Yao CH, Chen YS. Biodegradable glutaraldehyde-crosslinked casein conduit promotes regeneration after peripheral nerve injury in adult rats. Macromol Biosci. 2011b;11:914–26.

Windebank AJ, Grisold W. Chemotherapy-induced neuropathy. J Peripher Nerv Syst. 2008;13:27–46.

Wolf S, Barton D, Kottschade L, Grothey A, Loprinzi C. Chemotherapy-induced peripheral neuropathy: prevention and treatment strategies. Eur J Cancer. 2008;44:1507–15.

Wong R, Sagar S. Acupuncture treatment for chemotherapy-induced peripheral neuropathy—a case series. Acupunct Med. 2006;24:87–91.

Wong AM, Leong CP, Su TY, Yu SW, Tsai WC, Chen CP. Clinical trial of acupuncture for patients with spinal cord injuries. Am J Phys Med Rehabil. 2003;82:21–7.

Xinjia W, Kangmei K, Weili Q. Influence of acupuncture on the expression of BDNF and TrkB in chronic spinal cord injury of rats. J Shantou Univ Med Coll. 2002;1:006.

Yan Q, Ruan JW, Ding Y, Li WJ, Li Y, Zeng YS. Electro-acupuncture promotes differentiation of mesenchymal stem cells, regeneration of nerve fibers and partial functional recovery after spinal cord injury. Exp Toxicol Pathol. 2011;63:151–6.

Yao CH, Chang RL, Chang SL, Tsai CC, Tsai FJ, Chen YS. Electrical stimulation improves peripheral nerve regeneration in streptozotocin-induced diabetic rats. J Trauma Acute Care Surg. 2012;72:199–205.

Yoo S, Nguyen MP, Fukuda M, Bittner GD, Fishman HM. Plasmalemmal sealing of transected mammalian neurites is a gradual process mediated by Ca^{2+}-regulated proteins. J Neurosci Res. 2003;74:541–51.

Young MJ, Boulton AJ, Macleod AF, Williams DR, Sonksen PH. A multicentre study of the prevalence of diabetic peripheral neuropathy in the United Kingdom hospital clinic population. Diabetologia. 1993;36:150–4.

Younger DS. Diabetic peripheral neuropathy. Drug Today. 1998;34:699.

Zhang X, Wu B, Nie K, Jia Y, Yu J. Effects of acupuncture on declined cerebral blood flow, impaired mitochondrial respiratory function and oxidative stress in multi-infarct dementia rats. Neurochem Int. 2014;65:23–9.

The Effect of Acupuncture on Stroke

7

Chin-Yi Cheng and Jaung-Geng Lin

Abstract

Thrombolytic therapy is of proven benefit in ischemic stroke but its associated risk of intracerebral hemorrhage has encouraged the search for alternative medicines, including acupuncture treatment. In clinical research, acupuncture has exhibited significant effects on motor dysfunction, shoulder-hand syndrome, balance impairment, cognitive impairment, and dysphagia in the subacute or chronic stage of stroke. During cerebral ischemia, pathological processes including inflammatory response, oxidative stress, and apoptosis are evoked, which exacerbate cerebral ischemia-reperfusion (I/R) injury. In animal models of cerebral ischemia, acupuncture (electroacupuncture [EA] or manual acupuncture) stimulation provides neuroprotective effects through the downregulation of inflammation-related molecules (including tumor necrosis factor-α [TNF-α], interleukin [IL] -1β, IL-6, matrix metalloproteinases [MMPs], chemokines, and aquaporins) and enzymes (cyclooxygenase-2 [COX-2] and myeloperoxidase [MPO]), and modulation of oxidative stress-related molecules (including malondialdehyde [MDA], superoxide dismutase [SOD], glutathione peroxidase [GSH-Px], and gamma-glutamylcysteine synthetase [γ-GCS]) in the ischemic area. The anti-apoptotic effect of acupuncture can be attributed to the upregulation of anti-apoptotic proteins (Bcl-2 and Bcl-xL), and downregulation of pro-apoptotic proteins (Bad and Bax) and caspases (including caspase-3, 8,

C.-Y. Cheng
School of Chinese Medicine, College of Chinese Medicine, China Medical University, Taichung, Taiwan

Department of Chinese Medicine, Hui-Sheng Hospital, Taichung, Taiwan

J.-G. Lin (✉)
School of Chinese Medicine, College of Chinese Medicine, China Medical University, Taichung, Taiwan
e-mail: jglin@mail.cmu.edu.tw

© Springer Nature Singapore Pte Ltd. 2018
J.-G. Lin (ed.), *Experimental Acupuncturology*,
https://doi.org/10.1007/978-981-13-0971-7_7

95

and 9) through various signaling pathways. Acupuncture stimulation also induces neurogenesis through modulation of BrdU/nestin, collapsin response mediator protein-4 (CRMP-4), microtubule-associated protein-2 (MAP-2), retinaldehyde dehydrogenases, dopamine D_2 receptors, astrocytes, and glycogen synthase kinase-3β (GSK-3β) protein phosphatase 2A (PP2A) expression in the ischemic area.

Until now, acupuncture has exhibited promising effects in ischemic stroke in clinical and basic research. High-quality studies are required to clarify these effects, which could potentially be applied clinically in the future.

Keywords

Acupuncture · Cerebral ischemia-reperfusion injury · Inflammatory response · Oxidative stress · Apoptosis · Neurogenesis

7.1   Introduction

Stroke is the third leading cause of death worldwide and a leading cause of serious long-term disability in the elderly (Wu et al. 2006). Due to an aging population and high-fat diets, the incidence of stroke is rising and the average age of first stroke is becoming ever younger (Wu et al. 2010; Zhuang et al. 2014). The long-term disability associated with stroke places a heavy financial burden on the family and wider society (Zhuang et al. 2014; Mapulanga et al. 2014; Wang et al. 2014). Stroke can be classified into two major categories: ischemia and hemorrhage, with ischemic stroke accounting for about 80–85% of all strokes (Wang et al. 2012b). In clinical practice, the optimization of management of patients with acute ischemic stroke is an integrated and systematic approach with thrombolysis, which provides a higher rate of improved early outcome, including pre-existing disabilities (Wang et al. 2012b; Gumbinger et al. 2014). Intravenous administration of recombinant tissue plasminogen activator has been approved to treat eligible patients with acute ischemic stroke within a 4.5 h time window of stroke symptom onset (Gumbinger et al. 2014; Dharmasaroja and Pattaraarchachai 2011). Clinical trial results indicate that the effects of thrombolytic therapy are time-dependent with a strong association between earlier treatment and favorable outcome (Gumbinger et al. 2014). In contrast, thrombolytic therapy beyond the 4.5 h time window is associated with a marked increase in mortality and serious side effects, including intracerebral hemorrhage, brain edema, and angioedema (Gumbinger et al. 2014; Balami et al. 2013b). Statistical approaches for detecting the treatment of acute ischemic stroke revealed that only 1.8–2.1% of patients in the USA receive thrombolytic therapy within the therapeutic time window (Kleindorfer et al. 2008). The limitations of thrombolytic therapy in acute ischemic stroke have fueled the search for alternative treatments (Balami et al. 2013a; Elijovich and Chong 2010).

7.2   The Clinical Efficacy of Acupuncture in Stroke

Chinese physicians have used acupuncture to treat various disorders, including post-stroke disabilities, for centuries (Wu et al. 2010; Park et al. 2001). Like many other traditional Chinese medicines, acupuncture has been shown to be effective for the treatment of stroke, and it has long been used by Chinese doctors to improve motor, sensory, speech, and neurological functional recovery after stroke (Liu 2006; Wu et al. 2006; Liu et al. 2014). Nowadays, a large number of studies have evaluated the efficacy of acupuncture in adult patients with disability after stroke. Post-stroke spasticity is more commonly formed in upper limbs and causes difficulties in walking and activities of daily living. Therefore, treatment of post-stroke spasticity is the main goal of rehabilitation (Park et al. 2014). Wang et al. (2014) reported that electroacupuncture (EA) at the Zeqian (EX-UE, A32), Shounizhu (EX-UE), Shaohai (HT 3), and Neiguan (PC 6) (50 Hz, 20 min per session, twice per week) for 6 weeks effectively reduced upper-extremity spasticity in chronic stroke patients (Wang et al. 2014). A meta-analysis of randomized controlled trials evidence revealed that acupuncture plays an adjuvant role in modulation of spasticity induced by alpha-motor neuron activity (Park et al. 2014). A study by Zhou et al. (2014) showed that the floating-needle therapy performed through the needles inserting at sites 5–10 cm away from myofascial trigger points, combined with routine rehabilitation training, exerts beneficial effects in post-stroke shoulder-hand syndrome (Zhou et al. 2014). Warm acupuncture stimulation at the Waiguan acupoint (TE 5), combined with acupuncture stimulation at the Jianyu (LI 15), Jianjing (GB 21), Quchi (LI 11), Wangu (SI 4), Yangchi (TE 4), and Hegu (LI 4) acupoints, with routine rehabilitation training, significantly improves post-stroke shoulder-hand syndrome (Meng and Wen 2014). Zhao et al. (2014) demonstrated that acupuncture at the Shuigou (GV 26), Baihui (GV 20), Neiguan (PC 6), and Baxie (EX-UE 9) acupoints effectively improve the activities of the hemiplegic hand and daily life (Zhao et al. 2014). A systematic review and meta-analysis conducted by Wu et al. (2010) revealed that acupuncture may help in post-stroke rehabilitation and provides benefit in the reorganization process by increasing perfusion within peri-infarct areas (Wu et al. 2010). Another study found that acupuncture, inserted into acupoints located on the extensor of the upper limbs and flexor of the low limbs, combined with scalp acupuncture, applied to dingzhongxian (MS 5) and dingnie qianxiexian (MS 6) on the affected side exerted satisfactory effects on motor dysfunction in the subacute phase of ischemic stroke (Chen et al. 2014c). A similar study conducted by Tang et al. (2012) revealed that scalp acupuncture (MS 6) combined with acupuncture stimulation at the Neiguan, Jianyu, and Sanyinjiao (SP 6) acupoints (once daily and 20 days' duration) improved upper limb movement and function in stroke patients (Tang et al. 2012). Liu et al. (2012) reported that acupuncture applied to the Sanyinjiao, Taixi (KI 3) (located on the extensor side), Jiexi (ST 41), Shenmai (BL 62), and Yanglingquan (GB 34) (located on the flexor side) acupoints (once daily and for 1 month's duration) improved motor function and daily living activities among patients with drop foot after stroke (Liu et al. 2012). A meta-analysis of scalp acupuncture in the treatment of acute ischemic stroke showed that scalp acupuncture therapy improves neurological deficit scores and the clinical effective rate when compared with Western conventional medicines (Wang et al. 2012b). Balance plays a critical role in maintaining an independent daily life. Muscle weakness, spasticity, and hemiplegia caused by stroke will result in impaired balance, which critically affects quality of life (Liu et al. 2009; Huang et al. 2014). Therefore, balance is one of the most powerful prognostic indicators of functional independence after stroke and is a very important issue during rehabilitation processes (Huang et al. 2014; Liu et al. 2009). One study found that acupuncture stimulation at the Baihui and 4 spirit acupoints (1.5 cun anterior, posterior, left and right laterals from the Baihui acupoint, respectively) increased muscle strength of knee extensors and hip flexors in paralyzed limbs, indicating an immediate effect on the improvement of balance function in stroke patients (Liu et al. 2009). Acupuncture stimulation at the Yanglingquan and Zusanli (ST 36) acupoints for 20 min (twice a week, with the course lasting for 3–4 weeks) combined with conventional physiotherapy exerted beneficial effects on static balance for stroke patients with a low Brunnstrom stage (Huang et al. 2014). Patients with stroke in the basal ganglia have an obvious deficiency in the sensorimotor function on the contralesional side of the body (Chen et al. 2014a). Previous studies have demonstrated that acupuncture can regulate the function and connectivity of sensorimotor areas of normal healthy people (Hui et al. 2009; Fang et al. 2009). Chen et al. (2014a) reported that acupuncture stimulation at the Waiguan acupoint regulates the functional connectivity between the sensorimotor areas of the intra-hemisphere and inter-hemisphere, and that it provides beneficial effects by enhancing the cooperation between the left (unaffected) thalamus and the right (affected) motor areas to promote the regulation of the sensorimotor function on the right side of the body (Chen et al. 2014a). Another study conducted by Xie et al. (2014) found that acupuncture stimulation at the Yanglingquan acupoint (120 times per min and for 1 min in duration) induces a strong connectivity between the cerebellum and primary sensorimotor cortex in stroke patients, and which may improve integration of movement and motor learning (Xie et al. 2014). Cognitive impairment is one of the most common disorders caused by stroke (Haring 2002; Yang et al. 2014). Approximately 25–35% of stroke survivors presents with cognitive impairments within the initial 3 months and up to 32% of patients exhibits persistent cognitive deficits for up to 3 years after a first-ever stroke (Liu et al. 2014). Therefore, pos-stroke cognitive impairment is becoming a major public health problem worldwide (Yang et al. 2014). A recently published meta-analysis suggests that acupuncture has a positive effect on restoring cognitive function after stroke, and that this effect is closely related to the increased velocity of blood flow (Liu et al. 2014). Yang et al. (2014) demonstrated that acupuncture stimulation at the Baihui and Shenting (GV 24) acupoints, combined with computer-based cognitive training, is more effective than conventional treatment in the management of cognitive dysfunction after stroke (Yang et al. 2014). A systematic review and meta-analysis suggest that acupuncture has no effect on post-stroke mortality and disability (Zhang et al. 2014a). However, acupuncture may provide beneficial effects in treatment of post-stroke neurological impairment and dysfunction, particularly post-stroke dysphagia (Zhang et al. 2014a). In contrast, several studies have concluded that there is no evidence that acupuncture improves motor function in patients with stroke (Wu et al. 2006; Kong et al. 2010; Zhu et al. 2013b). Reviews and evaluations of acupuncture (body and scalp acupuncture) and post-stroke rehabilitation found no clear evidence of the effectiveness of acupuncture in the subacute or chronic phase after stroke (Wu et al. 2006; Zhu et al. 2013b). A systematic review conducted by Kong et al. (2010) also found no effectiveness of acupuncture on promoting functional recovery after stroke (Kong et al. 2010).

Despite ongoing debate concerning the effect of acupuncture on rehabilitation following stroke, generally speaking, acupuncture provides positive effects in motor dysfunction, spasticity, shoulder-hand syndrome, hemiplegia, balance impairment, cognitive impairment, and dysphagia during the subacute or chronic stage of stroke.

7.3   The Effects of Acupuncture in Cerebral Ischemic Models

7.3.1   The Anti-inflammatory Effects of Acupuncture

Inflammatory response has been shown to play a detrimental role in brain damage after acute cerebral ischemia-reperfusion (I/R) injury (Lan et al. 2013). During cerebral ischemia, blood-brain barrier (BBB) dysfunction promotes leukocytes trafficking into the central nervous system (CNS), resulting in blood-borne leukocytes adhesion to the endothelial surface and then infiltration into brain parenchyma (Cayrol et al. 2008). The transmigration and invasion of the ischemic territory by leukocytes is closely related to the activation of microglia/macrophages and astrocytes (Iadecola and Alexander 2001). Activated microglia/macrophages migrate toward brain parenchyma and undergo further activation in the ischemic core, and then release proinflammatory mediators, including proinflammatory cytokines, chemokines, nitric oxide (Bonomini and Rezzani), superoxide free radicals, and proinflammatory transcription factors (Loane and Byrnes 2010; Iadecola and Alexander 2001). During post-ischemic inflammatory responses, the transcription factor nuclear factor (NF)-κB upregulates proinflammatory cytokines production. Increased inflammatory cytokines, such as tumor necrosis factor (TNF)-α and interleukin (IL)-1β, subsequently upregulate the expression of adhesion molecules, including intercellular adhesion molecule-1, selectins, and integrins, which further facilitate leukocyte migration and infiltration, leading to exacerbation of ischemic brain damage (Oeckinghaus and Ghosh 2009; Iadecola and Alexander 2001). Lan et al. (2013) reported that cerebral I/R injury is tightly regulated by the Toll-like receptor 4 (TLR4)/NF-κB pathway, and inhibition of TLR4/NF-κB signaling is a promising target for anti-inflammatory therapy. EA stimulation at the Quchi and Zusanli acupoints (1/20 Hz and 0.01 mA) markedly reduced infarct volume and neurological deficits after 2 h of middle cerebral artery occlusion (MCAo) followed by 24 h of reperfusion. EA provides neuroprotective effects against cerebral I/R injury by suppressing the expression of TLR4, NF-κB, TNF-α, IL-1β, and IL-6 in the ischemic area (Lan et al. 2013). Proinflammatory mediators, such as cytokines and matrix metalloproteinases (MMPs), are released by resident microglia and infiltrating leukocytes, and play a critical role in the disruption of the BBB and development of brain edema in the early stage of cerebral ischemia. Aquaporin (AQP)-4 and AQP-9 both induce brain edema by accelerating water transport across the BBB into the brain parenchyma (Bonomini and Rezzani 2010; Xu et al. 2014). A previous study conducted by Xu et al. (2014) demonstrated that EA stimulation at the Baihui and Zusanli acupoints (2 Hz, 1 mA, for 20 min duration) significantly reduced brain infarction volume and neurological scores after 2 h of MCAo followed by 24 h of reperfusion. EA exerts beneficial effects against brain edema through downregulation of MMP2, AQP-4, and AQP-9 expression in the ischemic boundary zone (Xu et al. 2014). Elango and Devaraj (2010) demonstrated that cerebral I/R injury can initiate inflammatory cell activation and infiltration (detected by myeloperoxidase [MPO] assay) in the penumbra area, whereas pharmacological inhibition of MPO activity attenuates proinflammatory cytokine expression (Elango and Devaraj 2010). Xiao et al. (2012) found that heat-sensitive moxibustion at the Dazhui (GV 14) acupoint (once daily, 35 min duration, for 3 consecutive days) provides neuroprotection against cerebral infarction by suppressing MPO, IL-1β, and IL-2 expression in the ischemic area after 2 h of MCAo followed by 72 h of reperfusion (Xiao et al. 2012). A previous study conducted by Qin et al. (2013) aimed to investigate the effect of EA against inflammation in the hippocampus and found that EA stimulation at the Baihui, Hegu, and Taichong (LR 3) acupoints (2/100 Hz, 1 mA, for 20 min duration) exerts neuroprotective effects against cerebral I/R injury via downregulation of IL-1β and inhibitor of NF-κB kinase β (IKK-β) (required for activation of NF-κB) expression in the hippocampus at 12, 24, and 48 h after MCAo (Qin et al. 2013). A similar study conducted by Chen et al. (2012b) revealed that EA stimulation at the Baihui and Zusanli acupoints (20 min duration, once daily) significantly decreased IL-1β and TNF-α expression in the ischemic regions at 12, 24, 48, 72, 96, and 144 h after MCAo (Chen et al. 2012b). Wang et al. (2012c) showed that EA stimulation at the Shuigou and Neiguan acupoints significantly decreased IL-1 receptor (IL-1R) and TNF receptor (TNFR) mRNA and protein expression in the ischemic area after 1 h of MCAo followed by 6 and 12 h of reperfusion (Wang et al. 2012c). A previous study of scalp-acupuncture conducted by Zhou et al. (2008) also found that EA stimulation at the MS 6 and Dingnie Houxiexian (MS 7) (2/100 Hz, 2 mA, for 20 min duration) ameliorated neurological deficits and decreased expression of the proinflammatory cytokines IL-1β and TNF-α in the plasma and ischemic regions after 1 h of MCAo followed by 24, 48, or 72 h of reperfusion (Zhou et al. 2008). Another study of scalp acupuncture conducted by Zhang et al. (2009) demonstrated that EA stimulation at the Baihui and Qubin (GB 7) acupoints (2/100 Hz, 2 mA, 30 min duration, once daily) significantly decreased neurological deficits and downregulated the expression of cyclooxygenase-2 (COX-2) and NF-κB in the ischemic area after 1 h of MCAo followed by 24, 48, and 72 h of reperfusion (Zhang et al. 2009). In a previous study of MCAo, acupuncture stimulation at the Shuigou and Neiguan acupoints markedly reduced levels of the IL receptor, type 1 (IL-1R1) and TNF receptor, type 1 (TNFR-1) mRNA and protein in the ischemic regions 3 h after cerebral ischemia (Wang et al. 2012c). Chemokines are a type of cytokines that have the ability to induce chemotaxis on target cells and act as a critical enhancer during the post-ischemic inflammatory response (Shichita et al. 2012; Jin et al. 2013). Monocyte chemotactic protein-induced protein 1 (MCPIP1) has been shown to be a negative regulator of macrophage activation (Liang et al. 2008). Therefore, MCPIP1 plays an anti-inflammatory role in suppression of pro-inflammatory cytokine production (Jin et al. 2013). A preconditioning study conducted by Jin et al. (2013) showed that EA stimulation at the Baihui acupoint (2/15 Hz, 1 mA, 30 min duration, for 2 consecutive days) significantly reduced cerebral infarction and induced MCPIP1 expression in the ischemic area after 1.5 h of MCAo followed by 24 or 48 h of reperfusion, indicating that MCPIP1 plays a role in cerebral ischemic tolerance (Jin et al. 2013). It is known that $\alpha 7$ nicotinic acetylcholine receptor ($\alpha 7$nAChR)-dependent cholinergic signaling can downregulate the release of high mobility group box 1 (HMGB1), which enhances the inflammatory response in acute cerebral ischemia (Wang et al. 2004; Kim et al. 2008). Another preconditioning study conducted by Wang et al. (2012a) revealed that EA stimulation at the Baihui acupoint (2/15 Hz, 1 mA, 30 min duration, for 5 consecutive days) reduced cerebral infarct size and neurological deficits after 2 h of MCAo followed by 72 h of reperfusion. EA exerts beneficial effects against HMGB1 release through the activation of $\alpha 7$nAChR in the ischemic penumbra (Wang et al. 2012a). During the acute stage of cerebral ischemia, excitatory neurotransmitter glutamate release and causes excitotoxicity by initiating high levels of calcium influx, exacerbating the inflammatory response and cerebral ischemic injury (Lee et al. 2000). Glutamate transporters play a vital role in homeostasis of extracellular glutamate and excitatory amino-acid transporter 2 (EAAT2) is the most abundant form of glutamate transporter in the brain (Fang et al. 2002). Zhu et al. (2013a) found that EA preconditioning at the Baihui acupoint (2/15 Hz, 1 mA, 30 min duration, once daily for 5 consecutive days) decreased neurological scores and infarct volume and increased EAAT2 expression in the ischemic area at 24 h after reperfusion. The results indicate that EA preconditioning protects against cerebral infarction by activating EAAT2 (Zhu et al. 2013a).

From this evidence, we conclude that the neuroprotective effects of EA stimulation against cerebral I/R injury might be mediated by downregulation of proinflammatory mediators (including TNF-α, IL-1β, IL-6, MMPs, chemokines, and aquaporins), enzymes (including COX-2 and MPO), receptors (including IL-1R1, TNFR-1, and TLR4), and the transcription factor NF-κB, and by upregulation of $\alpha 7$nAChR and EAAT2 expression in the ischemia area (Fig. 7.1).

7.3.2   The Antioxidative Stress Effects of Acupuncture

Cerebral ischemia and reperfusion generate large amounts of reactive oxygen species (ROS), which disrupt antioxidant defense, and directly impair mitochondrial homeostasis and energy production (Seo et al. 2010; Zhang et al. 2014b). The generation of ROS, such as the superoxide anion radical, involves the

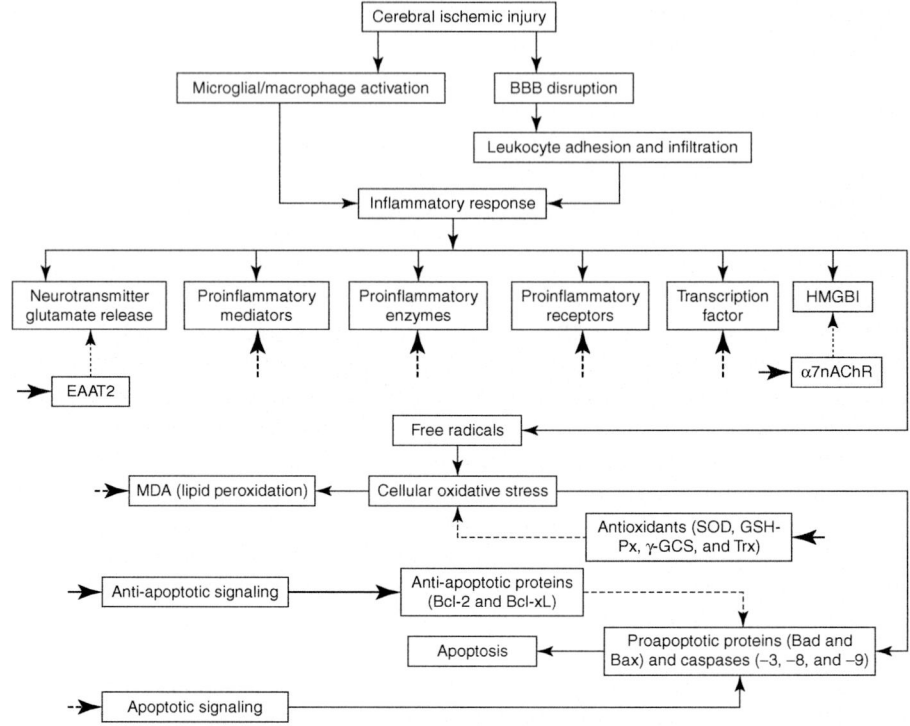

Fig. 7.1 The flowchart shows the anti-inflammatory, antioxidative, and anti- apoptotic effects of acupuncture in cerebral ischemic injury. *BBB* blood brain barrier, *HMGB1* high mobility group box 1, *EAAT2* excitatory amino-acid transporter 2, *α7nAChR* α7 nicotinic acetylcholine receptor, *MDA* malondialdehyde, *SOD* superoxide dismutase, *GSH-Px* glutathione peroxidase, *γ-GCS* gamma-glutamylcysteine synthetase, *Trx* thioredoxin. Thin solid lines with arrowheads indicate the pathological processes of cerebral ischemic injury. Thin dotted lines with arrowheads indicate downregulation. Thick solid lines with arrowheads indicate upregulation of protein expression induced by acupuncture. Thick dashed lines with arrowheads indicate downregulation of protein expression induced by acupuncture

mitochondrial electron transport chain and plays a critical role in brain damage after cerebral I/R (Zhang et al. 2014b; Noh et al. 2011). Under conditions of oxidative stress, free radicals attack macromolecules, including nucleic acid, lipids, and protein, and then generate deoxyguanosine (a marker of oxidative stress to DNA), malondialdehyde (MDA) (a marker of lipid peroxidation) and 4-hydroxy-trans-2-nonenal (a marker of lipid peroxidation) in the acute stage of cerebral ischemia (Chen et al. 2011; Cheng et al. 2008). Oxidative stress triggers apoptosis and exacerbates cerebral infarction during cerebral I/R injury (Chen et al. 2011). In contrast, endogenous antioxidant enzymes, including superoxide dismutase (SOD), glutathione peroxidase (GSH-Px) and catalase play a pivotal role in decreasing oxidant production and preventing oxidative stress during cerebral ischemia (Chen et al. 2011; Guo et al. 2011). An increased in SOD activity catalyses dismutation of the superoxide anion into H_2O_2. Subsequently, the increase in GSH-Px breaks down H_2O_2 into water molecules, preventing H_2O_2-induced hydroxyl radical formation (Liu et al. 2006). Vascular dementia is the second most common form of dementia in the elderly (Roman et al. 2002). Research findings suggest that decreased blood flow to the brain and oxidative stress might contribute to the brain damage associated with vascular dementia (Liu et al. 2006). Liu et al. (2006) demonstrated that EA stimulation at the Danzhong (CV17), Zhongwan (CV12), Qihai (CV6), Xuehai (SP10), and Zusanli acupoints markedly increased the activation of SOD and GSH-Px in the hippocampus 21 days after MCAo in an experimental model of multi-infarct dementia (Liu et al. 2006). A similar study conducted by Zhang et al. (2014b) found that EA stimulation improves cognitive function and cerebral blood flow in multi-infarct dementia. Furthermore, EA stimulation provides neuroprotection against oxidative stress by upregulating the expression of mitochondrial SOD and GSH and downregulating MDA expression and superoxide anion production in the ischemic area (Zhang et al. 2014b). Gamma-glutamylcysteine synthetase (γ-GCS) is involved in GSH synthesis and plays a role in neuroprotection (Pocernich and Butterfield 2012). A previous study conducted by Shen et al. (2012) reported that EA stimulation at Baihui and Dazhui acupoints (3 Hz, 1–3 mA, for 30 min duration) protects neurons against oxidative stress via the enhancement of γ-GCS protein, and human γ-GCS mRNA and protein expression in the ischemic cortex after 2 h of MCAo followed by 24 h of reperfusion (Shen et al. 2012). In a review study, He et al. (2009) concluded that acupuncture stimulation at Jing acupoints reduces cerebral infarction by scavenging free radicals in cerebral ischemia (He et al. 2009). The thioredoxin system (TS), comprised of thioredoxin (Trx) and Trx reductase and nicotinamide adenine dinucleotide phosphate as the electron donor, is involved in many cellular function and plays an important role against oxidative stress through the suppression of disulphide group formation (Silva-Adaya et al. 2014; Siu et al. 2005). Trx is a regulator of cellular function in response to oxidative stress, playing a role in cell survival after focal cerebral I/R injury (Siu et al. 2005). Siu et al. (2005) reported that EA stimulation at the Fengchi (GB 20) and Zusanli acupoints (2 Hz, 0.7 V, and 0.5 ms duration) upregulates the activation of TS, thereby preventing ROS-induced disulphide group formation in the ischemic area after 1 h of MCAo followed by 4 days of reperfusion (Siu et al. 2005).

Based on these results, we conclude that EA stimulation provides neuroprotection against oxidative stress by scavenging free radicals, downregulating the expression of MDA, and upregulating the expression of SOD, GSH-Px, γ-GCS, and TS in the cerebral ischemic area (Fig. 7.1).

7.3.3   The Anti-apoptotic Effects of Acupuncture

The apoptotic mode of cell death is an active and defined process that requires activation of associated genes and synthesis of pathogenesis-related proteins (Chen et al. 2014b). Apoptosis in the penumbra, occurring through various signaling pathways, is considered to be the major cause of cerebral infarct expansion following I/R injury (Cheng et al. 2014a, b; Feng et al. 2013). During the cerebral I/R period, the number of apoptotic cells observed in the ischemic region peaks at 24–48 h and lasts for up to 7 days of reperfusion (Zhao et al. 2011). There are two major caspase-dependent apoptotic pathways: the intrinsic apoptotic pathway, which involves the cytochrome c-mediated caspase cascade, and the extrinsic pathway, which is activated by the death receptors (TNF-α and Fas ligand receptors) and caspase-8 (Elmore 2007; Cheng et al. 2014b). In the mitochondrial pathway, ischemic insults activate and oligomerize Bax and Bak, which subsequently cause the release of cytochrome c. The release of cytochrome c and dATP-dependent formation of apoptotic protease activating factor-1/caspase-9 complex (apoptosome) then initiates the activation of caspase-3-mediated apoptosis (Cheng et al. 2014b; Imao and Nagata 2013). The Bcl-2 family proteins, including Bcl-2, Bcl-xL, Bax, and Bad play pivotal roles in regulating the mitochondria-mediated apoptotic pathway. Neuronal death or survival is determined by the balance between proapoptotic (Bax and Bad) and anti-apoptotic (Bcl-2 and Bcl-xL) proteins during cerebral ischemia (Sun et al. 2011; Zhu et al. 1999; Wang et al. 2009b). A reduced Bcl-2 (Bcl-xL)/Bax ratio shifts the balance toward apoptosis by triggering the release of cytochrome c, whereas an increased Bcl-2 (Bcl-xL)/Bax ratio will shift the balance toward anti-apoptotic effects by suppressing the release of apoptogenic factors from the mitochondria (Huang et al. 2010). Phosphorylated Bad inhibits its proapoptotic properties and enhances the anti-apoptotic action of Bcl-2 (Yip et al. 2008). The phosphoinositide 3-kinase/protein kinase B (PI3K/Akt) signaling pathway is a pivotal mediator that modulates cellular activation, inflammatory response, and apoptosis in cerebral ischemic injury (Chen et al. 2014b; Xue et al. 2014). Previous studies have identified that PI3K/Akt/glycogen synthase kinase 3β signaling plays a vital role in regulating cellular survival/death during I/R injury (Arslan et al. 2013; Li et al. 2012; Mullonkal and Toledo-Pereyra 2007). Xue et al. (2014) found that EA stimulation at the Zusanli and Quchi acupoints (4/20 Hz, 30 min duration, once daily for 3 consecutive days) significantly reduced neurological deficits and infarct volume after 2 h of MCAo followed by 72 h of reperfusion. EA protects against cerebral I/R injury by upregulating the expression of phospho-Akt (p-Akt), phospho-bad (p-Bad) and Bcl-2, and increased the ratio of Bcl-2/Bax, while simultaneously downregulating the expression of Bad and Bax in the ischemic area, thereby preventing caspase-3 activation (Xue et al. 2014). Members of the inhibitor of apoptosis protein (IAP) family, including X-linked IAP (XIAP), c-IAP1, c-IAP2, and survivin, participate in apoptosis regulation by directly binding to caspases (-3, -7, and -9), and suppressing caspase-3 activation and apoptosis following transient cerebral ischemia (Siegelin et al. 2005). Death receptor 5 (DR5) is a proapoptotic protein and its expression is mediated by NF-κB (Shetty et al. 2005). Kim et al. (2013) showed that EA stimulation at acupoints (2 Hz and 1 mA) markedly decreased the expression of caspase-3, -8, -9, and DR5, while simultaneously increasing the expression of Bcl-2, Bcl-xL, c-IAP1, and c-IAP2 in the ischemic area in a rat model of MCAo. These results suggest that EA protects against mitochondria-mediated apoptosis through the inhibition of DR5 expression (Kim et al. 2013). Protein kinase A (PKA) is a second messenger-dependent enzyme that controls a number of cellular functions by phosphorylating many substrates, such as cyclic AMP response element binding protein (CREB). CREB has been shown to play a pivotal role in synaptic plasticity and neuroprotection against apoptosis in cerebral ischemia (Tanaka 2001). A previous study using manual acupuncture showed that acupuncture stimulation at the Baihui, Shuigou, Quchi, Hegu, Neiguan, Zusanli, Sanyinjiao, and Taichong acupoints (30 min duration, once daily for 3, 7, or 14 days) exerts neuroprotective effects against apoptosis by increasing PKA expression in the ischemic cortex after 2 h of MCAo followed by 3, 7, and 14 days of reperfusion (Li et al. 2013). Brain-derived neurotrophic factor (BDNF) is a member of the neurotrophin family that plays a key role in neuronal survival. The binding of BDNF to the specific tyrosine kinase B receptor on neurons activates two signal transduction pathways: the PI3K and mitogen-activated protein kinase (MAPK) signaling (Sun et al. 2008). BDNF protects against apoptosis through the activation of Raf-1/MEK1/2/ERK1/2 signaling, which subsequently phosphates the 90 kDa ribosomal S6 kinase (p90RSK), leading to the phosphorylation of Bad and the inhibition of caspase-3-mediated apoptosis (Cheng et al. 2014a; Sung et al. 2011). Cheng et al. (2014a) reported that EA-like stimulation at the Baihui and Dazhui acupoints (5 Hz, 2.7-3 mA, 25 min duration, once daily for 2 consecutive days) markedly reduced the infarct area and improved neurological function, while also increasing the expression of BDNF, phospho-Raf-1, phospho-MEK1/2, phospho-ERK1/2, phospho-p90RSK, and p-Bad, and decreasing the expression of cleaved caspase-3 and apoptosis in the ischemic cortex after 15 min of MCAo followed by 3 days of reperfusion. Results suggest that EA-like stimulation provides neuroprotection against apoptosis by activation of BDNF-mediated MEK1/2/ERK1/2/p90RSK/Bad signaling in mild transient MCAo (Cheng et al. 2014a). S100B exerts its neurotoxic effect at micromolar concentrations and is an effective biomarker in predicting the extent of brain edema and the severity of infarction (Cheng et al. 2014b; Tanaka et al. 2007). In mild transient focal cerebral ischemia, astrocytic S100B interaction with the receptor for advanced glycation end products induces inflammation (cytokine)-mediated apoptosis in the ischemic penumbra, which triggers a delayed infarct expansion during the subacute stage (Cheng et al. 2014b). The extrinsic apoptotic pathway can be triggered by the binding of TNFα to the TNF receptor-1 (TNFR1), which activates the apoptotic TNFR1-associated death domain (TRADD)/Fas-associated death domain (FADD)/caspase-8 pathway and thereby elicits the cleavage of caspase-3, leading to apoptosis (Yu et al. 2006). Cheng and colleagues (2014) further examined the effect of EA-like stimulation on delayed infarct expansion and found that EA-like stimulation effectively downregulates astrocytic S100B expression to provide neuroprotective effects against delayed infarct expansion through the modulation of p38 MAPK-mediated NF-κB expression. The regulatory effects contribute to the downregulation of the TNFα/TRADD/FADD/cleaved caspase-8/cleaved caspase-3 signaling in the cortical penumbra 7 days after reperfusion (Cheng et al. 2014b). Previous studies also reported that BDNF inhibits neuronal apoptosis through upregulation of SOD and GSH after cerebral ischemia (Zhao et al. 2013). Zhao et al. (2013) demonstrated that EA stimulation at the Shenshu (BL 23), Geshu

(BL 17), and Baihui acupoints enhances endogenous BDNF mRNA expression, which may contribute to the inhibition of apoptosis in the hippocampus at 1 and 7 days after MCAo (Zhao et al. 2013). Under unstimulated conditions, NF-κB is held inactive in the cytosol by the inhibitor of κB (IκB), whereas under pathological conditions, IκB is phosphorylated by the IKK complex, which initiates proteolytic degradation of IκB, leading to the release of NF-κB (Clark and Coopersmith 2007). During cerebral ischemia, activated NF-κB translocates to the nucleus, where it binds to specific sequences of DNA and induces the expression of various target genes involved in apoptosis (Feng et al. 2013). Feng et al. (2013) reported that EA stimulation at the Baihui and Shenting acupoints (1/20 Hz, 30 min duration, once daily for 10 consecutive days) reduced neurological deficits and infarct volume and ameliorated cognitive impairment after 2 h of MCAo followed by 14 days of reperfusion. EA protects against apoptosis through the inhibition of NF-κB-induced Bax and Fas expression in the ischemic area (Feng et al. 2013). The protein kinase C (PKC) family consists of 10 isozymes. In the CNS, isozymes PKCα, PKCβ1, PKCβ2, PKCγ, PKCδ, PKCε, PKCζ, PKCη, and PKCθ are present (Bright and Mochly-Rosen 2005). Results from previous studies suggest that PKC is activated and plays a detrimental role in the development of neurotoxicity in *in vitro* and *in vivo* models (Maiese et al. 1993; Hara et al. 1990). In a previous study of scalp acupuncture conducted by Wang et al. (2012d), EA stimulation at MS 5 and Dingpangxian (MS 8) (2/15 Hz and 1 mA) decreased PKCγ and PKCδ expression, as well as numbers of apoptotic neuronal cells in the ischemic cortex at 4, 12, 24, and 72 h after cerebral I/R (Wang et al. 2012d). Another study of scalp acupuncture showed that EA stimulation at MS 6 and MS 7 reduced neuronal apoptosis in the ischemic area after 2 h of MCAo followed by 24 h of reperfusion. The anti-apoptotic effect of EA can be attributed to the upregulation of Bcl-2 and downregulation of caspase-3 expression in the ischemic area (Chen et al. 2009). It is already known that PI3K can be activated by neurotrophic factors, such as BDNF and glial cell line-derived neurotrophic factor (GDNF). In addition, activation of PI3K/Akt signaling provides neuroprotection against apoptosis by increasing the Bcl-2/Bax ratio in cerebral ischemia (Janelidze et al. 2001; Noshita et al. 2001). Chen et al. (2012a) demonstrated that EA stimulation at the Quchi and Zusanli acupoints decreased neurological deficits and infarct volume after 2 h of MCAo followed by 24 h of reperfusion. Furthermore, EA at these acupoints increased BDNF, GDNF, PI3K, p-Akt, and Bcl-2, and decreased Bax and TUNEL expression in the ischemic area. The data show that EA protects against apoptosis by activating PI3K/Akt signaling, and the anti-apoptotic effect of PI3K/Akt signaling can be further attributed to the increase of the Bcl-2/Bax ratio (Chen et al. 2012a). Zhao et al. (2011) reported that EA stimulation at the Shenshu, Geshu, and Baihui acupoints provides beneficial effects against apoptosis in the ischemic hippocampal and cortical areas 7 days after cerebral ischemia (Zhao et al. 2011). A similar study conducted by Chung et al. (2007) showed that acupuncture stimulation at the Zusanli and Hegu acupoints alleviates ischemia-induced apoptosis in the hippocampal dentate gyrus (Chung et al. 2007). In a previous study of multi-infarct dementia, results concluded that manual acupuncture stimulation at the Tanzhong

(CV 17), Zhongwan, Qihai, Zusanli, and Xuehai acupoints exerts neuroprotection against apoptosis through the increase of Bcl-2/Bax in the hippocampus 21 days after MCAo (Wang et al. 2009b). Chen et al. (2008) found that EA stimulation at the Shuigou and Baihui acupoints (2/15 Hz, 1 mA, 30 min duration) exerts an anti-apoptotic effect by upregulating the mitochondrial membrane potential in the ischemic cortex (Chen et al. 2008). Heat shock protein 70 (HSP70) and HSP90 are the major molecular chaperones in the eukaryotic cytosol. HSP70 is known to regulate apoptotic cell death directly by inhibiting the expression of proapoptotic factors as well as indirectly by increasing the expression of anti-apoptotic factors, such as Bcl-2. HSP70 and HSP90 cooperate in a multichaperone complex in the regulation of misfolded or abnormal proteins for degradation (Giffard and Yenari 2004; Yamamoto et al. 2014). Sun et al. (2003) concluded that EA stimulation protects against apoptosis through the enhancement of HSP70 and restoration of HSP90 expression in the ischemic area in a rat model of MCAo (Sun et al. 2003). During cerebral ischemia, c-Fos protein plays a vital role in the initiation of apoptosis in the hippocampus (Jiang et al. 2001; Jang et al. 2003). In a previous study, results showed that EA stimulation at the Zusanli and Hegu acupoints markedly decreased the number of c-Fos-, TUNEL-, and caspase-3-postive cells in the hippocampal CA1 region 10 days after bilateral common carotid artery occlusion, indicating that EA protects against apoptosis by suppressing c-Fos expression in the hippocampus (Jang et al. 2003). Tropomyosin receptor kinase A (TrkA) is a member of the growth factor receptor family that controls synaptic strength and plasticity in the CNS (Stoleru et al. 2013). Previous studies reported that TrkA mediates the anti-apoptotic effect of nerve growth factor (NGF) in neural tissue (Yoon et al. 1998; Emanueli et al. 2002). Shi (1999) found that acupuncture stimulation reduced infarct volume and increased the expression of TrkA following cerebral ischemia, indicating that EA protects against apoptosis by enhancing TrkA expression in the ischemic area after cerebral I/R injury (Shi 1999). Active p-Akt promotes cell survival by suppressing apoptotic signaling and plays a pivotal role in modulating the balance between survival and apoptosis (Wang et al. 2002). Wang et al. (2002) showed that EA stimulation at the Baihui and Renzhong (GV 26) acupoints (3/20 Hz and 3 mA) upregulated Akt but downregulated caspase-9 expression in the penumbra area after 90 min of MCAo followed by 8 and 24 h of reperfusion. The results showed that EA provides neuroprotection by activation of Akt-mediated anti-apoptotic signaling (Wang et al. 2002). Several studies have shown that acupuncture preconditioning inhibits apoptosis by modulating various components of cellular signaling pathways. In the CNS, endocannabinoids: N-arachidonoyl-ethanolamine (anandamide; AEA) and 2-arachidonoylglycerol (2-AG) act mainly through the activation of the central cannabinoid receptor type 1 (CB1), which is involved in the mechanisms of neuroprotection of cerebral ischemic preconditioning (Schomacher et al. 2006; Wang et al. 2011). Wang et al. (2009a) demonstrated that EA pretreatment (preconditioning) at the Baihui acupoint (2/15 Hz, 1 mA, 30 min duration) reduced neurological deficits and infarct volume after 2 h of MCAo and 1 or 7 days of reperfusion. EA pretreatment increased AEA, 2-AG, and CB1 expression in the ischemic area and decreased neuronal apoptosis in the penumbra, indicating that the anti-apoptotic effect of EA preconditioning is mediated by the endocannabinoids system following cerebral I/R injury (Wang et al. 2009a). Wang et al. (2011) further investigated the precise mechanism of EA pretreatment in modulating the endocannabinoids system and found that EA pretreatment exerts neuroprotection against apoptosis by activating εPKC (PKCε)/CB1 signaling, then increases the Bcl-2/Bax ratio in the ischemic penumbra 24 h after reperfusion (Wang et al. 2011). The oncogenic signal transducers and activators of transcription 3 (STAT3) is a transcription factor and also an intracellular signal transducer (Darnell Jr. 1997). During cerebral ischemic insult, phospho-STAT3 (p-STAT3) translocates into the nucleus and regulates expression of anti-apoptotic genes, such as Bcl-2. Thus, STAT3 plays a pivotal role in neuronal survival in response to cerebral ischemia (Wang et al. 2013b; Zhou et al. 2013). In a similar study of EA preconditioning (Zhou et al. 2013), EA stimulation increased the expression of p-STAT3 in the penumbra at 6 h, decreased neuronal apoptosis in the penumbra at 24 h, and reduced neurological deficits and infarct volume at 72 h after reperfusion. The data suggest that the anti-apoptotic effect of EA pretreatment can be attributed to the activation of STAT3 signaling, which subsequently increases the ratio of Bcl-2/Bax in the peri-infarct area 24 h after reperfusion. The N-myc downstream- regulated gene 2 (NDRG2) is a specific marker that is highly expressed in astrocyte of the adult brain; NDRG2 is a novel p53-associated regulator of apoptosis in cerebral ischemia (Li et al. 2014). EA pretreatment at the Baihui acupoint significantly decreased neurological scores, infarct volume and neuronal apoptosis after 2 h of MCAo followed by 24 h of reperfusion. The data suggest that the anti-apoptotic effect of EA pretreatment downregulates NDRG2 in astrocytes in the ischemic area (Wang et al. 2013a). A previous study of global cerebral ischemia (4-vessel occlusion) conducted by Zhou et al. (2011) reported that acupuncture preconditioning at the Baihui acupoint (15 Hz, 2 mA, 30 min duration, once daily for 5 days) protects against apoptosis via the inhibition of caspase-3 expression in the hippocampal CA1 region (Zhou et al. 2011).

On the basis of the above data, we conclude that EA stimulation exhibits beneficial effects against apoptosis through upregulation of anti-apoptotic proteins (including Bcl-2 and Bcl-xL), and downregulation of proapoptotic proteins (including Bad and Bax) and caspases (including caspase-3, 8, and 9). The modulation of apoptosis can be further attributed to the upregulation of IAP, BDNF/MEK1/2/ERK1/2/p90RSK/Bad, PI3K/Akt, HSP70/HSP90, Trk/NGF, AEA/2-AG/CB1, and STAT3 anti-apoptotic signaling pathways, and downregulation of DR5, TNFα/TRADD/FADD, NF-κB/Bax, PKC, c-Fos, and NDRG2 apoptotic signaling pathways in the cerebral ischemic area (Fig. 7.1).

7.3.4   The Effect of Acupuncture on Neurogenesis

Animal studies have demonstrated that endogenous neurogenesis occurs in the subventricular zone (SVZ) and dentate gyrus of the subgranular zone (SGZ) in response to cerebral ischemia (Luo et al. 2014). Glycogen synthase kinase-3 (GSK-3) exists as two isoforms, GSK-3α and GSK-3β. GSK-3β is involved in the modulation of various cellular functions, including differentiation, growth, proliferation, protein synthesis, and apoptosis (Jacobs et al. 2012). Protein phosphatase 2A (PP2A) negatively regulates GSK-3β, and regulatory interventions to maintain a balance between increased GSK-3β and decreased PP2A activity exerts neuroprotective and neurogenesis effects after cerebral ischemia (Luo et al. 2014). BrdU is commonly used to investigate cell proliferation in living tissue. The intermediate filament protein nestin can be used as a marker for the proliferative state of neural precursors (Wei et al. 2002; Luo et al. 2014). Luo et al. (2014) reported that acupuncture stimulation at the Shuigou acupoint increased blood flow 3 days after MCAo, and increased BrdU/ nestin and PP2A but decreased GSK-3β expression in the ischemic area 7 days after MCAo. The data suggest that delivering acupuncture at this acupoint leads to neurogenesis through regulation of GSK-3β/PP2A expression in permanent focal cerebral ischemia (Luo et al. 2014). In another study, EA stimulation at the Fengfu (GV 16) and Jinsuo (GV 8) acupoints (2/60 Hz, 10 mA, 20 min duration) increased the expression of BrdU, collapsin response mediator protein-4 (CRMP-4, a marker for immature neurons), and microtubule-associated protein-2 (MAP-2, a marker for mature neurons) in the ischemic striatum after a transient MCAo. The data indicate that EA at these acupoints improves neuronal regeneration during the period of cerebral ischemia (Yang et al. 2005). Retinoic acid (RA) plays an important role in the normal development of the CNS and influences the early stages of forebrain development (Jung et al. 2007; Hong et al. 2013). Three retinaldehyde dehydrogenases (Raldh1, Raldh2, and Raldh3) may control the synthesis of RA needed for retina development (Niederreither et al. 2002; Mic et al. 2004). A previous study performed on RA signaling found that EA stimulation at the Zusanli and Quchi acupoints (5/20 Hz, 2–4 mA, 20 min duration) reduced neurological deficits and infarct volume, and increased Raldh1 and Raldh2 mRNA expression in the ischemic area after 2 h of MCAo followed by 7 and 14 days of reperfusion, indicating that EA stimulation exerts its beneficial effect on neurogenesis by activating RA signaling in the ischemic area following cerebral I/R injury (Hong et al. 2013). Numerous studies have reported that dopaminergic nigrostriatal projections regulate neural precursor cell proliferation in the SVZ and SGZ (Veena et al. 2011; Baker et al. 2004; O'Keeffe et al. 2009). Dopaminergic neurons play an important role in the modulation of neuroplasticity of corticostriatal synapse after cerebral ischemia, and dopamine D_2 receptor activation affects motor cortex plasticity (Valjent et al. 2005; Xu et al. 2013; Fresnoza et al. 2014). Xu et al. (2013) demonstrated that EA stimulation at the Fengchi acupoint (2 Hz, 3 mA, 20 min duration) decreased neurological scores and infarct volume after 90 min of MCAo and 7 days of reperfusion. EA stimulation also increased the expression of growth-associated protein 43, which indicates developing neural connections and neuroplasticity in dopaminergic neurons. The data show that EA stimulation exerts its influences on neuroplasticity through the activation of dopamine D_2 receptors (Xu et al. 2013). Xiao et al. (2013) reported that EA stimulation at the Quchi and Zusanli acupoints (30 min duration, once daily for 5 consecutive days) at the frequencies of 15 and 30 Hz decreased neurological deficits and increased the number of glial fibrillary acidic protein immunoreactive cells in the ischemic area 5 days after MCAo. Experimental findings suggest that EA stimulation exerts regulatory effects on neurogenesis through astrocyte-mediated synaptic plasticity (Xiao et al. 2013).

In consideration of all of these experimental results, we conclude that EA stimulation provides its effects on neurogenesis through the upregulation of BrdU/nestin, CRMP-4, MAP-2, retinaldehyde dehydrogenases, dopamine D_2 receptors, astrocytes expression, and regulation of GSK-3β/PP2A expression in the cerebral ischemic area.

Conclusions

According to clinical trial evidence in ischemic stroke, acupuncture provides beneficial effects in motor dysfunction, shoulder-hand syndrome, balance impairment, cognitive impairment, and dysphagia. In several animal models of cerebral ischemia, acupuncture has shown promising effects including an anti-inflammatory response, inhibition of oxidative stress, anti-apoptotic effects, and enhancement of stroke recovery through neurogenesis. High-quality clinical trials are urgently needed to further identify the efficacy of acupuncture in the field of ischemic stroke.

Acknowledgment This study was supported by grants from China Medical University (CMU 103-N-07), Taichung, Taiwan.

References

Arslan F, Lai RC, Smeets MB, Akeroyd L, Choo A, Aguor EN, Timmers L, van Rijen HV, Doevendans PA, Pasterkamp G, et al. Mesenchymal stem cell-derived exosomes increase ATP levels, decrease oxidative stress and activate PI3K/Akt pathway to enhance myocardial viability and prevent adverse remodeling after myocardial ischemia/reperfusion injury. Stem Cell Res. 2013;10:301–12.

Baker SA, Baker KA, Hagg T. Dopaminergic nigrostriatal projections regulate neural precursor proliferation in the adult mouse subventricular zone. Eur J Neurosci. 2004;20:575–9.

Balami JS, Chen R, Sutherland BA, Buchan AM. Thrombolytic agents for acute ischaemic stroke treatment: the past, present and future. CNS Neurol Disord Drug Targets. 2013a;12:145–54.

Balami JS, Sutherland BA, Buchan AM. Complications associated with recombinant tissue plasminogen activator therapy for acute ischaemic stroke. CNS Neurol Disord Drug Targets. 2013b;12:155–69.

Bonomini F, Rezzani R. Aquaporin and blood brain barrier. Curr Neuropharmacol. 2010;8:92–6.

Bright R, Mochly-Rosen D. The role of protein kinase C in cerebral ischemic and reperfusion injury. Stroke. 2005;36:2781–90.

Cayrol R, Wosik K, Berard JL, Dodelet-Devillers A, Ifergan I, Kebir H, Haqqani AS, Kreymborg K, Krug S, Moumdjian R, et al. Activated leukocyte cell adhesion molecule promotes leukocyte trafficking into the central nervous system. Nat Immunol. 2008;9:137–45.

Chen XY, Zhang QL, Bai B. Effect of electroacupuncture on mitochondrial membrane potential and apoptosis in the cerebral cortex in rats with focal cerebral ischemia/reperfusion injury. Zhen Ci Yan Jiu. 2008;33:107–10.

Chen F, Yan ZK, Yang B. Effects of electroacupuncture on cerebral Bcl-2 and caspase-3 expression after cerebral ischemia reperfusion in rats. Zhen Ci Yan Jiu. 2009;34:363–7.

Chen H, Yoshioka H, Kim GS, Jung JE, Okami N, Sakata H, Maier CM, Narasimhan P, Goeders CE, Chan PH. Oxidative stress in ischemic brain damage: mechanisms of cell death and potential molecular targets for neuroprotection. Antioxid Redox Signal. 2011;14:1505–17.

Chen A, Lin Z, Lan L, Xie G, Huang J, Lin J, Peng J, Tao J, Chen L. Electroacupuncture at the Quchi and Zusanli acupoints exerts neuroprotective role in cerebral ischemia-reperfusion injured rats via activation of the PI3K/Akt pathway. Int J Mol Med. 2012a;30:791–6.

Chen SH, Sun H, Xu H, Zhang YM, Gao Y, Li S. Effects of acupuncture of "Baihui"(GV 20) and "Zusanli"(ST 36) on expression of cerebral IL-1beta and TNF-alpha proteins in cerebral ischemia reperfusion injury rats. Zhen Ci Yan Jiu. 2012b;37:470–5.

Chen J, Wang J, Huang Y, Lai X, Tang C, Yang J, Wu J, Zeng T, Qu S. Modulatory effect of acupuncture at Waiguan (TE5) on the functional connectivity of the central nervous system of patients with ischemic stroke in the left basal ganglia. PLoS One. 2014a;9:e96777.

Chen L, Wei X, Hou Y, Liu X, Li S, Sun B, Liu H. Tetramethylpyrazine analogue CXC195 protects against cerebral ischemia/reperfusion-induced apoptosis through PI3K/Akt/GSK3beta pathway in rats. Neurochem Int. 2014b;66:27–32.

Chen LF, Fang JQ, Wu YY, Ma RJ, Xu SY, Shen LH, Luo KT, Gao F, Bao YH, Ni KF, Li LP. Motor dysfunction in stroke of subacute stage treated with acupuncture: multi-central randomized controlled study. Zhongguo Zhen Jiu. 2014c;34:313–8.

Cheng CY, Su SY, Tang NY, Ho TY, Chiang SY, Hsieh CL. Ferulic acid provides neuroprotection against oxidative stress-related apoptosis after cerebral ischemia/reperfusion injury by inhibiting ICAM-1 mRNA expression in rats. Brain Res. 2008;1209:136–50.

Cheng CY, Lin JG, Su SY, Tang NY, Kao ST, Hsieh CL. Electroacupuncture-like stimulation at Baihui and Dazhui acupoints exerts neuroprotective effects through activation of the brain-derived neurotrophic factor-mediated MEK1/2/ERK1/2/p90RSK/bad signaling pathway in mild transient focal cerebral ischemia in rats. BMC Complement Altern Med. 2014a;14:92.

Cheng CY, Lin JG, Tang NY, Kao ST, Hsieh CL. Electroacupuncture-like stimulation at the Baihui (GV20) and Dazhui (GV14) acupoints protects rats against subacute-phase cerebral ischemia-reperfusion injuries by reducing S100B-mediated neurotoxicity. PLoS One. 2014b;9:e91426.

Chung JH, Lee EY, Jang MH, Kim CJ, Kim J, Ha E, Park HK, Choi S, Lee H, Park SH, et al. Acupuncture decreases ischemia-induced apoptosis and cell proliferation in dentate gyrus of gerbils. Neurol Res. 2007;29(Suppl 1):S23–7.

Clark JA, Coopersmith CM. Just the right amount of JNK: how nuclear factor-kappaB and downstream mediators prevent burn-induced intestinal injury. Crit Care Med. 2007;35:1433–4.

Darnell JE Jr. STATs and gene regulation. Science. 1997;277:1630–5.

Dharmasaroja PA, Pattaraarchachai J. Low vs standard dose of recombinant tissue plasminogen activator in treating East Asian patients with acute ischemic stroke. Neurol India. 2011;59:180–4.

Elango C, Devaraj SN. Immunomodulatory effect of Hawthorn extract in an experimental stroke model. J Neuroinflammation. 2010;7:97.

Elijovich L, Chong JY. Current and future use of intravenous thrombolysis for acute ischemic stroke. Curr Atheroscler Rep. 2010;12:316–21.

Elmore S. Apoptosis: a review of programmed cell death. Toxicol Pathol. 2007;35:495–516.

Emanueli C, Salis MB, Pinna A, Graiani G, Manni L, Madeddu P. Nerve growth factor promotes angiogenesis and arteriogenesis in ischemic hindlimbs. Circulation. 2002;106:2257–62.

Fang H, Huang Y, Zuo Z. The different responses of rat glutamate transporter type 2 and its mutant (tyrosine 403 to histidine) activity to volatile anesthetics and activation of protein kinase C. Brain Res. 2002;953:255–64.

Fang J, Jin Z, Wang Y, Li K, Kong J, Nixon EE, Zeng Y, Ren Y, Tong H, Wang P, Hui KK. The salient characteristics of the central effects of acupuncture needling: limbic-paralimbic-neocortical network modulation. Hum Brain Mapp. 2009;30:1196–206.

Feng X, Yang S, Liu J, Huang J, Peng J, Lin J, Tao J, Chen L. Electroacupuncture ameliorates cognitive impairment through inhibition of NF-kappaB-mediated neuronal cell apoptosis in cerebral ischemia-reperfusion injured rats. Mol Med Rep. 2013;7:1516–22.

Fresnoza S, Stiksrud E, Klinker F, Liebetanz D, Paulus W, Kuo MF, Nitsche MA. Dosage-dependent effect of dopamine D2 receptor activation on motor cortex plasticity in humans. J Neurosci. 2014;34:10701–9.

Giffard RG, Yenari MA. Many mechanisms for hsp70 protection from cerebral ischemia. J Neurosurg Anesthesiol. 2004;16:53–61.

Gumbinger C, Reuter B, Stock C, Sauer T, Wietholter H, Bruder I, Rode S, Kern R, Ringleb P, Hennerici MG, Hacke W. Time to treatment with recombinant tissue plasminogen activator and outcome of stroke in clinical practice: retrospective analysis of hospital quality assurance data with comparison with results from randomised clinical trials. BMJ. 2014;348:g3429.

Guo H, Hu LM, Wang SX, Wang YL, Shi F, Li H, Liu Y, Kang LY, Gao XM. Neuroprotective effects of scutellarin against hypoxic-ischemic-induced cerebral injury via augmentation of antioxidant defense capacity. Chin J Physiol. 2011;54:399–405.

Hara H, Onodera H, Yoshidomi M, Matsuda Y, Kogure K. Staurosporine, a novel protein kinase C inhibitor, prevents postischemic neuronal damage in the gerbil and rat. J Cereb Blood Flow Metab. 1990;10:646–53.

Haring HP. Cognitive impairment after stroke. Curr Opin Neurol. 2002;15:79–84.

He F, Yang J, Zhang QP, Cui XY. Progress of experimental studies on acupuncture treatment of ischemic cerebral injury with Jing (Well)-points. Zhen Ci Yan Jiu. 2009;34:279–82.

Hong J, Wu G, Zou Y, Tao J, Chen L. Electroacupuncture promotes neurological functional recovery via the retinoic acid signaling pathway in rats following cerebral ischemia-reperfusion injury. Int J Mol Med. 2013;31:225–31.

Huang CY, Liou YF, Chung SY, Lin WY, Jong GP, Kuo CH, Tsai FJ, Cheng YC, Cheng FC, Lin JY. Role of ERK signaling in the neuroprotective efficacy of magnesium sulfate treatment during focal cerebral ischemia in the gerbil cortex. Chin J Physiol. 2010;53:299–309.

Huang SW, Wang WT, Yang TH, Liou TH, Chen GY, Lin LF. The balance effect of acupuncture therapy among stroke patients. J Altern Complement Med. 2014;20:618–22.

Hui KK, Marina O, Claunch JD, Nixon EE, Fang J, Liu J, Li M, Napadow V, Vangel M, Makris N, et al. Acupuncture mobilizes the brain's default mode and its anti-correlated network in healthy subjects. Brain Res. 2009;1287:84–103.

Iadecola C, Alexander M. Cerebral ischemia and inflammation. Curr Opin Neurol. 2001;14:89–94.

Imao T, Nagata S. Apaf-1- and Caspase-8-independent apoptosis. Cell Death Differ. 2013;20:343–52.

Jacobs KM, Bhave SR, Ferraro DJ, Jaboin JJ, Hallahan DE, Thotala D. GSK-3beta: a bifunctional role in cell death pathways. Int J Cell Biol. 2012;2012:930710.

Janelidze S, Hu BR, Siesjo P, Siesjo BK. Alterations of Akt1 (PKBalpha) and p70(S6K) in transient focal ischemia. Neurobiol Dis. 2001;8:147–54.

Jang MH, Shin MC, Lee TH, Lim BV, Shin MS, Min BI, Kim H, Cho S, Kim EH, Kim CJ. Acupuncture suppresses ischemia-induced increase in c-Fos expression and apoptosis in the hippocampal CA1 region in gerbils. Neurosci Lett. 2003;347:5–8.

Jiang L, Ding Y, Tang Y. Relationship between c-fos gene expression and delayed neuronal death in rat neonatal hippocampus following hypoxic-ischemic insult. Chin Med J. 2001;114:520–3.

Jin Z, Liang J, Wang J, Kolattukudy PE. Delayed brain ischemia tolerance induced by electroacupuncture pretreatment is mediated via MCP-induced protein 1. J Neuroinflammation. 2013;10:63.

Jung DS, Baek SY, Park KH, Chung YI, Kim HJ, Kim CD, Cho MK, Han ME, Park KP, Kim BS, et al. Effects of retinoic acid on ischemic brain injury-induced neurogenesis. Exp Mol Med. 2007;39:304–15.

Kim JB, Lim CM, Yu YM, Lee JK. Induction and subcellular localization of high-mobility group box-1 (HMGB1) in the postischemic rat brain. J Neurosci Res. 2008;86:1125–31.

Kim YR, Kim HN, Jang JY, Park C, Lee JH, Shin HK, Choi YH, Choi BT. Effects of electroacupuncture on apoptotic pathways in a rat model of focal cerebral ischemia. Int J Mol Med. 2013;32:1303–10.

Kleindorfer D, Lindsell CJ, Brass L, Koroshetz W, Broderick JP. National US estimates of recombinant tissue plasminogen activator use: ICD-9 codes substantially underestimate. Stroke. 2008;39:924–8.

Kong JC, Lee MS, Shin BC, Song YS, Ernst E. Acupuncture for functional recovery after stroke: a systematic review of sham-controlled randomized clinical trials. CMAJ. 2010;182:1723–9.

Lan L, Tao J, Chen A, Xie G, Huang J, Lin J, Peng J, Chen L. Electroacupuncture exerts anti-inflammatory effects in cerebral ischemia-reperfusion injured rats via suppression of the TLR4/NF-kappaB pathway. Int J Mol Med. 2013;31:75–80.

Lee JM, Grabb MC, Zipfel GJ, Choi DW. Brain tissue responses to ischemia. J Clin Invest. 2000;106:723–31.

Li Y, Zhu W, Tao J, Xin P, Liu M, Li J, Wei M. Fasudil protects the heart against ischemia-reperfusion injury by attenuating endoplasmic reticulum stress and modulating SERCA activity: the differential role for PI3K/Akt and JAK2/STAT3 signaling pathways. PLoS One. 2012;7:e48115.

Li ZB, Liu FM, Liu WJ. Influence of acupuncture intervention on neurologic deficits, cerebrocortical cell apoptosis and protein kinase A expression in rats with focal cerebral ischemia. Zhen Ci Yan Jiu. 2013;38:106–11.

Li X, Luo P, Wang F, Yang Q, Li Y, Zhao M, Wang S, Wang Q, Xiong L. Inhibition of N-myc downstream-regulated gene-2 is involved in an astrocyte-specific neuroprotection induced by sevoflurane preconditioning. Anesthesiology. 2014;121:549–62.

Liang J, Wang J, Azfer A, Song W, Tromp G, Kolattukudy PE, Fu M. A novel CCCH-zinc finger protein family regulates proinflammatory activation of macrophages. J Biol Chem. 2008;283:6337–46.

Liu M. Acupuncture for stroke in China: needing more high-quality evidence. Int J Stroke. 2006;1:34–5.

Liu CZ, Yu JC, Zhang XZ, Fu WW, Wang T, Han JX. Acupuncture prevents cognitive deficits and oxidative stress in cerebral multi-infarction rats. Neurosci Lett. 2006;393:45–50.

Liu SY, Hsieh CL, Wei TS, Liu PT, Chang YJ, Li TC. Acupuncture stimulation improves balance function in stroke patients: a single-blinded controlled, randomized study. Am J Chin Med. 2009;37:483–94.

Liu ZP, Zeng MP, Xie H, Lou BD, Zhang W. Effect of muscle-tension-balance acupuncture therapy on the motor function and living ability of patients with drop foot and strephenopodia after stroke. Zhongguo Zhen Jiu. 2012;32:293–6.

Liu F, Li ZM, Jiang YJ, Chen LD. A meta-analysis of acupuncture use in the treatment of cognitive impairment after stroke. J Altern Complement Med. 2014;20:535–44.

Loane DJ, Byrnes KR. Role of microglia in neurotrauma. Neurotherapeutics. 2010;7:366–77.

Luo D, Fan X, Ma C, Fan T, Wang X, Chang N, Li L, Zhang Y, Meng Z, Wang S, Shi X. A study on the effect of neurogenesis and regulation of GSK3beta/PP2A expression in acupuncture treatment of neural functional damage caused by focal ischemia in MCAO rats. Evid Based Complement Alternat Med. 2014;2014:962343.

Maiese K, Boniece IR, Skurat K, Wagner JA. Protein kinases modulate the sensitivity of hippocampal neurons to nitric oxide toxicity and anoxia. J Neurosci Res. 1993;36:77–87.

Mapulanga M, Nzala S, Mweemba C. The socio-economic impact of stroke on households in Livingstone District, Zambia: a cross-sectional study. Ann Med Health Sci Res. 2014;4:S123–7.

Meng FY, Wen J. Effect of warm acupuncture stimulation of Waiguan (TE 5) on post-stroke shoulder-hand syndrome. Zhen Ci Yan Jiu. 2014;39:228–31, 251.

Mic FA, Molotkov A, Molotkova N, Duester G. Raldh2 expression in optic vesicle generates a retinoic acid signal needed for invagination of retina during optic cup formation. Dev Dyn. 2004;231:270–7.

Mullonkal CJ, Toledo-Pereyra LH. Akt in ischemia and reperfusion. J Investig Surg. 2007;20:195–203.

Niederreither K, Fraulob V, Garnier JM, Chambon P, Dolle P. Differential expression of retinoic acid-synthesizing (RALDH) enzymes during fetal development and organ differentiation in the mouse. Mech Dev. 2002;110:165–71.

Noh SJ, Lee SH, Shin KY, Lee CK, Cho IH, Kim HS, Suh YH. SP-8203 reduces oxidative stress via SOD activity and behavioral deficit in cerebral ischemia. Pharmacol Biochem Behav. 2011;98:150–4.

Noshita N, Lewen A, Sugawara T, Chan PH. Evidence of phosphorylation of Akt and neuronal survival after transient focal cerebral ischemia in mice. J Cereb Blood Flow Metab. 2001;21:1442–50.

Oeckinghaus A, Ghosh S. The NF-kappaB family of transcription factors and its regulation. Cold Spring Harb Perspect Biol. 2009;1:a000034.

O'Keeffe GC, Tyers P, Aarsland D, Dalley JW, Barker RA, Caldwell MA. Dopamine-induced proliferation of adult neural precursor cells in the mammalian subventricular zone is mediated through EGF. Proc Natl Acad Sci U S A. 2009;106:8754–9.

Park J, Hopwood V, White AR, Ernst E. Effectiveness of acupuncture for stroke: a systematic review. J Neurol. 2001;248:558–63.

Park SW, Yi SH, Lee JA, Hwang PW, Yoo HC, Kang KS. Acupuncture for the treatment of spasticity after stroke: a meta-analysis of randomized controlled trials. J Altern Complement Med. 2014;20:672–82.

Pocernich CB, Butterfield DA. Elevation of glutathione as a therapeutic strategy in Alzheimer disease. Biochim Biophys Acta. 2012;1822:625–30.

Qin WY, Luo Y, Yu C. Influence of electroacupuncture intervention on hippocampal IL-1beta content and I kappa B kinase beta expression in focal cerebral ischemia/reperfusion rats. Zhen Ci Yan Jiu. 2013;38:271–6.

Roman GC, Erkinjuntti T, Wallin A, Pantoni L, Chui HC. Subcortical ischaemic vascular dementia. Lancet Neurol. 2002;1:426–36.

Schomacher M, Muller HD, Sommer C. Short-term ischemia usually used for ischemic preconditioning down-regulates central cannabinoid receptors in the gerbil hippocampus. Acta Neuropathol. 2006;111:8–14.

Seo AY, Joseph AM, Dutta D, Hwang JC, Aris JP, Leeuwenburgh C. New insights into the role of mitochondria in aging: mitochondrial dynamics and more. J Cell Sci. 2010;123:2533–42.

Shen MH, Xiang XR, Li Y, Pan JL, Ma C, Li ZR. Effect of electroacupuncture on expression of gamma-glutamylcysteine synthetase protein and mRNA in cerebral cortex in rats with focal cerebral ischemia-reperfusion. Zhen Ci Yan Jiu. 2012;37:25–30.

Shetty S, Graham BA, Brown JG, Hu X, Vegh-Yarema N, Harding G, Paul JT, Gibson SB. Transcription factor NF-kappaB differentially regulates death receptor 5 expression involving histone deacetylase 1. Mol Cell Biol. 2005;25:5404–16.

Shi J. A study on the effect and mechanism of acupuncture suppression of neuronal apoptosis following cerebral ischemia. Sheng Li Ke Xue Jin Zhan. 1999;30:326–9.

Shichita T, Sakaguchi R, Suzuki M, Yoshimura A. Post-ischemic inflammation in the brain. Front Immunol. 2012;3:132.

Siegelin MD, Kossatz LS, Winckler J, Rami A. Regulation of XIAP and Smac/DIABLO in the rat hippocampus following transient forebrain ischemia. Neurochem Int. 2005;46:41–51.

Silva-Adaya D, Gonsebatt ME, Guevara J. Thioredoxin system regulation in the central nervous system: experimental models and clinical evidence. Oxidative Med Cell Longev. 2014;2014:590808.

Siu FK, Lo SC, Leung MC. Electro-acupuncture potentiates the disulphide-reducing activities of thioredoxin system by increasing thioredoxin expression in ischemia-reperfused rat brains. Life Sci. 2005;77:386–99.

Stoleru B, Popescu AM, Tache DE, Neamtu OM, Emami G, Tataranu LG, Buteica AS, Dricu A, Purcaru SO. Tropomyosin-receptor-kinases signaling in the nervous system. Maedica (Buchar). 2013;8:43–8.

Sun N, Shi J, Chen L, Liu X, Guan X. Influence of electroacupuncture on the mRNA of heat shock protein 70 and 90 in brain after cerebral ischemia/reperfusion of rats. J Huazhong Univ Sci Technolog Med Sci. 2003;23:112–5.

Sun X, Zhou H, Luo X, Li S, Yu D, Hua J, Mu D, Mao M. Neuroprotection of brain-derived neurotrophic factor against hypoxic injury in vitro requires activation of extracellular signal-regulated kinase and phosphatidylinositol 3-kinase. Int J Dev Neurosci. 2008;26:363–70.

Sun M, Gu Y, Zhao Y, Xu C. Protective functions of taurine against experimental stroke through depressing mitochondria-mediated cell death in rats. Amino Acids. 2011;40:1419–29.

Sung JH, Kim MO, Koh PO. Nicotinamide prevents the down-regulation of MEK/ERK/p90RSK signaling cascade in brain ischemic injury. J Vet Med Sci. 2011;74:35–41.

Tanaka K. Alteration of second messengers during acute cerebral ischemia—adenylate cyclase, cyclic AMP-dependent protein kinase, and cyclic AMP response element binding protein. Prog Neurobiol. 2001;65:173–207.

Tanaka Y, Koizumi C, Marumo T, Omura T, Yoshida S. Serum S100B indicates brain edema formation and predicts long-term neurological outcomes in rat transient middle cerebral artery occlusion model. Brain Res. 2007;1137:140–5.

Tang X, Tang CL, Xu FM, Xie HW, Li LM, Song YE. Effect of scalp acupuncture combined with body acupuncture on limb function in subacute stroke patients. Zhen Ci Yan Jiu. 2012;37:488–92.

Valjent E, Pascoli V, Svenningsson P, Paul S, Enslen H, Corvol JC, Stipanovich A, Caboche J, Lombroso PJ, Nairn AC, et al. Regulation of a protein phosphatase cascade allows convergent dopamine and glutamate signals to activate ERK in the striatum. Proc Natl Acad Sci U S A. 2005;102:491–6.

Veena J, Rao BS, Srikumar BN. Regulation of adult neurogenesis in the hippocampus by stress, acetylcholine and dopamine. J Nat Sci Biol Med. 2011;2:26–37.

Wang SJ, Omori N, Li F, Jin G, Zhang WR, Hamakawa Y, Sato K, Nagano I, Shoji M, Abe K. Potentiation of Akt and suppression of caspase-9 activations by electroacupuncture after transient middle cerebral artery occlusion in rats. Neurosci Lett. 2002;331:115–8.

Wang H, Liao H, Ochani M, Justiniani M, Lin X, Yang L, Al-Abed Y, Metz C, Miller EJ, Tracey KJ, Ulloa L. Cholinergic agonists inhibit HMGB1 release and improve survival in experimental sepsis. Nat Med. 2004;10:1216–21.

Wang Q, Peng Y, Chen S, Gou X, Hu B, Du J, Lu Y, Xiong L. Pretreatment with electroacupuncture induces rapid tolerance to focal cerebral ischemia through regulation of endocannabinoid system. Stroke. 2009a;40:2157–64.

Wang T, Liu CZ, Yu JC, Jiang W, Han JX. Acupuncture protected cerebral multi-infarction rats from memory impairment by regulating the expression of apoptosis related genes Bcl-2 and Bax in hippocampus. Physiol Behav. 2009b;96:155–61.

Wang Q, Li X, Chen Y, Wang F, Yang Q, Chen S, Min Y, Xiong L. Activation of epsilon protein kinase C-mediated anti-apoptosis is involved in rapid tolerance induced by electroacupuncture pretreatment through cannabinoid receptor type 1. Stroke. 2011;42:389–96.

Wang Q, Wang F, Li X, Yang Q, Xu N, Huang Y, Zhang Q, Gou X, Chen S, Xiong L. Electroacupuncture pretreatment attenuates cerebral ischemic injury through alpha7 nicotinic acetylcholine receptor-mediated inhibition of high-mobility group box 1 release in rats. J Neuroinflammation. 2012a;9:24.

Wang Y, Shen J, Wang XM, Fu DL, Chen CY, Lu LY, Lu L, Xie CL, Fang JQ, Zheng GQ. Scalp acupuncture for acute ischemic stroke: a meta-analysis of randomized controlled trials. Evid Based Complement Alternat Med. 2012b;2012:480950.

Wang ZK, Ni GX, Liu K, Xiao ZX, Yang BW, Wang J, Wang S. Research on the changes of IL-1 receptor and TNF-alpha receptor in rats with cerebral ischemia reperfusion and the chronergy of acupuncture intervention. Zhongguo Zhen Jiu. 2012c;32:1012–8.

Wang ZK, Zhang LC, Zhao SH, Zhang JW, Shang LH, Zhang YL, Lin CR, Guo JK. Effect of electroacupuncture on cerebral PKC isozyme expression levels in cerebral ischemia-reperfusion rats. Zhen Ci Yan Jiu. 2012d;37:312–7.

Wang F, Gao Z, Li X, Li Y, Zhong H, Xu N, Cao F, Wang Q, Xiong L. NDRG2 is involved in anti-apoptosis induced by electroacupuncture pretreatment after focal cerebral ischemia in rats. Neurol Res. 2013a;35:406–14.

Wang JP, Yang ZT, Liu C, He YH, Zhao SS. L-carnosine inhibits neuronal cell apoptosis through signal transducer and activator of transcription 3 signaling pathway after acute focal cerebral ischemia. Brain Res. 2013b;1507:125–33.

Wang BH, Lin CL, Li TM, Lin SD, Lin JG, Chou LW. Selection of acupoints for managing upper-extremity spasticity in chronic stroke patients. Clin Interv Aging. 2014;9:147–56.

Wei LC, Shi M, Chen LW, Cao R, Zhang P, Chan YS. Nestin-containing cells express glial fibrillary acidic protein in the proliferative regions of central nervous system of postnatal developing and adult mice. Brain Res Dev Brain Res. 2002;139:9–17.

Wu HM, Tang JL, Lin XP, Lau J, Leung PC, Woo J, Li YP. Acupuncture for stroke rehabilitation. Cochrane Database Syst Rev. 2006;(3):CD004131.

Wu P, Mills E, Moher D, Seely D. Acupuncture in poststroke rehabilitation: a systematic review and meta-analysis of randomized trials. Stroke. 2010;41:e171–9.

Xiao A, Chen R, Kang M, Tan S. Heat-sensitive moxibustion attenuates the inflammation after focal cerebral ischemia/reperfusion injury. Neural Regen Res. 2012;7:2600–6.

Xiao Y, Wu X, Deng X, Huang L, Zhou Y, Yang X. Optimal electroacupuncture frequency for maintaining astrocyte structural integrity in cerebral ischemia. Neural Regen Res. 2013;8:1122–31.

Xie Z, Cui F, Zou Y, Bai L. Acupuncture enhances effective connectivity between cerebellum and primary sensorimotor cortex in patients with stable recovery stroke. Evid Based Complement Alternat Med. 2014;2014:603909.

Xu MS, Zhang SJ, Zhao D, Liu CY, Li CZ, Chen CY, Li LH, Li MZ, Xu J, Ge LB. Electroacupuncture-induced neuroprotection against cerebral ischemia in rats: role of the dopamine D2 receptor. Evid Based Complement Alternat Med. 2013;2013:137631.

Xu H, Zhang Y, Sun H, Chen S, Wang F. Effects of acupuncture at GV20 and ST36 on the expression of matrix metalloproteinase 2, aquaporin 4, and aquaporin 9 in rats subjected to cerebral ischemia/reperfusion injury. PLoS One. 2014;9:e97488.

Xue X, You Y, Tao J, Ye X, Huang J, Yang S, Lin Z, Hong Z, Peng J, Chen L. Electro-acupuncture at points of Zusanli and Quchi exerts anti-apoptotic effect through the modulation of PI3K/Akt signaling pathway. Neurosci Lett. 2014;558:14–9.

Yamamoto S, Subedi GP, Hanashima S, Satoh T, Otaka M, Wakui H, Sawada K, Yokota S, Yamaguchi Y, Kubota H, Itoh H. ATPase activity and ATP-dependent conformational change in the co-chaperone HSP70/HSP90-organizing protein (HOP). J Biol Chem. 2014;289:9880–6.

Yang ZJ, Shen DH, Guo X, Sun FY. Electroacupuncture enhances striatal neurogenesis in adult rat brains after a transient cerebral middle artery occlusion. Acupunct Electrother Res. 2005;30:185–99.

Yang S, Ye H, Huang J, Tao J, Jiang C, Lin Z, Zheng G, Chen L. The synergistic effect of acupuncture and computer-based cognitive training on post-stroke cognitive dysfunction: a study protocol for a randomized controlled trial of 2 × 2 factorial design. BMC Complement Altern Med. 2014;14:290.

Yip WK, Leong VC, Abdullah MA, Yusoff S, Seow HF. Overexpression of phospho-Akt correlates with phosphorylation of EGF receptor, FKHR and BAD in nasopharyngeal carcinoma. Oncol Rep. 2008;19:319–28.

Yoon SO, Casaccia-Bonnefil P, Carter B, Chao MV. Competitive signaling between TrkA and p75 nerve growth factor receptors determines cell survival. J Neurosci. 1998;18:3273–81.

Yu L, Miao H, Hou Y, Zhang B, Guo L. Neuroprotective effect of A20 on TNF-induced postischemic apoptosis. Neurochem Res. 2006;31:21–32.

Zhang HX, Wang Q, Zhou L, Liu LG, Yang X, Yang M, Liu YN, Li X. Effects of scalp acupuncture on acute cerebral ischemia-reperfusion injury in rats. Zhong Xi Yi Jie He Xue Bao. 2009;7:769–74.

Zhang JH, Wang D, Liu M. Overview of systematic reviews and meta-analyses of acupuncture for stroke. Neuroepidemiology. 2014a;42:50–8.

Zhang X, Wu B, Nie K, Jia Y, Yu J. Effects of acupuncture on declined cerebral blood flow, impaired mitochondrial respiratory function and oxidative stress in multi-infarct dementia rats. Neurochem Int. 2014b;65:23–9.

Zhao JX, Tian YX, Xiao HL, Hu MX, Chen WR. Effects of electroacupuncture on hippocampal and cortical apoptosis in a mouse model of cerebral ischemia-reperfusion injury. J Tradit Chin Med. 2011;31:349–55.

Zhao J, Xu H, Tian Y, Hu M, Xiao H. Effect of electroacupuncture on brain-derived neurotrophic factor mRNA expression in mouse hippocampus following cerebral ischemia-reperfusion injury. J Tradit Chin Med. 2013;33:253–7.

Zhao YL, Li WC, Huang J, Fu ZL, Tan LQ, Tang ZA, He JF. Effects of jingjin acupuncture on fine activity of hemiplegic hand in recovery period of stroke. Zhongguo Zhen Jiu. 2014;34:120–4.

Zhou L, Zhang HX, Liu LG, Huang H, Li X, Yang M. Effect of scalp-acupuncture on plasma and cerebral TNF-alpha and IL-1beta contents in acute cerebral ischemia/reperfusion injury rats. Zhen Ci Yan Jiu. 2008;33:173–8.

Zhou HP, Wang MS, Shi F, Ma SL, Li HO, Bi YL, Liu YQ, Liu H. Effects of acupuncture preconditioning on apoptosis in hippocampal neurons following ischemia-reperfusion injury in aged rats. Zhonghua Yi Xue Za Zhi. 2011;91:1203–6.

Zhou H, Zhang Z, Wei H, Wang F, Guo F, Gao Z, Marsicano G, Wang Q, Xiong L. Activation of STAT3 is involved in neuroprotection by electroacupuncture pretreatment via cannabinoid CB1 receptors in rats. Brain Res. 2013;1529:154–64.

Zhou ZH, Zhuang LX, Chen ZH, Lang JY, Li YH, Jiang GH, Xu ZQ, Liao MX. Post-stroke shoulder-hand syndrome treated with floating-needle therapy combined with rehabilitation training: a randomized controlled trial. Zhongguo Zhen Jiu. 2014;34:636–40.

Zhu Y, Prehn JH, Culmsee C, Krieglstein J. The beta2-adrenoceptor agonist clenbuterol modulates Bcl-2, Bcl-xl and Bax protein expression following transient forebrain ischemia. Neuroscience. 1999;90:1255–63.

Zhu X, Yin J, Li L, Ma L, Tan H, Deng J, Chen S, Zuo Z. Electroacupuncture preconditioning-induced neuroprotection may be mediated by glutamate transporter type 2. Neurochem Int. 2013a;63:302–8.

Zhu Y, Zhang L, Ouyang G, Meng D, Qian K, Ma J, Wang T. Acupuncture in subacute stroke: no benefits detected. Phys Ther. 2013b;93:1447–55.

Zhuang L, He J, Zhuang X, Lu L. Quality of reporting on randomized controlled trials of acupuncture for stroke rehabilitation. BMC Complement Altern Med. 2014;14:151.

Experimental Study of Electroacupuncture Therapy in Diabetes Mellitus

8

Shih-Liang Chang, Yu-Chen Lee, and Jaung-Geng Lin

Abstract

Aim and Background: Acupuncture and moxibustion was applied in the treatment of diabetes mellitus (DM), which was termed the *Xiao-Ke* syndrome in traditional Chinese medicine (TCM). Also, the metabolic syndrome (MS) is associated with an increased risk of cardiovascular disease and diabetes. Persistent hyperglycemia may exhaust beta cells, leading to their demise. Loss of beta cell mass and function are central to the development of both type I and II DM. Therefore, treating insulin resistance is important. Recently, the electric stimulation was combined with acupuncture named electroacupuncture (EA) in the treatment of diseases and there were serial experimental studies in DM from basic animal to clinical studies and recent investigations have explored the efficacy of EA for enhancing insulin sensitivity and suggested a hypoglycemic effect of EA for insulin resistance. This chapter will review and summarize the related studies. Materials and Methods: Firstly, the use of acupuncture in DM is introduced in ancient traditional Chinese medicine, and the using acupoints for treating DM in animal studies is summa-

S.-L. Chang
Department of Medicinal Botanicals and Health Applications, College of Biotechnology and Bioresources, Da-Yeh University, Changhua, Taiwan

School of Chinese Medicine, College of Chinese Medicine, China Medical University, Taichung, Taiwan

Y.-C. Lee
Graduate Institute of Acupuncture Science, College of Chinese Medicine, China Medical University, Taichung, Taiwan

Department of Acupuncture, China Medical University Hospital, Taichung, Taiwan

J.-G. Lin (✉)
School of Chinese Medicine, College of Chinese Medicine, China Medical University, Taichung, Taiwan
e-mail: jglin@mail.cmu.edu.tw

© Springer Nature Singapore Pte Ltd. 2018
J.-G. Lin (ed.), *Experimental Acupuncturology*,
https://doi.org/10.1007/978-981-13-0971-7_8

rized from modern basic experimental studies. Secondary, the classification of DM and experimental animal models in EA studies is illustrated and listed into type I & type II DM, then to illustrate DM animal models apply in the study of plasma glucose regulation. Finally, the passible mechanisms of EA in the regulation of plasma glucose then is hypothesized also use the hypoglycemic effect to explore the interaction between EA and Drugs. Results: A serial animal studies had been studied in the EA regulating the plasma glucose in diabetic animal models or animal in insulin resistance state. Hypoglycemic activity of EA on the Zhongwan (CV12) and Zusanli acupoints (ST36) was obtained under anesthesia by the serial studies. EA stimulating cholinergic nerve via adrenal grand secreting EOPs for encourage insulin secretion from pancreas. Then, activating insulin signaling pathway or non-insulin dependent by opioid receptor activation for lowering plasma glucose. Also, serotonin, NO and FFA might involve in the EA stimulation for improving hypoglycemic effect or insulin sensitivity and depended on different acupoints or different frequencies induced different pathway of mechanism. Furthermore, there was certain interaction between EA and drugs (oral hypoglycemic agent, steroids, volatile anesthetics…etc.).

Conclusion: Although there were serial of animal studies and small samples size randomized control clinical trial (RCT) in human of combined therapy, large sample size and multiple centers of RCTs should be further studied for the lowering plasma glucose or improving insulin sensitivity effect of EA stimulating on DM patients.

Keywords

Diabetes mellitus (DM) · Metabolic syndrome (MS) · Electroacupuncture (EA) · Experimental animal models · Mechanisms of hypoglycemic effect · Interaction between EA and drugs

8.1   The Use of Acupuncture in Diabetes Mellitus

In ancient China, acupuncture was used in the treatment of DM, which was termed the *Xiao-Ke* syndrome, characterized by the presence of polyuria (abnormally large production or passage of urine), polydipsia (abnormally great thirst) and polyphagia (excessive eating or appetite). In the Jin dynasty (265–420 AD), the "A-B classic of Acupuncture and Moxibustion" publication recorded acupoint locations used in the treatment of DM. In the Tang dynasty (618–907 AD), the acupoints were increased from 6 to 35, as recorded in the classic book, The Immortal Sun's Precious Formulary. Before the Ming and Chin dynasty of China, By the time of the Ming dynasty (1368–1744 AD), the meridian theory was well developed, encompassing 12 clinical channels and 2 other channels (Ren and Du) defining 361 acupoints. In historical clinical experience, the Lung, Spleen and Kidney channels, as well as some important acupoints such as Zhongwan (CV14), Zusanli (ST36) and … etc., all of which were involved in treatment of the *Xiao-Ke* syndrome (DM). The stimulation of the acupoints depended upon the instruction of Traditional Chinese Medicine (TCM) theory.

Since the end of the Chinese dynasties in 1912, many technologies (e.g., electrical, laser) have been combined with acupuncture treatment. Electroacupuncture (EA) has recently received much research attention for its ability to enhance the activity of acupuncture (Lin and Chen 2011). Investigations into pain relief have demonstrated that different frequencies, i.e., high (100 Hz), middle (15 Hz) and low (2 Hz), have different effects on the opioid receptors (Han 2004). Opioid receptors have been found in pancreas cells and are closely related to the secretion of insulin. EA stimulation at the Zhongwan acupoint (CV12) lowers plasma glucose level in normal wistar rats and rat models with type 2 diabetes mellitus (NIDDM) (Chang et al. 1999). Investigations into the role of the adrenal gland in this hypoglycemic response to EA at middle frequency (15 Hz) in adrenalectomized normal rats (ADX) demonstrate that multiple sources of endogenous opioid peptides (EOPs) participate in the lowering of plasma glucose (Lin et al. 2004).

The MS is associated with an increased risk of DM and cardiovascular disease. In the USA, an estimated 34% of the adult population have MS; the prevalence increases with age (Saad et al. 2014). The exact mechanisms of the complex pathways of MS are yet to be determined. Most patients are older, obese, sedentary, and have a degree of insulin resistance. Insulin resistance plays a key role in the pathophysiology of MS. In insulin-resistant states, pancreatic islets usually increase insulin secretion to maintain normoglycemia, via expansion of the beta cell mass and enhanced beta cell function. Persistent hyperglycemia may exhaust beta cells, leading to their demise. Loss of beta cell mass and function are central reason to the development of both type 1 and II DM (Cerf 2013). Therefore, treating insulin resistance is important. Recent investigations have explored the efficacy of EA for enhancing insulin sensitivity and suggest a hypoglycemic effect of EA for insulin resistance (Yin et al. 2014).

8.2   Using Acupoints for Treating DM in Animal Studies

According to the meridian theory, certain acupoints can be used to treat DM. Traditional Chinese medicine (TCM) divides Xiao-Ke syndrome (DM) into three types: upper, middle and lower. Each type reflects the predominance of one of the three main symptoms (polydipsia, polyphagia and polyuria) and is intimately related to the viscera state of TCM, lung, spleen and kidneys, respectively. A clinical analysis of a patient's overall symptoms should reveal which viscera state (i.e., lung, spleen, or kidneys) is predominantly involved and the focus of acupuncture treatment is on which acupoints are associated with the principal clinical manifestations (Covington 2001). In contrast, modern medicine theory analyses signs such as nerves and hormones to select the appropriate acupoints. When both aspects are considered, the prescription of acupoints should fit both TCM and modern medicine theory.

The Zhongwan acupoint (CV12) is located vertically on the conception vessel meridian along the median of the abdomen and horizontally 9 units above the upper

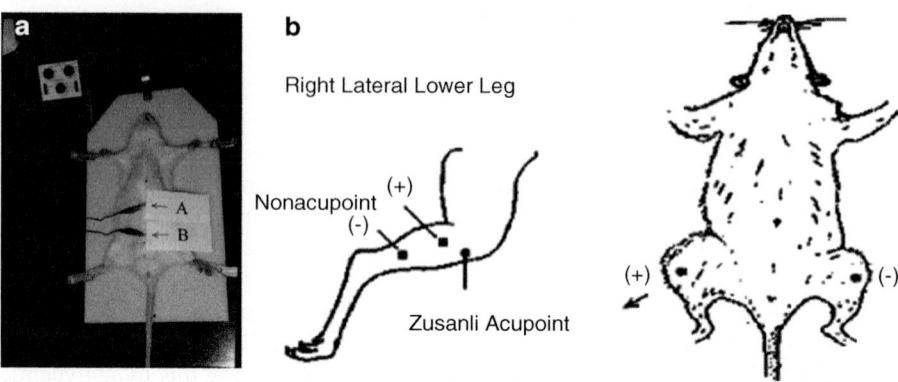

Fig. 8.1 (**a**) EA on the *A*: Zhongwan (CV12) and *B*: Guanyuan (CV4) acupoints of the rat (Chang et al. 1999); (**b**) Locations of acupoints and sham acupoints in the animal: (+) shows the positive charge connecting to the EA instrument; (−) indicates the negative charge connected to the EA instrument (Chang et al. 2005) (Reprint with permission from Diabetologia)

crest of the pubis bond. It is near the gastric organs, the pancreas in particular, and thus can be considered as stimulating insulin secretion. Moreover, the Zhongwan acupoints is located near the stomach Mu point, which has a marked regulating effect on stomach function. The Guanyuan (CV4) acupoint is located 2 units above the CV2 (the upper crest of the pubis bond) (Fig. 8.1a), also CV4 is the Small Intestine Mu point that has the regulating effect of small intestine on the absorption of nutrition including glucose (Chang et al. 1999). The Zusanli acupoint (ST36) is located on the anterior tibia muscle, approximately upper 1/6 to the length of lower leg below the knee, and belongs to the stomach meridian, which regulates gastric function (Chang et al. 2005). It is used to tonify deficient Qi or Blood. In TCM, treatment of all abdominal complaints involve the Zusanli acupoint (ST36) (Fig. 8.2). These three acupoints are usually selected in experimental studies exploring the mechanisms and searching for evidence. Besides these three acupoints, others may be selected as according to both TCM and modern medicine theory (Covington 2001) (see Table 8.1).

8.3 The Classification of Diabetes Mellitus and Experimental Animal Models in EA Studies

8.3.1 Classification of Diabetes Mellitus

DM is defined as a metabolic disease characterized by hyperglycemia resulting from defects in insulin secretion, insulin action, or both (Alberti and Zimmet 1998). Chronic hyperglycemia of DM is associated with long-term damage, dysfunction, and failure of various organs, especially the kidneys, eyes, nerves, heart and blood

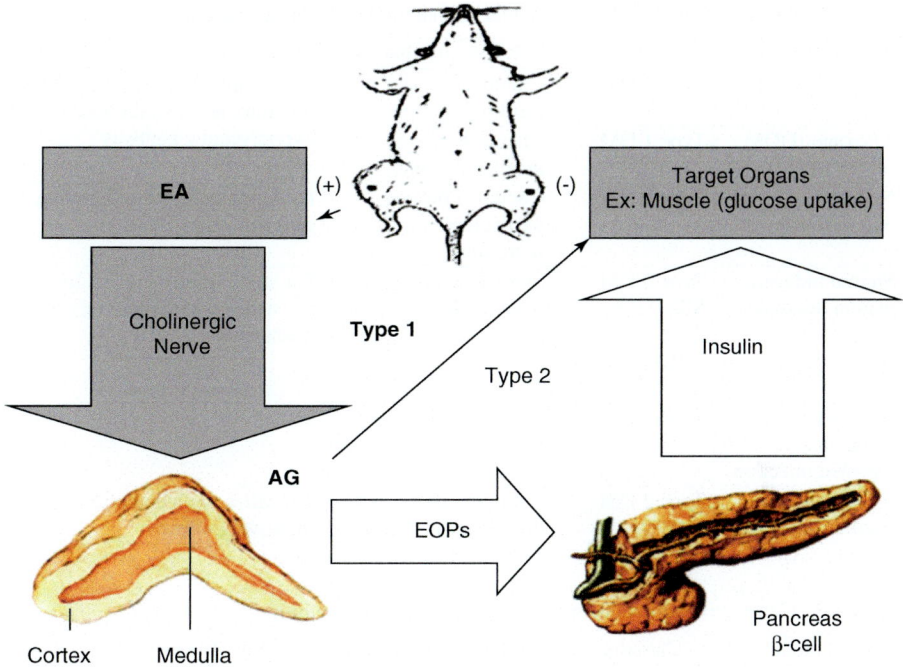

Fig. 8.2 Hypoglycemic effect of EA in different types of DM. The gray block and arrow indicate the main pathway of insulin-dependent DM (Type 1); the open arrows summarize the pathway suggested from previous study in non-insulin-dependent DM (type 2); the solid thin arrow indicates the direction of stimulation. Type 1: insulin-dependent DM; Type 2: non-insulin-dependent DM; AG: adrenal gland; EOPs: endogenous opioid peptides; (+) (−): bilateral zusanli acupoints (ST-36) connected to the positive and negative pole of the EA apparatus (Lee et al. 2011b) (Reprint with permission from Evid Based Complement Alternat Med)

Table 8.1 Acupoints used to treat DM in rat studies

Acupoints	Location	Meridian	Function
Zhongwan (CV12)	1 unit in acupuncture is defined as 1/14 of the distance between the top of xiphoid process and the upper crest of pubis bond. The CV12 acupoint is oriented vertically on the CV median of the abdomen and horizontally 9 units above the upper crest of the pubis bond (Chang et al. 1999)	Conception vessel	Meeting points Front mu points (stomach)
Guanyuan (CV4)	Located at 2 units above the upper crest of pubis bond (Chang et al. 1999)	Conception vessel	Front mu points (small intestine)
Zusanli (ST36)	The ST36 acupoint is located approximately upper 1/6 to the length of the lower leg on the anterior tibia muscle below the knee (Chang et al. 2005)	Stomach	Tonify deficient Qi or blood

Table 8.2 Chemically induced experimental animal models of diabetes mellitus

Animal models	Classification	Induction mechanism	Possible use
STZ-IDDM rat	Type 1 DM	Chemical broken insulin secretion	Simple model of hyperglycemic for study non-insulin dependent hypoglycemic pathway
Alloxane-IDDM	Type 1 DM	Chemical broken insulin secretion	
Neonatal STZ-NIDDM rat	Type 2 DM	Chemical broken partial insulin secretion	For study the insulin secreting function
Steroid induced insulin resistance	Type 2 DM SBR-large dose SIIR-clinical dose	Steroid elevated plasma FFA	For study improving insulin resistance and explore relative mechanisms
Human long-acting insulin repeated injection	Type 2 DM	Induce insulin antibody	To realized insulin-related action
Fructose-induced insulin resistance	Type 2 DM	Inhibition of pyruvate dehydrogenase kinase	To realize the metabolic improving effect

Table 8.3 Genetic experimental animal models of diabetes mellitus

Animal models	Classification	Induction mechanism	Possible use
BB-rat	Type 1 DM	Genetic and spontaneous model autoimmune induce insulitis	Understanding mechanisms of type 1 DM
Fat Sand-rat *Psammomys obesus*	Type 2 DM	High fat diet induced insulin resistance Genetic and spontaneous model	For study improving insulin resistance and explore relative mechanisms
Zucker Diabetic Fatty rat (ZDF)	Type 2 DM	Genetic model is resistant to insulin without being hyperglycemic	For research on obesity and hypertension with insulin resistance.
Otsuka Long-Evans Tokushima Fatty rat (OLETF)	Type 2 DM	Hereditary disorder	As a model resemble those of human NIDDM with hereditary disorder
Goto-Kakizaki rats (GK)	Type 2 DM	Genetic spontaneous type 2 DM Non-obese type 2 diabetic animal model	To inspect various pathologic mechanisms of T2DM

vessels. The pathogenesis of DM usually classifies the disease into two classes, Type 1 diabetes: associated with beta cell destruction, usually leading to absolute insulin deficiency, and Type 2 diabetes: this is associated with predominantly impair insulin sensitivity with relative insulin deficiency, or predominantly an defect of insulin secretory with insulin resistance. Commonly used experimental models in DM relating to acupuncture research are listed in Tables 8.2 and 8.3.

8.3.2   Type 1 Diabetes Animal Model in Acupuncture Research

In the type 1 DM model, streptozotocin or alloxane destroy beta cells. Large doses of chemical agents with free radicals induce severe broken DNA for secreting insulin that will form type 1 DM model (Oberley 1988). When used in low doses, or combined with a reducing agent such as nicotinamide, these agents induce less broken DNA for secreting insulin and thereby form the type 2 DM model (Szkudelski 2012). The chemically-induced models of type 1 DM are usually more commonly used in the experimental lab, as they offer advantages of cost and time savings as compared with the genetic animal model. The main characteristic of type 1 DM is the autoimmune destruction of the pancreatic beta cells, leading to lack of insulin production, as observed in genetically-engineered strains of rodents that spontaneously develop autoimmune diabetes, such as the diabetes-prone BB rat (Chang et al. 1999; Koevary et al. 1983).

Animal models of Type I DM lacking insulin are commonly used to study acupuncture or EA treatment involving the non-insulin dependent hypoglycemic pathway, or to study the hypoglycemic effect of injected insulin. For example, use of 15 Hz EA at the bilateral ST36 acupoints enhance the hypoglycemic effect of injected insulin in streptozocin (STZ)-induced diabetic rats (Chang et al. 2006). Animals in the EA experimental group were anesthetized and subjected to the insulin challenge test (ICT) and EA for 60 min. The control group was subjected to the ICT treatment, without EA stimulation. EA augmented the blood glucose-lowering effects of EA by activating the cholinergic nerves in rats that had been exposed to injected insulin i.p. This phenomenon may be related to the enhancement of insulin signaling transduction (Lee et al. 2011b).

The major hypoglycemic effect of EA focuses on the non-insulin dependent DM (type 2 DM). For example, a decrease in plasma glucose was observed in both normal rats and type 2 DM (NIDDM) rats after EA (15 Hz, 10 mA) for 30 min at the Zhongwan acupoint (CV12). In contrast, no significant effect on plasma glucose was observed in Type 1 (insulin-dependent) DM models (i.e., STZ-diabetic rats and genetic BB/W rats) (Chang et al. 1999). Application of EA to different acupoints STZ rats with type 1 DM has demonstrated a stronger hypoglycemic effect of the Zusanli acupoint (ST36) compared with that of the Zhongwan acupoint (Lin et al. 2014). Further studies provide further support (Lee et al. 2011a, b). In another study, 2 Hz EA was applied to bilateral ST36 acupoints in the experimental group for 30 min, and to a non-acupoint area in the control group for 30 min, to compare the specific characters of these acupoints with non-acupoint in the hypoglycemic effect of EA (Chang et al. 2005). And this investigation into the insulin-dependent mechanism of the hypoglycemic effect in STZ diabetic rats suggested that serotonin is involved in the hypoglycemic action of 2 Hz EA at bilateral ST36 acupoints in normal rats. This phenomenon was not found with EA at the CV12 acupoint, which contributes to the hypoglycemic effect by stimulating the adrenal gland to release EOPs (Lin et al. 2002, 2004).

8.3.3   Type 2 Diabetes Animal Models in Acupuncture Research

Type 2 DM accounts for ~90–95% of diabetes cases and involves individuals who have insulin resistance as well as relative (rather than absolute) insulin deficiency (at least initially). In the clinical experience, the treatment of EA may prevent developing type 2 diabetes. Acupuncture or EA is used for lowering plasma glucose to stimulate insulin secretion via opioid receptor activation (Chang et al. 1999). Moreover, EA therapy can enhance insulin sensitivity, which is appropriate in the treatment of type 2 DM (Chang et al. 2006). Nitric oxide, serotonin and cholinergic nerve involvement, lowering free fatty acid effect that may elevating insulin sensitivity (Lin et al. 2011). In the study that investigated this hypothesis, the intravenous glucose tolerance test (IVGTT) and ICT examined the influence of EA on insulin sensitivity in rats. 15 Hz EA at bilateral ST36 acupoints improved glucose tolerance. Thus, EA should be considered as an alternative method of pharmacological therapy for improving insulin resistance and/or increasing insulin-hypoglycemic activity in rats.

However, the type 2 DM model with the characters, relative insulin deficiency and/or insulin resistance are applied to study the treatments including acupuncture or EA that can improve insulin sensitivity and/or enhance insulin secretion for lowering the plasma glucose. For example, a neonatal STZ-induced non-insulin dependent diabetic rat (NIDDM-rat) is an insulin deficiency model. The Zhongwan acupoint (CV12) EA was applied to this NIDDM-rat model and conclude that EA stimulation at the CV12 acupoint induces secretion of endogenous beta-endorphin which reduces plasma glucose concentration in an insulin-dependent manner (Chang et al. 1999). In this case, the hypoglycemic activity of EA stimulation disappeared in rats with insulin-resistance induced by an injection of human long-acting insulin repeated daily to cause the loss of tolbutamide-induced hypoglycemia. This insulin resistance model will help to realized insulin-related action. Also, a high fat diet induced induce insulin resistance Psammomys obesus report from the middle east, the diabetic Psammomys randomly into three groups: abdominal EA (real), back EA (placebo) and control (anaesthesia). Comparison of the decline in plasma glucose, throughout the 3 weeks, between the real and placebo groups by ANOVA statistic analysis was highly significant. Animal weight gain, fructosamine, serum insulin, triglycerides and cholesterol were not significantly different between real and placebo groups. The study concluded that the CV12 acupoint EA induces a sustained hypoglycaemic effect in diabetic Psammomys compared with EA at non-specific points, without weight loss (Shapira et al. 2000).

There are still some chemical induced insulin resistance models like fructose induced insulin resistance model, steroid induced insulin resistance model even the gas anesthesia agent that will simulate different clinical situations and research the methods of clinical treatment. For example, a previous study reported the use of a large dose of steroid prednisolone to evaluate the effects of EA in a state of insulin resistance. The plasma levels of free fatty acids (FFAs) were estimated in steroid-background rats (SBRs) and compared with those in healthy rats treated with normal saline. In addition, plasma glucose levels and plasma insulin levels were assayed to calculate the homeostasis model assessment index (HOMA). The IVGTT was carried out to compare glucose tolerance. The normal Wistar was injected a single intraperitoneal of large-dose prednisolone (40 mg/kg) forming the SBRs were randomly divided into EA-treatment and non-EA treatment groups and 15-Hz EA was applied to the bilateral Zusanli acupoints (ST36) to investigate its effects on insulin resistance. In addition to an ICT and IVGTT, the plasma levels of FFAs were measured and western blot was performed to help determine the effects of EA on the insulin resistant state. This study concluded that the insulin resistance was successfully induced by a large dose of prednisolone in male rats. This insulin resistance can be improved by 15 Hz EA at the bilateral ST36 acupoints, as shown by decreased plasma levels of FFAs and the elevated signal proteins, insulin receptor substrate 1 (IRS-1) and GLUT-4 also recovered by this EA (Lin et al. 2009).

Besides, a similar to clinical dose of dexamethasone 1 mg/kg/day for 5 days, steroid induced insulin resistance was applied to explore the effect of EA on this common hyperglycemic situation by steroid induction. The SIIR rats were randomly divided into the SIIR+EA group, which received 15 Hz EA at ST36 for 60 min, and the SIIR group, which remained untreated. Plasma glucose and free fatty acid (FFA) levels were measured in serial blood samples taken without further manipulation and during ICT and IVGTT. IRS-1 and GLUT-4 were measured using Western blotting and expressed relative to β-actin. This study concluded that EA decreased the plasma FFA level and increased insulin sensitivity in SIIR rats and relative expression of IRS-1 and GLUT-4 were significantly increased by EA (Tzeng et al. 2016).

8.4 DM Animal Models Apply in the Study of Plasma Glucose Regulation

8.4.1 Chemically Induced Diabetic Animal Models

High-Dose Chemicals induce Type 1 DM: STZ [2-deoxy-2-(3-(methyl-3-nitrosoureido)-d-glucopyranose] is synthesized by *Streptomycetes achromogenes*. After administration by i.p. or i.v., it enters the pancreatic beta cell through the GLUT-2 transporter and causes alkylation of the DNA. For induction of STZ-induced experimental diabetes in male adult rats weighted 250–300 g (75–90 days), 60 mg/kg of STZ i.v. was injected after a fasting period. Three days after degeneration of beta cells, DM was induced in all animals. The diabetic and normal animals were kept in the metabolic cages separately and their body weight, consumption of water and food, urine volume, the levels of plasma glucose, plasma insulin and plasma C-peptide quantities in all animals were measured and then these quantities were compared. The weight loss, polyphagia, drink a lot of water and polyuria will be observed after STZ induction (Dufrane et al. 2006). Besides, the diabetic effect of alloxane (2,4,5,6-tetraoxypyrimidine; 5,6-dioxyuracil) is mainly attributed to the formation of free radicals and rapid uptake by the beta cells, which will break the insulin secretion to form type 1 DM animal model. Because the insulin secretion function is totally blocked by the high-dose chemical, this model can be used to explore the treatment with non-insulin dependent hypoglycemic effect (Lenzen 2008).

Neonatal Low Dose induce Type 2 DM: STZ injected in rats during the neonatal period has usually led to the major features (polydipsia, polyphagia, polyuria, hyperglycemia and abnormal glucose tolerance) in a short period. Male Wistar rats (5-day old) were injected with STZ (150 mg/kg, i.p.) that apart of a decrease in pancreatic insulin content, this experimental diabetic model may promote a remarkable and sustained picture of insulin resistance in adulthood that is strongly related to a loss in adipose mass. This experimental models of DM has been useful in understanding the complex pathogenesis of DM. Due to this model exist the partial insulin secretion function that can be used to explore the treatment with stimulating insulin secretion (Chang et al. 1999; Pai et al. 2009).

Steroid induced insulin resistance (SIIR) rat: Glucocorticoids, such as prednisolone, dexamethasone exerts their impact on metabolism through several different tissues in the body. In the presence of glucocorticoids there is an increase in adiposity as well as an increase in lipolysis, leading to elevated plasma FFA level in the circulation and an increase in insulin resistance. Post receptor insulin signaling defects such as a decrease in IRS-1 and GLUT-4 also contribute to insulin resistance, there is increased steatosis, causing insulin resistance in the liver, which is compounded by increased gluconeogenesis and hyperglycemia (Lin et al. 2009; Tzeng et al. 2016). In order to enhance the effect of insulin resistance in a short period, a large single dose of prednisolone 40 mg/kg i.p. after the rats had fasted for 12 h was applied to explore the hypoglycemic effect of EA. The study concluded that the insulin resistance can be improved by 15 Hz EA at the bilateral ST36 acupoints, as shown by decreased plasma FFA levels and elevating the decreased IRS-1 and GLUT-4 (Lin et al. 2009). A low dose of dexamethasone (1 mg/kg/day, i.p.) for 5 days was applied to simulate the clinical use. EA decreased the plasma FFA level and elevated the decreased insulin sensitivity and the decreased IRS-1 and GLUT-4 in this SIIR rats (Tzeng et al. 2016).

Human long-acting insulin repeated injection: this insulin resistance was induced by the repeated i.p. injections of long-acting human insulin (Monotard HM; 0.5 IU/kg) three times daily into adult male Wistar rats and was identified using the loss of tolbutamide-induced plasma glucose lowering action. The model with exogenous insulin resistance feature is facile to check the action like tolbutamide for lowering the plasma glucose and to realize insulin-relative action (Chang et al. 1999).

Fructose-induced insulin resistance: as we know consuming fructose-sweetened, not glucose-sweetened, beverages increases plasma lipids and visceral adiposity and decreases insulin sensitivity in overweight/obese humans. Therefore, Sprague-Dawley (SD) rats were fed a diet containing fructose 66% as a percentage of total calories for approximately 2 weeks. The hypertriglyceridemia and hyperinsulinemia were associated with hypertension in fructose-fed rats. This animal model is facile to realize the metabolic improving effect (Padiya et al. 2011).

8.4.2 Genetic and Spontaneous Models

BB (Biobreeding)-rat was derived from outbred Wistar rats, and usually develop DM just after puberty and have similar incidence in females and males. The Diabetes-Prone BB (BBDP) rat spontaneously develops autoimmune Type 1 DM between 50 and 90 days of age. Spontaneous autoimmune DM in a Canadian colony was first identified in 1974 and lead to the creation of two founder colonies from which all substrains have derived, one inbred (BBDP/Wor) and one outbred (BBdp). Diabetes-resistant BB rats (BBDR) have also been bred to act as controls. The BBDR rat has similar diabetes-susceptible genes as the BBDP, but does not become diabetic in viral antibody-free conditions. However, the BBDR rat can be induced to develope Type 1 DM in response to certain treatments such as regulatory T cell (T(reg)) depletion, virus infection or toll-like receptor ligation. These rat strains are invaluable models for studying autoimmune DM and the role of environmental factors in its development, of particular importance due to the influx of studies associating virus infection and human Type 1 DM (Bortell and Yang 2012; Chang et al. 1999).

Psammomys obesus **(fat sand rat)** is a model of nutritionally induced Type 2 diabetes mellitus (T2DM). Diabetes development and progression is very fast in *Psammomys obesus*. *Psammomys* is prone to developing hyperinsulinemia, hyperglycemia and obesity when transferred to a high-energy diet, also primary insulin resistance is a species characterization of *Psammomys*. They are four stages (1) normal glucose/normal insulin (2) hyperglycemia/normal insulin (3) hyperglycemia/hyperinsulinemia (4) hyperglycemia/hypoinsulinemia. The animal will reach the irreversible hypoinsulinemic end stage of the disease, in which a marked reduction of β-cell mass is apparent, within 4–6 weeks of high caloric diet. The present review describes the *Psammomys obesus* of the Hebrew University colony, with emphasis on its use for the study of β-cell dysfunction in T2DM (Shapira et al. 2000).

Zucker Diabetic Fatty rat (ZDF) a mutation occurred in a colony of outbred Zucker rats in the laboratory of Dr. Walter Shaw at Eli Lilly Research Laboratories in Indianapolis, inbreeding of selected pairs from this re-derivation was done in the laboratory of Dr. Richard Peterson at Indiana University Medical School (IUMS). An inbred line of ZDF rat was established in 1985. It's a Genetic Model and resistant to insulin without being hyperglycemic that is fed special diet (Purina #5008) to induce programmed and consistent development of Type 2 DM, which has emerged as a standard model of human type 2 DM. This model is applied for research on obesity and hypertension with insulin resistance that is helpful to study the influence of EA on a genetic defect developing into insulin resistance and in the gene encoding the leptin receptor, resulting in severe dysregulation of appetite and body weight (Peplow 2015b; Peplow and Han 2014).

Otsuka Long-Evans Tokushima Fatty rat (OLETF) The characteristic features of OLETF rats are: (1) late onset of hyperglycemia (age 18 weeks); (2) mild obesity; (3) clinical onset of DM mostly in males; (4) a chronic course of disease; (5) hereditary disorder; (6) the changes of pancreatic islets can be classified into three stages from the primary inflammation to islets failure; (7) diabetic nephropathy; These clinical and pathologic features of disease in OLETF rats are similar to those of human NIDDM. In OLETF rats, acupuncture treatment on the acupoint of abdominal and back significantly reduced plasma glucose levels, but not their body weight, suggesting that acupuncture therapy was effective in preventing the development of type 2 DM (Kim et al. 2007).

Goto-Kakizaki rat (GK) it is a spontaneous type 2 DM and has been considered as one of the best non-obese type 2 diabetic animal model. GK rats exhibit valuable characteristic tools that are more or less common and functionally present in human DM patients. This animal model is considered appropriate to inspect various pathologic mechanisms of T2DM. Recently, a study applied the GK rat to explore the impact of plasma glucose and insulin. A significant decrease in fasting plasma glucose levels and an increase in plasma insulin levels were observed during the fasting period in GK rats treated with abdominal EA (CV12 acupoint). Plasma glucose levels after glucose load were also significantly lower in GK rats treated with EA compared with controls (Ishizaki et al. 2009).

8.5   The Possible Mechanisms of EA in the Regulation of Plasma Glucose

8.5.1   Mechanisms of Hypoglycemic Effect

Since the 1999, an insulin dependent hypoglycemic effect was reported while using EA on the Zhongwan (CV12) and Guanyuan acupoints (CV4). This hypothesis is supported by an increase in plasma insulin after EA stimulation in normal wistar rats and type 2 diabetic rats. Participation of glucagon was ruled out because there was no change in plasma glucagon resulting from EA stimulation. In addition to an increase in plasma beta-endorphin, the plasma glucose lowering action of EA stimulation at CV12 and CV4 acupoints was abolished by naloxone in a sufficient dose to block opioid receptors. Thus this study suggested that EA stimulation at the CV12 and CV4 acupoint induces secretion of endogenous beta-endorphin which reduces plasma glucose concentration in an insulin-dependent manner.

A whole picture had been reported in 2011 entitled "Electroacupuncture at the Zusanli (ST-36) Acupoint Induces a Hypoglycemic Effect by Stimulating the Cholinergic Nerve in a Rat Model of Streptozotocine-Induced Insulin-Dependent DM" (Lee et al. 2011a). The cholinergic blocking agents and adrenalectomy method has been applied in exploring the mechanisms of hypoglycemic effect by EA stimulation on the acupoints of STZ induced type 1 DM. 15-Hz EA was applied for 30 min to bilateral ST-36 acupoints after administration of Atropine (0.1 mg/kg, i.p.), or Hemicholinium-3 (5 µg/kg, i.p.) in non-adrenalectomized rats. Atropine and hemicholinium-3 completely blocked the plasma glucose lowering effects of EA. Also, a cholinesterase inhibitor, eserine was applied in this study, whereas eserine led to a significant hypoglycemic effect. Therefore, EA at the ST-36 acupoint reduces plasma glucose concentrations by stimulating the cholinergic nerves. This

EA was also applied to STZ-ADX rats. Plasma glucose levels did not change significantly. In addition, there were no significant differences in mean hypoglycemic activity between STZ-ADX rats with EA and without EA stimulation. The adrenal glands may play an important role in the hypoglycemic effect of this EA. Taken together, this finding indicate that hypoglycemic effect of EA is not only mediated by the cholinergic nerves but also by the adrenal glands (Fig. 8.2).

Furthermore, different acupoints or frequencies were compared and with different hypoglycemic mechanisms. The different acupoints stimulation had been compared the hypoglycemic activity between CV12 and ST36 acupoints. The EA stimulation on bilateral ST36 acupoint with higher hypoglycemic effect than stimulating on CV12 and CV2 acupoint because of more complication neurotransmitters take part in. for example: serotonin involvement was obtained in the 2 Hz EA stimulation (Chang et al. 2005); Also, different frequencies (2 and 15 Hz) stimulation on the same acupoints, Zhongwan acupoint (CV12) had been compared that was obtained the beta-endorphin come from adrenal gland by 2 Hz EA stimulation for lowering the plasma glucose (Lin et al. 2002) and multiple sources of EOPs was encouraged by 15 Hz EA stimulation (Lin et al. 2004).

8.5.2 Mechanisms of Improving Insulin Sensitivity

Can EA Stimulation improve the insulin sensitivity, especially in the insulin resistant state? In 2000, a high-fat diet induced insulin resistant non-insulin-dependent DM model, *Psammomys obesus* was applied in the hypoglycemic effect of CV12 acupoints EA study and proposed a sustained, non-insulin related, hypoglycemic effect of EA that implied not only stimulating insulin secretion but also enhancing insulin sensitivity for lowering plasma glucose (Shapira et al. 2000).

Further, the ICT and IVGTT were used to explore the insulin sensitivity on the Zusanli acupoints (ST36) by 15 Hz EA. Enhanced insulin sensitivity using EA was reported in 2006. The rats were divided into the control group (CG) and experiment group (EG) randomly. After fasting, plasma glucose levels and plasma insulin levels were assayed in the normal Wistar rats undergoing IVGTT. Plasma glucose levels and hypoglycemic activity were also evaluated in the normal Wistar rats and STZ diabetic rats during ICT. As the data showed, EA improved the glucose tolerance from 15 to 90 min (p < 0.005 compared with the plasma glucose levels of the CG) during IVGTT. In addition, significant improvement in the Homeostasis Model Assessment (HOMA) index was found in the EG from 15 to 90 min (p < 0.005 compared with the CG). More hypoglycemic activity was achieved in normal Wistar and STZ diabetic rats in the EG than in the CG (from 30 to 60 min) during ICT (Chang et al. 2006).

After EA improving insulin sensitivity was proposed by the of experiment ICT and IVGTT and the experience from EA hypoglycemic effect study that the cholinergic nerve and NOS system may activate by 15 Hz EA on Zusanli acupoints (ST36) that can thus be hypothesized (Lin et al. 2014). A continuous study was further to realize the mechanism of EA in improving glucose tolerance (Fig. 8.3). The cholinergic (Atropine, HC-3) and nitric oxide blocking agent (L-NAME) were injected alone or simultaneously to explore the relationship with cholinergic nerve and/or NO. Plasma glucose levels differed significantly between the EA and non-EA control groups after the administration of atropine, HC-3 or L-NAME treatments alone, but there were no significant differences in plasma glucose with combined treatment of L-NAME and atropine or L-NAME and HC-3. This EA also decreased plasma FFA levels and enhanced insulin signal protein (IRS-1) and nNOS activities in skeletal muscle during IVGTT. Therefore, EA stimulated cholinergic nerves and nitric oxide synthase for lowering plasma FFA levels to improve glucose tolerance that can thus be summarized (Lin et al. 2011).

8.5.3   Mechanisms of Improve Insulin Resistance State

Is there any improving insulin sensitivity effect of EA under insulin resistant state? As we know the large single large dose or long-term clinical dose steroids treatment may induce insulin resistance by elevating internal plasma FFA levels that may impair insulin signal transduction. According to the previous experience in the study of improving insulin sensitivity of EA that may reduce the plasma FFA for improving the insulin sensitivity (Lin et al. 2011; Yin et al. 2014). Therefore, these studies implied EA with the potential to improve steroid induced insulin resistant (SIIR) state. In 2009, A report entitled "Acute effect of electroacupuncture at the Zusanli acupoints (ST36) on decreasing insulin resistance as shown by lowering plasma free fatty acid levels in steroid-background male rats" had been obtained the evidence of EA improving SIIR induced by a large single large dose of prednisolone (Lin et al. 2009). Further, in 2016, another report entitled "15 Hz electroacupuncture at ST36 improves insulin sensitivity and reduces free fatty acid levels in rats with chronic dexamethasone-induced insulin resistance" also had been obtain the evidence of EA improving SIIR induced by long-term clinical dose of dexamethasone treatment (Tzeng et al. 2016).

In these two studies, the insulin signaling proteins were also investigated. The large dose prednisolone suppressed the IRS-1 and GLUT-4 that recovered by 15 Hz EA on bilateral Zusanli acupoints (ST36). Also, these two signals were improved by this EA after long-term clinical dose of dexamethasone induced insulin resistance. Obesity and type 2 DM are associated with raised concentrations of insulin, saturated fatty acids (e.g., palmitate) and cytokines (e.g., tumor necrosis factor-α, TNF-α) both in the circulation and locally in the hypothalamus, which eventually lead to central insulin resistance. Palmitate activates the transcription factor NF-κB, which induces the expression of one of the main negative regulators of insulin signaling, suppressor of cytokine signaling 3. NF-κB induces endoplasmic reticulum stress that results in increased activity of c-jun N-terminal kinase (JNK), which in turn leads to inhibitory phosphorylation events on IRS proteins (Peplow 2015a). The EA also lowered plasma TNF-α in the obese ZDF rat, which exhibits insulin resistance and is a model of the MS (Peplow 2015b). That indicated EA with a close relationship to plasma FFA and cytokines for improving insulin resistance.

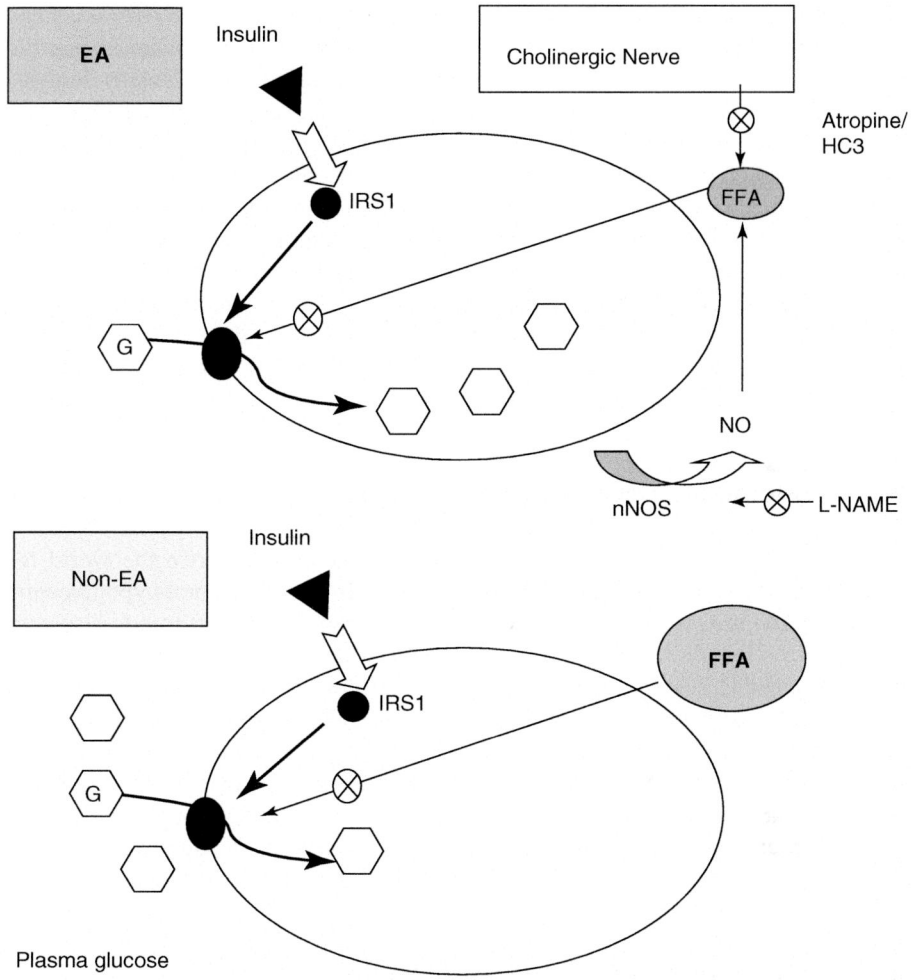

Fig. 8.3 The mechanism of EA significantly improved the glucose tolerance and/or insulin sensitivity. (1) The cholinergic antagonist or alone cannot block the improving effect. (2) Combined cholinergic antagonist with L-NAME blocks the improving effect. (3) EA decreased FFA and enhanced insulin signal protein (IRS-1) and nNOS activities. (4) EA stimulated cholinergic nerves and NOS to improve glucose tolerance *G* glucose, *IRS-1* insulin receptor substrate 1, *FFA* free fatty acid, l-*NAME* L-NG-Nitrosarginine methyl ester, *NO* nitric oxide, *nNOS* neuronal nitric oxide synthase (Lin et al. 2011) (Reprint with permission from Neurosci Lett)

8.5.4 Microarray Approached in the Hypoglycemic Effect of EA

Since the EA activating EOPs as the mechanism of analgesia was reported, the intracellular cellular activating pathways including gene expression may be thought as the passible activating target for controlling EOPs synthesis. But the intracellular network of signaling proteins even the gene expressions are too complicate to be approached until the DNA microarray technique had been proposed. The mass gene expressions can be screened at the same time that would be a tool for screen the change of EA for activating hypoglycemic effect. Recently, a microarray analysis was used to examine various signaling pathways that may contribute to the glucose-lowering effect of 15 Hz EA at ST36 bilaterally in streptozotocin-induced diabetic rats and to screen for relationships between gene sets and DM. It was found that cell adhesion molecules and type 1 DM pathways were significantly associated with the hypoglycemic effect (Tzeng et al. 2015). That indicated EA with a close relationship to immune response that may recover the inflammation and close relationship to hypoglycemic effect in STZ-induced diabetic rats. This is a pioneer approach the hypoglycemic activity of EA by DNA microarray, but a serial study should be further explored after this screening for ensure the control of intracellular network under EA stimulation.

8.5.5   Interaction Between EA and Drugs

In recent years, acupuncture therapy is more and more popular in the world for treating disease. The opportunity of using EA and drugs such as oral hypoglycemic agents (OHA) in DM patients at the same time is elevated by this trend. Also, steroids induced insulin resistance were recovered by EA stimulation in previous section mentioned (Lin et al. 2009; Tzeng et al. 2016) that is also a type of interaction between EA and drugs. Another example showed that electro stimulating on the acupoints by (TENS) improving *volatile anesthetics induced insulin resistance* that is also a type of interaction between EA and drugs, like as against the disadvantages of volatile anesthetics (Man et al. 2011). Can the EA therapy lower the dose of drugs? Is there any interaction such as: summation, synergism and against the disadvantages…etc.? That is an important issue worth for further investigations.

8.5.6   Interaction Between EA and Insulin

According to the theory of TCM, acupuncture has the effect of balance Yin-Yang and regulation in Chi and Blood. It is means that acupuncture can regulate the homeostasis even the bioability of drug via impact on the pharmacokinetic. In 2006, the EA and exogenous insulin were used on the normal Wistar rat and STZ-induced diabetic rat at the same time and compare with the control group without EA.

During the insulin background, more hypoglycemic activity in the 15 Hz bilateral ST36 acupoints EA group ($65 \pm 8\%$) was noted than in the non-EA control group ($30 \pm 15\%$) 30 min after the start of insulin injecting to the normal Wistar rats ($p < 0.05$). Sixty minutes after the start of insulin injection, the hypoglycemic activity of the EA group ($77 \pm 7\%$) still was significantly higher than that of the non-EA control group ($44 \pm 14\%$; $p < 0.001$ using Student's t-test). The STZ-induced diabetic rats showed the same trends as the normal Wistar rats, including that more hypoglycemic activity for the EA group ($32 \pm 17\%$) was noted than for the non-EA control group (15 ± 9%) 30 min after the start of insulin injection ($p < 0.05$). Sixty minutes after beginning insulin injection, the hypoglycemic activity of the EA group (55 ± 22%) was higher than that of the non-EA control group (25 ± 15%) ($p < 0.01$) (Chang et al. 2006). That would be thought as a summation or synergism effect while the EA and insulin were applied at the same time.

8.5.7   Interaction Between EA and Rosiglitazone

The OHA are usually used in the clinical management of plasma glucose of DM patient. A class of insulin sensitizer thiazolidinedione (TZD) by activating peroxisome proliferator-activated receptors (PPARs), a group of nuclear receptors, with greatest specificity for peroxisome proliferator-activated receptor γ (PPARγ), this type of OHA generally decrease triglycerides and increase high-density lipoprotein cholesterol (HDL-C) and low-density lipoprotein cholesterol (LDL-C) that is suit for MS and type 2 DM with high lipids induced insulin resistance. As the previous reports show that EA had multiple mechanisms including stimulating insulin secretion via EOPs. While combined both therapies TZD and EA may have a summation or synergism effect (Itoh et al. 1999).

In 2009, EA and Rosiglitazone were put together into normal Wistar and STZ-neonatal induced noninsulin dependent DM. A marked hypoglycemic activity was observed in the normal Wistar rat TZD, TZD + EA and EA groups, with the response more significant in the TZD + EA group than in the TZD group. Among the STZ-neonatal induced NIDDM rats, the hypoglycemic responses in the TZD + EA and EA groups were greater than in the TZD group. In both the normal and diabetic rats, plasma insulin levels was increased by EA or TZD + EA treatment, but not by TZD only (Pai et al. 2009).

Further in 2013, a randomized control clinical trial was report in the hypoglycemic effect of TZD + EA compared with that of TZD only for T2DM patients. A total of 31 newly diagnostic T2DM patients, who fulfilled the study's eligibility criteria, were recruited. The individuals were randomly assigned into two groups, the TZD group and the TZD + EA group. Changes in their plasma glucose, plasma FFA, and plasma insulin levels, together with their homeostasis model assessment (HOMA) indices, were statistically compared before and after treatment. Hypoglycemic activity (%) was also compared between these two groups. As the results showed that no significant difference was obtained in hypoglycemic activity between the TZD and TZD + EA group. The effectiveness of the combined therapy seems to derive from an improvement in insulin resistance and a significant lowering of the secreted plasma insulin rather than the effect of TZD alone on T2DM. The combined treatment had no significant adverse effects. A lower plasma FFA concentration is likely to be the mechanism that causes this effect (Lin et al. 2013).

Although no significant difference in hypoglycemic activity between the patients in the TZD + EA group and the patients in the TZD group was identified, a trend towards a lowering of plasma glucose levels was found for the patients in both groups. These results are different from previous animal studies, which showed that the plasma glucose lowering activity of TZD was increased by EA in both normal and T2DM rats (Pai et al. 2009). A number of conditions were different between the present study and the earlier animal studies, particularly in which the animal studies were carried out under general anesthesia, while the human subjects were fully conscious during the clinical trial. One possibility is that the plasma glucose lowering effect in patients from the TZD + EA group may have been masked by environmental factors, such as pain and stress during EA. Another possibility is that there may have been selection bias because a higher percentage of male patients were excluded because they were already being prescribed thiazolidinedione class drugs.

8.5.8   Interaction Between EA and Metformin

Metformin, marketed under the tradename Glucophage is the first-line medication for the treatment of T2DM. Metformin ameliorates hyperglycemia without promoting weight gain, stimulating insulin secretion, or causing hypoglycemia. In addition, metformin has beneficial effects on circulating lipids linked to increased cardiovascular risk. The molecular mechanism of metformin is inhibition of the mitochondrial respiratory chain (complex I), activation of AMP-activated protein kinase (AMPK). The AMPK is an enzyme that plays an important role in insulin signaling, metabolism of glucose and fats, and the whole body energy balance, was required for metformin's inhibitory effect on the production of glucose by liver cells for lowering plasma glucose (Zhou et al. 2001). The hypoglycemic mechanisms of EA including stimulating insulin secretion via EOP and intercellular insulin signaling pathway for lowering plasma glucose. Therefore, a hypothesis was proposed that EA combined metformin would have better hyperglycemic effect than treating metformin alone because of combined the hypoglycemic mechanism activating AMPK and activating insulin signaling protein for lowering the plasma glucose.

In 2015, a report entitled "Electroacupuncture plus metformin lowers glucose levels and facilitates insulin sensitivity by activating mitogen-activated protein kinase (M APK) in steroid-induced insulin-resistant rats" The whole picture of this study was summarized in the Fig. 8.4. This study showed that EA-metformin resulted in a better greater insulin sensitivity, glucose-lowering effect, lower plasma FFA levels and higher levels of MAPK than metformin alone ($p < 0.05$) and concluded that the glucose-lowering effect and increased insulin sensitivity associated with EA-metformin administration is governed, at least in part, by its ability to stimulate the activation of GLUT-4 via upregulation of MAPK expression.

8.5.9   Interaction Between EA and Sevoflurane

As we known that volatile anesthetics directly manipulate glucose homeostasis by affecting pancreatic insulin release and by inducing hyperglycemia (Desborough et al. 1998). Both sevoflurane and isoflurane anesthesia also impair glucose tolerance to the same degree are independent of agent and dosage up to 1.5 minimum

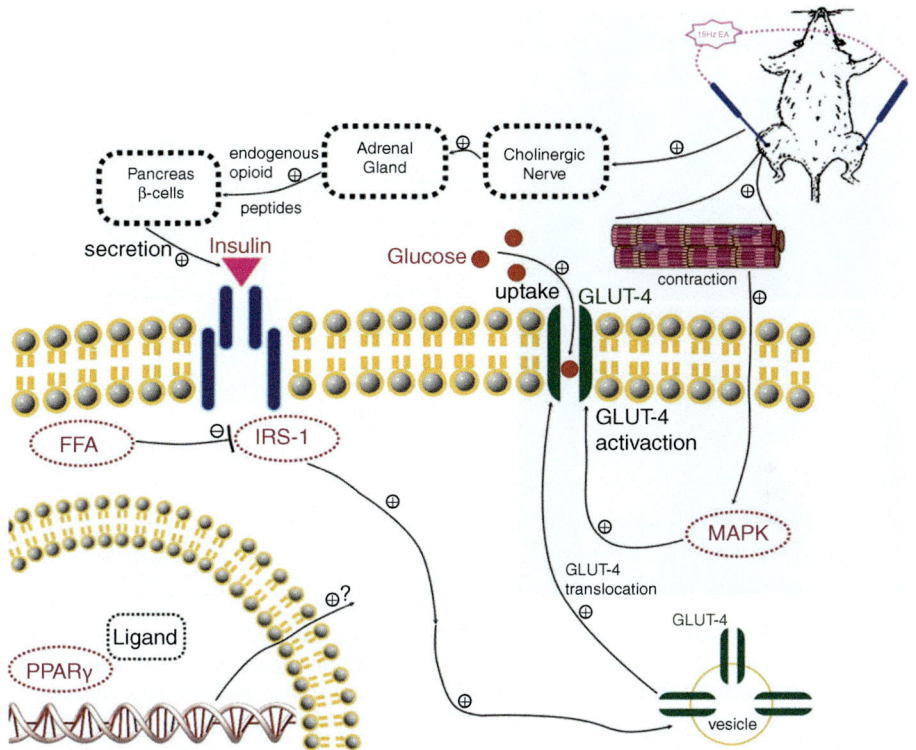

Fig. 8.4 Intracellular and extracellular insulin signaling factors in muscle cells. Diagram illustrating the intracellular GLUT-4 activation and translocation and extracellular (endocrine) mechanisms of insulin signaling. FFAs impair insulin sensitivity by decreasing the levels of IRS-1 and GLUT-4. Accumulation of IRS-1 facilitates GLUT-4 vesicle exocytosis GLUT-4 translocation to cell surface. In addition, PPAR-γ plays the role of a GLUT-4 promoter in primary adipocytes, making skeletal muscle cells more sensitive to insulin. Low-frequency EA causes muscle contraction and activates MAPK. Activation of MAPK leads to GLUT-4 expression. Key: plus signs indicate facilitation and minus signs indicate inhibition (Liao et al. 2015) (Reprint with permission from Acupunct Med)

alveolar concentration (Tanaka et al. 2005). In the animal studies, EA stimulation can encourage insulin secretion and improving glucose tolerance and/or insulin sensitivity (Chang et al. 1999, 2006). Therefore, there was certain interaction between EA and volatile anesthetics thus has been hypothesized that EA may against the disadvantages of volatile anesthetics in the impairment of glucose tolerance and insulin sensitivity.

In 2011, a small sample size RCT were reported entitled "Transcutaneous electrical nerve stimulation on ST36 and SP6 acupoints prevents hyperglycemic response during anesthesia: a randomized controlled trial" The protocol and acupoints are showed in Fig. 8.5. This study was designed a single-blind, randomized controlled clinical study of female patients, scheduled for elective hysterectomy. The 52 patients consented to enrolment and were assigned to receive either TENS

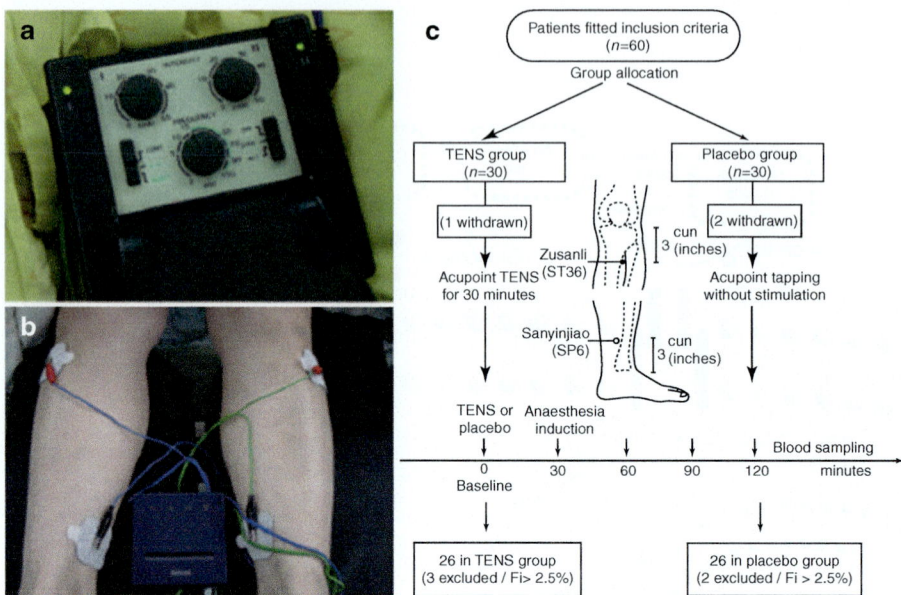

Fig. 8.5 Study of interaction between EA and Sevoflurane; (**a**) HANS electro stimulator; (**b**) TENS stimulation on the Zusanli (ST36) and Sanyinjiao (SP6) acupoints before Sevoflurane anesthesia (**c**) study protocol (Man et al. 2011) (Reprint with permission from Eur J Anaesthesiol)

(n = 26) on bilateral ST36 and SP6 acupoints with continuous mode at a frequency of 15 Hz and the intensity of 10 mA synchronously for 30 min or non-stimulation (placebo group, n = 26) preoperatively. Hemodynamics, plasma glucose and plasma insulin were measured during general anesthesia.

As the results of this study showed, the plasma glucose, plasma insulin and HOMA index increased during induction of general anesthesia, surgical incision, and throughout the operation in the placebo group. Plasma glucose and plasma insulin levels as well as HOMA index were significantly lower in the TENS group as compared to the placebo group at different time points after discontinuation of TENS application treating on bilateral ST36 and SP6 acupoint. These results indicate the positive effect of prevention of hyperglycemia and the increased sensitivity of plasma insulin in the TENS group that agreed the original hypothesis (Man et al. 2011).

Conclusions

A serial animal studies had been studied in the EA regulating the plasma glucose in diabetic animal models or animal in insulin resistance state (Lin et al. 2014). Hypoglycemic activity of EA on the Zhongwan (CV12) and Zusanli acupoints (ST36) was obtained under anesthesia by the serial studies. EA stimulating cholinergic nerve via adrenal grand secreting EOPs for encourage insulin secretion from pancreas. Then, activating insulin signaling pathway or non-insulin dependent by opioid receptor activation for lowering plasma glucose (Lee et al. 2011a).

Also, serotonin, NO and FFA might involve in the EA stimulation for improving hypoglycemic effect or insulin sensitivity and depended on different acupoints or different frequencies induced different pathway of mechanism (Lin et al. 2011). Furthermore, there was certain interaction between EA and drugs (OHA, steroids, volatile anesthetics…etc.).

Although there were serial of animal studies and small samples size randomized control clinical trial (RCT) in human of combined therapy, (Lin et al. 2013; Man et al. 2011) large sample size and multiple centers of RCTs should be further studied for the lowering plasma glucose or improving insulin sensitivity effect of EA stimulating on DM patients.

References

Alberti KG, Zimmet PZ. Definition, diagnosis and classification of diabetes mellitus and its complications. Part 1: diagnosis and classification of diabetes mellitus provisional report of a WHO consultation. Diabet Med. 1998;15:539–53.

Bortell R, Yang C. The BB rat as a model of human type 1 diabetes. Methods Mol Biol. 2012;933:31–44.

Cerf ME. Beta cell dysfunction and insulin resistance. Front Endocrinol. 2013;4:37.

Chang SL, Lin JG, Chi TC, Liu IM, Cheng JT. An insulin-dependent hypoglycaemia induced by electroacupuncture at the Zhongwan (CV12) acupoint in diabetic rats. Diabetologia. 1999;42:250–5.

Chang SL, Tsai CC, Lin JG, Hsieh CL, Lin RT, Cheng JT. Involvement of serotonin in the hypoglycemic response to 2 Hz electroacupuncture of zusanli acupoint (ST36) in rats. Neurosci Lett. 2005;379:69–73.

Chang SL, Lin KJ, Lin RT, Hung PH, Lin JG, Cheng JT. Enhanced insulin sensitivity using electroacupuncture on bilateral Zusanli acupoints (ST 36) in rats. Life Sci. 2006;79:967–71.

Covington MB. Traditional Chinese medicine in the treatment of diabetes. Diabetes Spectr. 2001;14:154–9.

Desborough JP, Knowles MG, Hall GM. Effects of isoflurane-nitrous oxide anaesthesia on insulin secretion in female patients. Br J Anaesth. 1998;80:250–2.

Dufrane D, van Steenberghe M, Guiot Y, Goebbels RM, Saliez A, Gianello P. Streptozotocin-induced diabetes in large animals (pigs/primates): role of GLUT2 transporter and beta-cell plasticity. Transplantation. 2006;81:36–45.

Han JS. Acupuncture and endorphins. Neurosci Lett. 2004;361:258–61.

Ishizaki N, Okushi N, Yano T, Yamamura Y. Improvement in glucose tolerance as a result of enhanced insulin sensitivity during electroacupuncture in spontaneously diabetic Goto-Kakizaki rats. Metabolism. 2009;58:1372–8.

Itoh H, Doi K, Tanaka T, Fukunaga Y, Hosoda K, Inoue G, Nishimura H, Yoshimasa Y, Yamori Y, Nakao K. Hypertension and insulin resistance: role of peroxisome proliferator-activated receptor gamma. Clin Exp Pharmacol Physiol. 1999;26:558–60.

Kim SK, Moon HJ, Park JH, Lee G, Shin MK, Hong MC, Bae H, Jin YH, Min BI. The maintenance of individual differences in the sensitivity of acute and neuropathic pain behaviors to electroacupuncture in rats. Brain Res Bull. 2007;74:357–60.

Koevary S, Rossini A, Stoller W, Chick W, Williams RM. Passive transfer of diabetes in the BB/W rat. Science. 1983;220:727–8.

Lee YC, Li TM, Tzeng CY, Chen YI, Ho WJ, Lin JG, Chang SL. Electroacupuncture at the Zusanli (ST-36) acupoint induces a hypoglycemic effect by stimulating the cholinergic nerve in a rat model of streptozotocine-induced insulin-dependent diabetes mellitus. Evid Based Complement Alternat Med. 2011a;2011:650263.

Lee YC, Li TM, Tzeng CY, Cheng YW, Chen YI, Ho WJ, Lin JG, Chang SL. Electroacupuncture-induced cholinergic nerve activation enhances the hypoglycemic effect of exogenous insulin in a rat model of streptozotocin-induced diabetes. Exp Diabetes Res. 2011b;2011:947138.

Lenzen S. The mechanisms of alloxan- and streptozotocin-induced diabetes. Diabetologia. 2008;51:216–26.

Liao HY, Sun MF, Lin JG, Chang SL, Lee YC. Electroacupuncture plus metformin lowers glucose levels and facilitates insulin sensitivity by activating MAPK in steroid-induced insulin-resistant rats. Acupunct Med. 2015;33:388–94.

Lin JG, Chen YH. The mechanistic studies of acupuncture and moxibustion in Taiwan. Chin J Integr Med. 2011;17:177–86.

Lin JG, Chang SL, Cheng JT. Release of beta-endorphin from adrenal gland to lower plasma glucose by the electroacupuncture at Zhongwan acupoint in rats. Neurosci Lett. 2002;326:17–20.

Lin JG, Chen WC, Hsieh CL, Tsai CC, Cheng YW, Cheng JT, Chang SL. Multiple sources of endogenous opioid peptide involved in the hypoglycemic response to 15 Hz electroacupuncture at the Zhongwan acupoint in rats. Neurosci Lett. 2004;366:39–42.

Lin RT, Tzeng CY, Lee YC, Ho WJ, Cheng JT, Lin JG, Chang SL. Acute effect of electroacupuncture at the Zusanli acupoints on decreasing insulin resistance as shown by lowering plasma free fatty acid levels in steroid-background male rats. BMC Complement Altern Med. 2009;9:26.

Lin RT, Chen CY, Tzeng CY, Lee YC, Cheng YW, Chen YI, Ho WJ, Cheng JT, Lin JG, Chang SL. Electroacupuncture improves glucose tolerance through cholinergic nerve and nitric oxide synthase effects in rats. Neurosci Lett. 2011;494:114–8.

Lin RT, Pai HC, Lee YC, Tzeng CY, Chang CH, Hung PH, Chen YI, Hsu TH, Tsai CC, Lin JG, Chang SL. Electroacupuncture and rosiglitazone combined therapy as a means of treating insulin resistance and type 2 diabetes mellitus: a randomized controlled trial. Evid Based Complement Alternat Med. 2013;2013:969824.

Lin RT, Tzeng CY, Lee YC, Chen YI, Hsu TH, Lin JG, Chang SL. Acupoint-specific, frequency-dependent, and improved insulin sensitivity hypoglycemic effect of electroacupuncture applied to drug-combined therapy studied by a randomized control clinical trial. Evid Based Complement Alternat Med. 2014;2014:371475.

Man KM, Man SS, Shen JL, Law KS, Chen SL, Liaw WJ, Lee CT, Lee YJ, Liao WL, Chang TM, et al. Transcutaneous electrical nerve stimulation on ST36 and SP6 acupoints prevents hyperglycaemic response during anaesthesia: a randomised controlled trial. Eur J Anaesthesiol. 2011;28:420–6.

Oberley LW. Free radicals and diabetes. Free Radic Biol Med. 1988;5:113–24.

Padiya R, Khatua TN, Bagul PK, Kuncha M, Banerjee SK. Garlic improves insulin sensitivity and associated metabolic syndromes in fructose fed rats. Nutr Metab (Lond). 2011;8:53.

Pai HC, Tzeng CY, Lee YC, Chang CH, Lin JG, Cheng JT, Chang SL. Increase in plasma glucose lowering action of rosiglitazone by electroacupuncture at bilateral Zusanli acupoints (ST.36) in rats. J Acupunct Meridian Stud. 2009;2:147–51.

Peplow PV. Electroacupuncture treatment of insulin resistance in diabetes mellitus. Acupunct Med. 2015a;33:347–9.

Peplow PV. Repeated electroacupuncture in obese Zucker diabetic fatty rats: adiponectin and leptin in serum and adipose tissue. J Acupunct Meridian Stud. 2015b;8:66–70.

Peplow PV, Han SM. Repeated application of electroacupuncture ameliorates hyperglycemia in obese Zucker diabetic fatty rats. J Acupunct Meridian Stud. 2014;7:1–5.

Saad MA, Cardoso GP, Martins Wde A, Velarde LG, Cruz Filho RA. Prevalence of metabolic syndrome in elderly and agreement among four diagnostic criteria. Arq Bras Cardiol. 2014;102:263–9.

Shapira MY, Appelbaum EY, Hirshberg B, Mizrahi Y, Bar-On H, Ziv E. A sustained, non-insulin related, hypoglycaemic effect of electroacupuncture in diabetic Psammomys obesus. Diabetologia. 2000;43:809–13.

Szkudelski T. Streptozotocin-nicotinamide-induced diabetes in the rat. Characteristics of the experimental model. Exp Biol Med (Maywood). 2012;237:481–90.

Tanaka T, Nabatame H, Tanifuji Y. Insulin secretion and glucose utilization are impaired under general anesthesia with sevoflurane as well as isoflurane in a concentration-independent manner. J Anesth. 2005;19:277–81.

Tzeng CY, Lee YC, Ho TY, Chen YI, Hsu TH, Lin JG, Lee KR, Chang SL. Intracellular signalling pathways associated with the glucose-lowering effect of ST36 electroacupuncture in streptozotocin-induced diabetic rats. Acupunct Med. 2015;33:395–9.

Tzeng CY, Lee YC, Chung JJ, Tsai JC, Chen YI, Hsu TH, Lin JG, Lee KR, Chang SL. 15 Hz electroacupuncture at ST36 improves insulin sensitivity and reduces free fatty acid levels in rats with chronic dexamethasone-induced insulin resistance. Acupunct Med. 2016;34:296.

Yin J, Kuang J, Chandalia M, Tuvdendorj D, Tumurbaatar B, Abate N, Chen JD. Hypoglycemic effects and mechanisms of electroacupuncture on insulin resistance. Am J Physiol Regul Integr Comp Physiol. 2014;307:R332–9.

Zhou G, Myers R, Li Y, Chen Y, Shen X, Fenyk-Melody J, Wu M, Ventre J, Doebber T, Fujii N, et al. Role of AMP-activated protein kinase in mechanism of metformin action. J Clin Invest. 2001;108:1167–74.

Experimental Models for Mechanistic Studies of Moxibustion

9

Jen-Hwey Chiu

Abstract

"Acupmoxa", a word meaning "acupuncture" and "moxibustion", combines ancient Chinese medical techniques that have maintained the well-being of Chinese people for many thousands years. The Western society is more familiar with acupuncture; moxibustion is less popular, most likely due to scant scientific data. Moxibustion reputably treats symptoms of "coldness" or "deficiency" and prevents various disorders.

Potential mechanisms underlying moxibustion include temperature- and non-temperature-related pathways. One type of moxibustion, local somato-thermal stimulation (LSTS), is performed by using a heat source to and above the acupoint. Experimental models have used LSTS on skin acupoints PC6 and LR 14 and measured the sphincter of Oddi's pressure to determine Hsp 70 expression in corresponding organs (heart and liver, respectively), to precondition the animals and protect visceral organs against ischemia-reperfusion injury. LSTS is a remote preconditioning method that has potential clinical implications. Efficacy and safety data are needed from large-scale, double-blind, randomized clinical trials to provide scientific data for Western researchers.

Keywords

Moxibustion · Thermal stimulation · Preconditioning · Heat shock proteins · LSTS

J.-H. Chiu
Institute of Traditional Medicine, School of Medicine, National Yang-Ming University, Taipei, Taiwan

Division of Surgery, Department of Surgery, Taipei Veterans General Hospital, Taipei, Taiwan
e-mail: chiujh@ym.edu.tw

9.1   Clinical Relevance

"Acupmoxa", a word meaning "acupuncture" and "moxibustion", combines ancient Chinese medical techniques that have maintained the well-being of Chinese people for thousands of years (Cheng et al. 1987). Instead of acupuncture, moxibustion is less known in western research, most likely due to lack of proved evidence.

Traditionally, moxibustion is applied with or without moxa-sticks, directly or indirectly onto acupoints of the human body (Lin 2009). Moxibustion reputably treats symptoms of "coldness" or "deficiency" and prevents various disorders. Moxibustion has proven efficacy in the treatment of cervical vertigo, dysmenorrhea, chemotherapy-induced leucopenia, vertigo, and various emergent conditions (Wang et al. 2012; Xiaoxiang 2006; Yang et al. 2008; Zhao et al. 2007). A meta-analysis of clinical data has highlighted the inadequate evidence in support of the efficacy of moxibustion in many kinds of diseases or disorders, such as external cephalic version for breech position (Coyle et al. 2012), stoke (Lee et al. 2010b), and ulcerative colitis (Lee et al. 2010a), amongst others. Large scaled randomized controlled trials (RCTs) in humans are mandatory to assess the efficacy and safety of moxibustion. Moreover, sound experimental animal models are urgently needed to elucidate the mechanisms underlying moxibustion.

9.2   Experimental Models

9.2.1   Manipulation-Local Somatothermal Stimulation in the Experimental Setting

All the animal experiments performed in this article have been approved by a committee for experimental animals organized in National Yang-Ming University and all animals were cared for according to the "Principles of Laboratory Animal Care" (DHHS publication No. [NIH], revised 1996) regulations. The application of heat to skin area (acupoints) through the burning herbals on the surface of the body surface implicates many factors such as smoke, herbs, and fluctuations in temperature in the possible mechanisms underlying moxibustion, complicating the interpretation of data with multisensory stimulations. Some researchers have overcome these difficulties by using temperature as the only stimulator (Chiu et al. 1998). In these experiments, LSTS was achieved via a heat generator above (at 0.5 cm) the acupoint without skin contact. Variations in skin temperature were achieved by 4 min on and 5 min off (3 courses) of the heat generator. It takes 27 min to complete one dose of LSTS. A 12-h interval is required to repeat ≥ 2 LSTS sessions. A temperature fluctuation above or below 42 °C was designed to avoid tolerance developing to heat-sensitive neural transmission. Beside, no skin burning or neural damage is observed.

9.2.2   Anesthesia for Experimental Animals

This study used New Zealand White rabbits and cats of either sex weighing 2.5–3.5 kg, or male Sprague-Dawley rats weighing 250–300 g, After fasting but with free access to water overnight, animals received adequate anesthesia. The depth of anesthesia was kept at steady status without affecting blood pressure, heart rate, or inducing a pain response to peritoneal traction. Respiration was controlled with a respirator through a tracheostomy tube.

9.2.3   Experimental Model for Measuring the Sphincter of Oddi Motility

Animals: Animals were placed in the supine position with a slow infusion of 5% dextrose in normal saline, and respiration was controlled with a respirator (model 141, New England Medical Instruments Inc.) through a tracheostomy tube. The gallbladder (GB) and biliary trees were identified through an upper midline incision, and gallbladder pressure and sphincter of Oddi (SO) motility were measured as described previously (Slivka et al. 1994; Thune et al. 1990). In brief, after identification of the GB and biliary trees, the cystic duct was isolated and ligated, then cannulated with a catheter (OD = 1.57 mm) from the GB neck and secured with purse-string ties to prevent bile leakage from the cannulation site. After aspiration of the bile in the GB, 3 mL of normal saline was introduced and GB pressure measured. A tube (OD = 1.57 mm) was inserted upward into the proximal part of the common bile duct for bile drainage and a constantly perfused open-tipped catheter (OD = 1.57 mm) was placed into the distal part of the common bile duct. The distal tube was passed downward to where resistance was encountered and then withdrawn 1 mm, where the SO pressure was measured. The abdomen was then closed in layers. The SO pressure was measured with an open-tipped catheter constantly perfused (0.3 mL/min) with physiologic warm saline (38 °C) and recorded on a multichannel polygraphic recorder. The bile output drained from the cannulated proximal common duct was collected with an autonomic sample collector and the amount recorded.

Parameter evaluation: Manometry tracings revealed a basal pressure superimposed by contraction (phasic contraction), inducing a maximum pressure. Occasionally, several peaks were summed together (i.e., summation peaks). Basal or tonic SO pressure was measured as the mean end-expiratory pressure during resting, while SO phasic contraction pressure was measured as the mean amplitude of the contractions above the tonic pressure as described previously (Thune et al. 1990). Notably, SO values of herbivorous animals, such as the possums and rabbits, differ considerably from those of carnivorous ones, such as humans and cats; SO responses to cholecystokinin 8 (CCK-8) are inhibitory in possums and rabbits, and excitatory in humans and cats (Chiu et al. 1998, 1999). Summation peak durations (expressed in seconds) were measured in rabbits, whereas in cats, the frequency distribution of phase contractions was given by plotting the peak-to-peak intervals (PPI), also expressed in seconds. The manometric method was validated by an increase in SO pressure in rabbits and a decrease in SO pressure in cats, observed soon after injection of 100 ng/kg cholecystokinin octapeptide (CCK-8) (Sigma C2175).

Drugs: The mechanistic studies used the following pharmacological agents: phentolamine (P7547) 1.5 mg/kg, atropine sulfate (A0257), proglumide (P-4160) 5 mg/kg/min, 30 µg/kg, propranolol (P0884) 2 mg/kg, and naloxone (N-7758) 640 µg/kg.

9.2.4   Experimental Model for Evaluation of Heat Shock Protein 70 (HSP70) Expression

Animals: After male Sprague-Dawley rats were adequately anesthetized, LSTS was applied at 0.5 cm above the PC 6 (Neiquan) acupoint left for three doses (Chiu et al. 2003) or to the LR 14 (Qimen) acupoint right (Lin et al. 2001) for one dose, as mentioned above. The liver and the heart were obtained for Western blot analysis using antibody against Hsp70.

Parameter evaluation: Tissues were homogenized on ice in the presence of protease inhibitors, and the proteins were assayed according to Bradford's method (Bradford 1976). Thirty micrograms of proteins was separated on a 7.5–10% SDS-polyacrylamide gel electrophoresis, transferred to a PVDF, blocked with 5% skim milk and then incubated with primary antibodies against Hsp70 (Hsp72). After washing and incubation with diluted biotin-conjugated secondary antibody, the proteins were detected using an enhanced chemiluminescence detection kit (ECL, Amersham Pharmacia Biotech., Inc., NJ, USA) and analyzed by autoradiography. Anti-β-actin antibody was used as the internal control. The optical density values of the various bands was analyzed using a computer that was equipped with image analysis software (PhotoCapt, Vilber Lourmat, Marne LuVallee Cedex, France).

9.2.5   Experimental Model for Preconditioning Organs with LSTS

In anesthetized mice, LSTS was applied at 0.5 cm above left PC 6 (Neiquan) for three doses (Chiu et al. 2003) or acupoint right LR 14 (Qimen) (Lin et al. 2001) for one dose as mentioned above, to study the modulatory effect of LSTS preconditioning on hepatic Hsp70 expression. Mice were divided into two preconditioning groups: LSTS or control (no LSTS). The LSTS group received different doses of LSTS separated by 12-h intervals, applied on left PC 6 acupoint or right of the LR 14 acupoint, followed by subsequent ischemia–reperfusion injury of the heart or the liver, as described in the following section.

9.2.6 Experimental Model for Preconditioning Organs with LSTS Against Ischemia-Reperfusion (I/R) Injury

Ischemic–reperfusion (I/R) injury of the liver. The I/R injury rat model was performed as described previously (Lin et al. 2001). In brief, male Sprague–Dawley rats were anesthetized and the liver was exposed through an upper midline incision. Two pieces of fine silk were looped along the right and left branches of the portal vein, hepatic artery, and bile duct. Ischemia of left/median lobes was maintained for 60 min, followed by reperfusion of left/median lobes with immediate occlusion of the right lobe vasculature for another 60 min. One hour after completion of the reperfusion procedure, the initial ischemic–reperfused left/median lobes were resected for further analysis.

Ischemia/reperfusion (I/R) injury of the heart. I/R injury of the heart was performed as described previously but with some modification (Lin et al. 2001). In brief, after undergoing tracheotomy under adequate anesthesia, the animals were ventilated by a small rodent respirator and the fourth and fifth ribs were sectioned. The heart was then quickly externalized, inverted and a 6/0 silk ligature was placed around the left main coronary artery. The heart was repositioned in the chest and the animal was allowed to recover for 15 min. Those animals surviving after the end of I/R injury were euthanized early with an anesthetic overdose and the heart was harvested for further analysis.

9.2.6.1 Parameter Evaluation

Infarction size: After 180 min of reperfusion, the coronary artery was re-occluded and Evan's blue (1%) was injected for 5 min into the aortic artery to mark the area at risk, which was excised and weighed. The occluded zone was expressed as the percentage of total ventricular weight. The excised ventricular tissue was sliced (1-mm) and incubated with tetrazolium dye (2,3,5-triphenyltetrazolium chloride 1% in normal saline) at 37 °C for 15 min in darkness, followed by immersion in a solution of 4% formaldehyde overnight and the infarcted tissue zone (white) was measured.

Hemodynamic index: During the ischemia and reperfusion periods, vital signs such as HR, BP and ECG changes were recorded continuously using WAVE FORM data analysis software (MacLab data acquisition system, AD Instruments, Castle Hill, NSW, Australia). The number of and the incidence and duration of ventricular tachyarrhythmias, such as fibrillation (VF), ventricular tachycardia (VT) and ventricular premature beats (VPB), were determined in the surviving animals.

Statistics: Data are presented as the mean ± S.E.M. All data were analyzed using GraphPad Prism V4.03 for Windows (GraphPad Software, San Diego California USA). Unpaired Student's t tests or Mann-Whitney U tests were used to analyze the differences between two groups; concentration-dependent and time effects were analyzed using repeated measures one-way analysis of variance (ANOVA) followed by Dunnett's test. The mortality rate was analyzed using Fisher's exact test. A p value less than 0.05 was considered to be statistically significant.

9.3   Results

9.3.1   LSTS on Acupoints Relaxes Oddi's Sphincter Through Neural Release of Nitric Oxide

When LSTS was applied onto and at 0.5 cm above acupoint GB 24, manometry of sphincter of Oddi (SO) revealed decreases in the tonic pressure and phasic contraction pressure. LSTS-induced relaxation of SO was not blocked by pre-treatment with atropine, phetolamine, or propanolol, but could be blocked by L-NAME, then reversed by L-arginine not by D-arginine, suggesting that LSTS relaxes SO pressure via activation of the neural L-arginine/NO pathway. These LSTS-induced effects upon SO relaxation were not only observed in carnivorous animals (cat), but also in a herbivorous species (rabbit) and in humans (Chiu et al. 1998). Other research has demonstrated that LSTS on certain acupoints (BL 36, BL 40) relaxes the hypertonic anal sphincter in humans (Jiang et al. 1999), possibly via nitrergic neural release of nitric oxide (Jiang et al. 2000). Responses with both the SO and anal sphincters were temperature-specific (42 °C) and acupoint-specific, and involved the nitric oxide neurotransmitter.

9.3.2   LSTS on Peripheral Acupoints Induces Hsp70 Expression

To test the hypothesis that application of LSTS to the peripheral acupoint without contacting the skin surface induces Hsp70 expression in the corresponding visceral organ, LSTS was applied onto and above the LR14 or PC 6 acupointsand HspP70 gene expressions in the liver and the heart were analyzed by Western blot and RT-PCR, respectively. Acupoints PC 6 and LR 14 are well-known in TCM for treatment of heart and hepatobiliary disease, respectively. The study findings demonstrated that LSTS at LR 14 induced Hsp70 expression in the liver, but not in the heart. In contrast, LSTS at PC 6 induced *de novo* Hsp70 expression in the heart, but not in the liver. These findings suggest that LSTS-induced visceral Hsp70 expression is meridian-specific (Chiu et al. 2003; Lin et al. 2001).

9.3.3   LSTS Preconditioning Protects the Organs Against Ischemia-Reperfusion Injury

When animals were preconditioned with three doses of LSTS on left PC 6 and the hearts were severed with I/R injury, significant decreases in the duration of arrhythmia and mortality rates were observed. Besides, an improvement in mitochondrial respiratory function compared with values seen in animals without prior LSTS preconditioning. Moreover, when animals were preconditioned with one dose of LSTS on right LR 14, followed by I/R injury of the liver, there were significant decreases in liver enzymes (ALT/AST) and MDA formation compared with those not treated with LSTS or with three doses of LSTS (Chiu et al. 2003;

Lin et al. 2001). These results suggest that LSTS preconditioning on peripheral acupoints in certain meridians protects animals against subsequent I/R injury of corresponding organs.

Conclusions

Moxibustion is an ancient Chinese medical technique. Temperature effects evoked by LSTS might partly explain how moxibustion works. Compared with whole-body hyperthermia or brief ischemia preconditioning, LSTS (an alternative to moxibustion without causing skin damage) is a preconditioning easy method that could apply for the prevention or treatment of I/R injury.

Acknowledgments This work was supported by grants from the National Science Council, ROC (NSC 98-2320-B-010-012-MY3, NSC 101-2320-B-010-051-MY3, MOST 104-2320-B-010-006-MY3).

References

Bradford MM. A rapid and sensitive method for the quantitation of microgram quantities of protein utilizing the principle of protein-dye binding. Anal Biochem. 1976;72:248–54.

Cheng XN, editor. Chinese acupuncture and moxibustion. Beijing: Foreign Languages Press; 1987.

Chiu JH, Lui WY, Chen YL, Hong CY. Local somatothermal stimulation inhibits the motility of sphincter of Oddi in cats, rabbits and humans through nitrergic neural release of nitric oxide. Life Sci. 1998;63:413–28.

Chiu JH, Kuo YL, Lui WY, Wu CW, Hong CY. Somatic electrical nerve stimulation regulates the motility of sphincter of Oddi in rabbits and cats: evidence for a somatovisceral reflex mediated by cholecystokinin. Dig Dis Sci. 1999;44:1759–67.

Chiu JH, Tsou MT, Tung HH, Tai CH, Tsai SK, Chih CL, Lin JG, Wu CW. Preconditioned somatothermal stimulation on median nerve territory increases myocardial heat shock protein 70 and protects rat hearts against ischemia-reperfusion injury. J Thorac Cardiovasc Surg. 2003;125:678–85.

Coyle ME, Smith CA, Peat B. Cephalic version by moxibustion for breech presentation. Cochrane Database Syst Rev. 2012;(5):CD003928.

Jiang JK, Chiu JH, Lin JK. Local thermal stimulation relaxes hypertonic anal sphincter: evidence of somatoanal reflex. Dis Colon Rectum. 1999;42:1152–9.

Jiang JK, Chiu JH, Lin JK. Local somatothermal stimulation inhibits motility of the internal anal sphincter through nitrergic neural release of nitric oxide. Dis Colon Rectum. 2000;43:381–8.

Lee DH, Kim JI, Lee MS, Choi TY, Choi SM, Ernst E. Moxibustion for ulcerative colitis: a systematic review and meta-analysis. BMC Gastroenterol. 2010a;10:36.

Lee MS, Shin BC, Kim JI, Han CH, Ernst E. Moxibustion for stroke rehabilitation: systematic review. Stroke. 2010b;41:817–20.

Lin JG. Newly edited color book of acupuncture and moxibustion. JYIN Publishing; 2009.

Lin YH, Chiu JH, Tung HH, Tsou MT, Lui WY, Wu CW. Preconditioning somatothermal stimulation on right seventh intercostal nerve territory increases hepatic heat shock protein 70 and protects the liver from ischemia-reperfusion injury in rats. J Surg Res. 2001;99:328–34.

Slivka A, Chuttani R, Carr-Locke DL, Kobzik L, Bredt DS, Loscalzo J, Stamler JS. Inhibition of sphincter of Oddi function by the nitric oxide carrier S-nitroso-N-acetylcysteine in rabbits and humans. J Clin Invest. 1994;94:1792–8.

Thune A, Friman S, Conradi N, Svanvik J. Functional and morphological relationships between the feline main pancreatic and bile duct sphincters. Gastroenterology. 1990;98:758–65.

Wang LL, Wang XJ, Zhang JB. To recognize the emergency and understand the value of moxibustion: book review of Bei ji Jiu fa (Moxibustion for emergency). Zhongguo Zhen Jiu. 2012;32:941–5.

Xiaoxiang Z. Jinger moxibustion for treatment of cervical vertigo-a report of 40 cases. J Tradit Chin Med. 2006;26:17–8.

Yang JJ, Sun LH, She YF, Ge JJ, Li XH, Zhang RJ. Influence of ginger-partitioned moxibustion on serum NO and plasma endothelin-1 contents in patients with primary dysmenorrhea of cold-damp stagnation type. Zhen Ci Yan Jiu. 2008;33:409–12.

Zhao XX, Lu M, Zhu X, Gao P, Li YL, Wang XM, Ma DY, Guo XH, Tong BY, Yang XL, et al. Multi-central clinical evaluation of ginger-partitioned moxibustion for treatment of leukopenia induced by chemotherapy. Zhongguo Zhen Jiu. 2007;27:715–20.

Acupuncture Elicits Neuroprotective Effect by Ameliorating Cognitive Deficits

10

Hsin-Ping Liu and Jaung-Geng Lin

Abstract

Dementia is a global epidemic, with the number of people with dementia steadily increasing worldwide each year. New therapeutic strategies are needed to treat cognitive impairment, to mitigate the growing demands this syndrome is placing on health and long-term care providers as the world's population ages. Increasing scientific evidence indicates that acupuncture may be a clinically effective intervention for people with cognitive impairment. In this study, we describe how acupuncture shows significant neuroprotective activity in the hippocampus of rodent models with impaired learning and memory ability. The evidence suggests that acupuncture may improve cognitive function in neurodegenerative diseases.

Keywords

Acupuncture · Cognitive impairment · Animal models · Neuroprotective effects

10.1 Chinese Medicine and Acupuncture

Chinese medicine has been practiced for thousands of years in ancient Chinese. The practice of acupuncture in clinic is growing in the worldwide. More than 64 symptoms have been endorsed by the World Health Organization (WHO) that can be

H.-P. Liu
Graduate Institute of Acupuncture Science, College of Chinese Medicine, China Medical University, Taichung, Taiwan

J.-G. Lin (✉)
School of Chinese Medicine, College of Chinese Medicine, China Medical University, Taichung, Taiwan
e-mail: jglin@mail.cmu.edu.tw

© Springer Nature Singapore Pte Ltd. 2018
J.-G. Lin (ed.), *Experimental Acupuncturology*,
https://doi.org/10.1007/978-981-13-0971-7_10

relief or beneficial effects from acupuncture treatment (WHO 2008). There are two major therapeutic strategies in traditional Chinese medicine (TCM); one is herbal medicine and the other is acupuncture and moxibustion. The therapeutic principles of TCM consist of the yin and yang theory, visceral manifestation theory, and the anatomical acupoints or meridians, which regulate bodily equilibrium (White and Ernst 2004). During acupuncture manipulation, practitioners stimulate trigger points (acupoints) by inserting fine needles into the skin, to regulate the circulation of qi and blood through meridians. The curative principles of qi and blood are characterized as central ideas in TCM. Qi is considered to be the body's energy that maintains vital essence and enhances blood circulation to remove wastes and increase nutritional supply, thereby promoting health. Acupuncture has been performed for many centuries as a nonpharmacological therapy. Advantages offered by acupuncture over pharmacological therapies include fewer adverse reactions and an obvious therapeutic effect, especially in some conditions including pain, neurodegenerative diseases, sleep disturbance, and cardiovascular disease, amongst others (Gamer 2012; Ho et al. 2014; Li et al. 2012b; Zhao 2013). Increasingly, patients are considering TCM in conjunction with Western medicine to reduce medication burden and relieve symptoms or treat disease.

While acupuncture has beneficial effects in the treatment of disease, various factors potentially influence therapeutic efficacy, including selection of acupoints, and parameters of needle manipulation, such as depth, frequency, and intensity (Goh et al. 2014; Lin and Chen 2008). Various techniques and animal models with homologous diseases are used to explore the underlying mechanisms of acupuncture. At the cellular level, Li et al. found that 1 Hz mechanical movement of needle inserted at the Zusanli (ST36) acupoint can elicit cytosolic Ca^{2+} oscillation and elevate β-endorphin levels in mouse hindlimb muscle fibers (Li et al. 2011). Other studies have shown that acupuncture treatment can change the expression of neurotransmitters, growth factors and neurotrophic factors (Li et al. 2015b; Wang et al. 2002), suggesting that acupuncture stimulation at specific acupoints may trigger Ca^{2+} signal propagation through meridian tracks to activate different signaling pathways and regulate physiological functions, such as gene expression, reproduction, endocrine homeostasis, and neural transmission. Functional magnetic resonance imaging (fMRI) studies demonstrate that acupuncture at Hegu (LI4) and Zusanli (ST36) mediates limbic system activity. Changes in activity have also been observed in sensorimotor cortices, thalamus and paralimbic regions when acupuncture is performed at the Taichong (LV3), Xingjian (LV2), and Neiting (ST44) acupoints, suggesting that the physiological effects of acupuncture action are exerted through the central nervous system (CNS) (Fang et al. 2009).

10.2 Cognitive Impairment

Aging is an irreversible and complex process that may involve many factors (genetics, environmental factors, life experience, and nutrition). As they age, people generally exhibit a progressive decline in cognitive behavior. In the brain, the aging process is at least partly correlated with higher oxidative stress, chronic inflammation or brain injury, and is usually accompanied by synaptic destruction and neuronal loss. Excessive synaptic destruction and selective regional neuronal loss are often correlated with cognitive dysfunction and memory loss, are common features that are observed in some types of neurodegenerative disorders, including Alzheimer's disease (AD), vascular dementia (VD), and Parkinson's disease (PD) (De Marco et al. 2014; Emre et al. 2014; Iadecola 2013). Compared with the normal aging process, patients with AD or VD after ischemic injury exhibit more severe behavioral impairment. Medical interventions including cholinesterase inhibitors, such as donepezil, rivastigmine and galantamine, can temporarily increase acetylcholine (Ach) concentrations at cholinergic synapses and significantly slow AD progression (Tan et al. 2014). However, up to now, no curative therapy exists for this disease, so both pharmacological and nonpharmacological forms of treatment are used in attempts to alleviate the problems accompanying the aging process or dementia. In older people, adverse drug events may outweigh the benefits of prescription drugs, so complementary and non-drug therapies that have fewer side effects, such as exercise, restriction of food uptake (also named caloric restriction), and social activities, have been seen as beneficial for delaying brain aging and potentially lowering the incidence of AD and age-related brain diseases (Horr et al. 2015; Lautenschlager et al. 2014). As increasing evidence identifies the efficiency and mechanisms underlying TCM therapy, acupuncture is being recognized as a powerful therapeutic technique that provides symptom relief without adverse effects.

10.3   Acupuncture Therapy for Treatment of Cognitive Impairment in the Clinic

Acupuncture treatments produce their therapeutic efficacies in neurological diseases through the CNS. Recently, fMRI has explored the central therapeutic mechanisms underlying acupuncture stimulation of the human brain. This noninvasive technique exhibits brain activity *in vivo* and provides interactive connection signals between different brain areas, to immediately measure the effects of acupuncture. The hippocampus is an important area with memory encoding and retrieval, and is also a highly sensitive region relating to the process of cognitive decline. In AD patients, fMRI scanning has observed hippocampal atrophy and lower glucose metabolism, even in the early stages of the disease (Allen et al. 2007). Some fMRI reports involving AD patients and age-matched healthy controls have shown that acupuncture stimulation at the Taichong (LR3) and Hegu (LI4) acupoints enhances hippocampal connectivity with the frontal and lateral temporal regions and increases impaired brain areas showing default mode network (DMN) activity (Liang et al. 2014; Wang et al. 2014b). Similar results have also been observed in patients with mild cognitive impairment (MCI) (Feng et al. 2012; Wang et al. 2012). Following acupuncture treatment, healthy human individuals appear to have a better working memory and less anxiety, as assessed by testing on the Automated Operation Span

Task (AOSPAN) and State-Trait Anxiety Inventory (STAI) (Bussell 2013). In addition, elderly patients with dementia given acupuncture treatment had significant improvements in sleep quality (Kwok et al. 2013). A recent review of clinical trial evidence demonstrates that acupuncture has therapeutic effects in neurodegenerative diseases (Hsieh 2012).

Patients suffering from stroke are at higher risk of vascular dementia (VD), and their quality of life correlates with the level of cognitive decline. Compared with healthy controls, patients with VD are subjected to high oxidative stress and have increased urinary 8-hydroxydeoxyguanosine (8-OHdG) levels, a potential marker of DNA oxidative stress due to free radical attack (Shi et al. 2012b). Acupuncture intervention can relieve VD-related symptoms, lowering 8-OHdG levels and increasing the Mini Mental State Examination (MMSE) score (Shi et al. 2012a), indicating that acupuncture stimulation increases antioxidative activity and improves cognitive function, resulting in better daily living abilities. Accumulating evidence supports the contention that acupuncture treatment increases activities in several brain regions which are closely related to memory and cognition. Thus, acupuncture treatment may become an alternative therapeutic medicine for patients with dementia and cognitive impairment.

10.4 Acupuncture Effects on Animal Models with Cognitive Impairment

10.4.1 Experimental Designs

Animal experiments must be conducted in accordance with the Guide for the Care and Use of Laboratory Animals and be approved by the Institutional Animal Care and Use Committee. Researchers can choose from various acupoints located on the specific track of each meridian. Needle stimulation is made by either manual twisting (manual acupuncture, MA) or electrical stimulation (electroacupuncture, EA). For clinical practice and to study mechanisms in animals, EA by electrical apparatus could have good repeatability and stable therapeutic efficacy because the intensity of acupuncture stimulation can be determined by the frequency setting and a pulsed current. Control intervention groups consist of needle insertion into acupoints located in different meridians or non-acupoints, such as at the tail and on the bilaterial hypochondrium.

The cognitive abilities of learning and memory can be assessed by performance on the passive avoidance test (PAT) and maze test. The PAT analyzes non-spatial ability of learning and memory. The apparatus composes of two adjoining compartments, one illuminated and one darkened, separated by a guillotine door. The test begins by placing a mouse in the light space, and the latency period for entering the dark one is recorded. When the animal enters the dark compartment, the guillotine door closes immediately and mouse's foot receives a slight electric shock. After training, mice are tested for their retention of the passive avoidance response. Typical studies into learning and memory behavior involve training rodents are put into the Morris water maze (MWM) or radial arm maze to evaluate spatial cognitive ability with or without EA application. The maze test is a particularly useful tool for assessment of spatial discrimination and learning and memory ability in rodents. For the radial arm maze test, food pellets are placed in the same region each time. A rat is placed alone in the center of the maze and the experiment ended when all food is empty or 5 min has elapsed. The numbers of times the animals visit the baited and unbaited arms evaluate memory formation. The MWM is another way of analyzing spatial learning and memory. In the hidden platform trial, escape latency, swimming distances and swimming speed are collected for analysis. For the probe test, animals are allowed to swim freely in the platform-free pool and the percentage of time spent on the target quadrant is recorded.

To investigate whether acupuncture can improve cognitive function and associated mechanisms, such as biochemical activity or mRNA and protein expression, tools such as Western blot, enzyme activities, immunohistochemistry and reverse transcription-polymerase chain reaction (RT-PCR) analysis can assess activity changes of molecules, for example, choline acetyltransferase (ChAT), acetylcholinesterase (AchE), and cAMP responsive element binding protein (CREB). Brain activity can be measured by the micro-positron emission tomography (micro-PET) scan, a functional brain imaging technique that monitors blood glucose uptake by certain brain areas *in vivo* using the isotope-labeled ^{18}F-fluorodeoxyglucose (^{18}F-FDG) tracer. These data reflect whether acupuncture stimulation enhances glucose metabolic activity and which brain areas mediate the effects of acupuncture.

10.4.2 Acupuncture and Animal Models

To study how to improve learning and memory, several animal models of cognitive impairments have been established. Some of these models focus on the potent neurotoxicant effects that damage vulnerable neuronal populations, increase the risk of neurodegeneration and cause further behavior deficits. Anatomical and behavioral findings have shown that these models are attractive for degenerative diseases such as AD, which is the most common cause of dementia. The effects of acupuncture on cognitive impairment in animal studies are summarized in Table 10.1.

10.4.2.1 Chronic Corticosterone (CORT)-Induced Cognitive Deficits

Chronic stress, characterized by sustained release of hormones from the adrenal gland, exerts wide ranging effects in areas of the brain and can influence immune function and psychological performance such as anxiety, depression and cognitive tasks (Luine 2015). Epidemiological findings indicate that stressed people at higher risk of developing MCI, or even AD, compared with non-stressed individuals (Elgh et al. 2006). A chronic stress model in rats involves repeated administration of exogenous CORT. Elevated levels of CORT cause hyperactivity and dysregulation of the hypothalamic-pituitary-adrenal (HPA) axis, and disturbance of the glucocorticoid receptor (GR)-negative feedback circuit, causing brain damage and dysfunction. Hippocampal neurons are highly expressed GR, so prolonged or excessive exposure

Table 10.1 Effects of acupuncture, EA, and moxibustion on rodent's models with cognitive impairment

Animal model	Model-induced methods	Treatment type	Acupoints	Functional outcomes	Experimental groups	References
CORT-induced memory deficit rats	SD male rats CORT 5 mg/kg s.c., for 21 days	ACU	HT7 (Sinmun), TE5 (Waiguan)	• Acupuncture at bilateral HT7 acupoints showed a reduction in escape latency and longer time in the probe trial of the MWM test • Acupuncture treatment restored the loss of cholinergic neurons hippocampus by ChAT and AchE immunohistochemistry • Acupuncture treatment increased BDNF and CREB mRNA expression levels, compared with CORT-injected group	Normal group, CORT-injected group, CORT-injected acupoint group (HT7), CORT-injected sham group (TE5), and CORT-injected nonacupoint group (tail)	Lee et al. (2012)
SCO-induced memory deficit rats	SD male rats SCO 2 mg/kg i.p., for 14 days	ACU	GV20 (Baihui), TE4 (Yangji)	• Acupuncture at GV20 acupoints showed recovery of memory dysfunction by the PAT and MWM tests • Acupuncture treatment restored the loss of cholinergic neurons in the hippocampus by ChAT immunohistochemistry • Acupuncture treatment increased BDNF- and CREB-immunopositive neurons, compared with SCO-injected group • Acupuncture treatment increased CHT1, VAChT1, BDNF, and CREB mRNA expression levels, compared with SCO-injected group	Normal group, SCO-injected group, SCO-injected acupoint group (GV20), SCO-injected sham group (TE4), and SCO-injected nonacupoint group (tail)	Lee et al. (2014)

SAMP8 mice	Autogenic senile strain	ACU	"Yiqitiaoxue and Fubenpeiyuan" acupuncture CV17 (Danzhong), CV12 (Zhongwan), CV6 (Qihai), bilateral SP10 (Xuehai), bilateral ST36 (Zusanli)	• Proliferated cells are detected in the hippocampal dentate gyrus (DG) region, and presented along the dorsum of alveus hippocampi (Alv), extending from lateral ventricle (LV) to corpus callosum (CC) by BrdU immunostaining analysis • Acupuncture at acupoints showed improvement of the memory ability by the MWM tests	SAMP8 acupoint group, SAMP8 non-acupoint group, SAMP8 control group, and SAMR1 group	Cheng et al. (2008)
SAMP8 mice	Autogenic senile strain	EA	GV20 (Baihui), GV26 (Shuigou), EX-NH3 (Yintang)	• EA treatment improved the spatial learning and memory ability by the MWM tests • EA treatment increased the uptake rate of glucose in the hippocampus by micro-PET test	SAMP8 EA group, SAMP8 control group, and SAMR1 group	Jiang et al. (2015)
SAMP8 mice	Autogenic senile strain	MOX	Whole mice exposed to moxa smoke generated by burning moxa sticks	• Using enzyme-linked immunosorbent assay (ELISA) kits of monoamine neurotransmitters, moxa smoke treatment significantly reversed the declined levels of 5-HT, NE, and DA in L2 and M1 groups, compared to the model group • Moxa smoke intervention for the M1 group, with 25–35 mg/m³ concentration and 15 min, manifested the highest effect on increasing cerebral monoamine neurotransmitters	SAMP8 six doses of moxa smoke groups (L1, L2, M1, M2, H1, or H2), SAMP8 group, and SAMR1 group	Xu et al. (2013)
AD rats	SD male rats 1 Aβ$_{25\text{-}35}$ 5 μg i.c.	EA, MOX	GV20 (Baihui), BL23 (Shenshu)	• Decreases in axin and increases in β-catenin expression were detected in three pretreatment groups, containing EA, moxibustion, and EA combined with moxibustion groups, by western blot and immunostaining analysis • Organelle disintegration, nuclear swelling, pyknosis and, dark heterochromatin were markedly reduced in three pretreatment groups	EA group, moxibustion group, model group, EA + moxibustion group, sham surgery group, and normal group	Zhou et al. (2014)

(continued)

Table 10.1 (continued)

				Findings	Groups	Reference
AD rats	SD male rats 2 $A\beta_{1-40}$ 5 μg i.c.	EA	GV20 (Baihui), BL23 (Shenshu)	• EA showed improvement of the learning and memory ability by the MWM tests • Neuronal apoptosis in the hippocampus was obviously attenuated in EA group by nuclear staining and western blot against proapoptotic proteins, Bcl-2 and Bax • EA had beneficial effects on synaptic function by immunohistochemistry and western blot of presynaptic protein expression, synapsin-1 and synaptophysin • EA regulated notch signaling pathway by decreasing Notch1 and Hes1 gene expression in the hippocampus	EA group, sham-EA group (tail), model group, and normal group	Guo et al. (2015)
AD rats	Wistar male rats 3 $A\beta_{1-42}$ 5 mg i.c.	MOX	GV20 (Baihui), BL23 (Shenshu)	• Moxibustion treatment prior to Aβ exposure reduced neuronal apoptotic features in the hippocampal ultrastructure observed by TEM • Improvement of learning and memory abilities in Aβ-exposed AD rats was better in pre-moxibustion group than moxibustion group by the MWM tests	Pre-moxibustion group, moxibustion group, model group, and control group	Du et al. (2013)

ACU acupuncture, *EA* electroacupuncture, *MOX* moxibustion, *CORT* corticosterone, *s.c.* subcutaneously injection, *SD* Sprague-Dawley, *MWM* Morris water maze, *ChAT* choline acetyltransferase, *AchE* acethylcholinesterase, *BDNF* brain-derived neurotrophic factor, *CREB* cAMP-response element-binding protein, *SCO* scopolamine, *i.p.* intraperitoneally injection, *PAT* passive avoidance test, *CHT1* choline transporter 1, *VAChT1* vesicular acetylcholine transporter, *BrdU* 5′-bromo-2′-deoxyuridine, *SAMP8* senescence-accelerated mouse prone 8, *SAMR1* senescence-resistant inbred strains 1, *micro-PET* micro-position emission tomography, *5-HT* serotonin, *NE* norepinephrine, *DA* dopamine, *AD* Alzheimer's disease, *Aβ* β-amyloid peptides, *i.c.* intracerebral injection, *TEM* transmission electron microscopy to exogenous CORT results in neuronal damages and impairs hippocampus-dependent cognitive abilities (Jameison and Dinan 2001; McEwen 2008; Wuppen et al. 2010; Zhu et al. 2006). Moreover, the number of proliferating and surviving new neurons in the dentate gyrus (DG) also decreases under high CORT stimulation (Brummelte and Galea 2010).

Acupuncture treatment at the bilateral Sinmun (HT7) acupoints significantly alleviated cognitive impairment induced by elevated levels of CORT in rats; acupuncture stimulation prior to CORT administration modulated CORT-induced decreases in cholinergic immunoreactivity and increased brain-derived neurotrophic factor (BDNF) and CREB mRNA expression (Lee et al. 2012). Notably, manipulating acupuncture at the Sinmun (HT7) acupoint alone can exhibit such significant responses, compared with at the sham acupoint, Waiguan (TE5), or nonacupoint at the tail. Acupuncture also has benefits in chronic CORT-induced mental illness, such as anxiety or depression. Acupuncture at the bilateral Neiguan (PC6) acupoints before CORT injection significantly relieved depression-like behavior and restored neuropeptide Y (NPY) expression in the hypothalamus (Lee et al. 2009). Although the biological mechanisms of acupuncture are not yet clear, a recent study suggested that acupuncture can promote GR expression in the hippocampus and hypothalamus and thereby reduces excessive activation of the HPA axis from stressful stimuli (Wang et al. 2014a). These results indicate that increased GR protein induces negative feedback inhibition to lower glucocorticoid secretion from the adrenal cortex. Thus, acupuncture has the potential to benefit mental disorders and stress-related memory impairment.

10.4.2.2   Trimethyltin (TMT)-Induced Cognitive Deficits

The organotin compound TMT has potent neurotoxicant effects. As a byproduct of plastic and heat stabilizers and pesticides, exposure to TMT results in abnormal neuropathological features, with profound impacts upon human health (Rey et al. 1984; Tang et al. 2010). TMT intoxication leads to selective neuronal loss in the limbic system and, in particular, in the hippocampus, as well as behavior alterations, including hyperactivity, aggression, seizure and impaired spatial memory performance (Geloso et al. 2011; Kreyberg et al. 1992). The mechanisms involved in TMT-induced neurodegeneration are not yet clarified. They probably correlate with mitochondrial dysfunction, calcium-induced cytotoxic response, and inflammation (Lattanzi et al. 2013). Rats injected with TMT show decreases in cholinergic neurons and dopamine receptors and transporters in the hippocampus (Mignini et al. 2012; Park et al. 2012), and inhibition of GSK-3 signaling by lithium-protected neurons against TMT-induced neurotoxicity (Kim et al. 2013). TMT-induced brain injury and impaired memory is therefore regarded as a useful tool for the study of neurodegenerative diseases, such as AD. However, scant evidence exists as to chemical entities, with no details on acupuncture treatment, as having neuroprotective effects on TMT-induced learning and memory deficits in the rat (Jung et al. 2013; Park et al. 2011; Shim et al. 2012).

10.4.2.3 Scopolamine (SCO)-Induced Cognitive Deficits

Lower Ach transmission has often been associated with AD. SCO is a tropane alkaloid compound that inhibits binding to muscarinic acetylcholine receptors (mAchRs). Repeated injection of SCO interferes with cholinergic synapses, causing neuronal injury and evoking cognitive dysfunction in the hippocampus (Burke 1986; Elvander et al. 2004).

Acupuncture stimulation at the Baihui (GV20) acupoint suppresses learning and memory deficits in rats with chronic SCO administration, as assessed by behavioral assessments such as PAT and MWM analysis. Acupuncture treatment also significantly restored memory-associated loss in cholinergic neurons by ChAT immunohistochemistry and increased BDNF and CREB expression in the hippocampus. These results demonstrate that performing acupuncture at the Baihui (GV20) acupoints prior to SCO administration exhibits significantly neuroprotective effects against SCO-induced neuronal toxicity and impaired cognitive dysfunction (Lee et al. 2014).

10.4.3 Cognitive Deficits in the Senescence-Accelerated Mouse

The senescence accelerated mouse (SAM) was originally established through phenotypic selection of the AKR/J strain from Professor Takeda of Kyoto University, and is often considered as an appropriate mouse model for studying the mechanism of aging (Takeda et al. 1981). Senescence-prone (SAMP) mice are mainly characterized by an earlier onset of several physiological disorders and age-related increases in the degree of senescence, including loss of hair and reactivity, shortened lifespan, increased incidence of cataract, emotional dysfunctions, and impaired learning and memory, compared with senescence-resistant (SAMR) mice. Age-dependent alterations of signal transduction also play roles in brain activity and aging process. For example, phosphorylation at serine 473 of Akt, which is involved in cell survival and anti-apoptotic effect, was significant decreased after 6 months in the hippocampus of senescence-accelerated mouse SAMP10, while aged SAMP10 mice showed obvious learning and memory impairments in the MWM test (Nie et al. 2009). In another series of SAMP mice, the SAM-prone 8 (SAMP8) is an autogenic senile murine strain with β-amyloid accumulation, characterized by upregulation of amyloid precursor protein (APP) expression with age (Butterfield and Poon 2005). Increases in Aβ production and decreases in hippocampal gene expression of neurotropic factors such as glial cell line-derived neurotrophic factor (GDNF), neurotrophin-3 (NT-3), and nerve growth factor (NGF), suggest that the molecular basis of the pathological changes induces brain dysfunction and age-related deficits in learning and memory. These phenomena are closely related to AD during the aging process, therefore SAMP8 is often used as an AD model to study the mechanism of aging and Aβ-mediated dementia (Butterfield and Poon 2005; Flood and Morley 1998; Tomobe and Nomura 2009). SAMP8 and its relative age-matched senescence-resistant inbred strains 1 (SAMR1) can be used to investigate whether acupuncture intervention can improve age-related deterioration of learning and memory.

Accumulating evidence suggests that acupuncture improves learning and memory of middle-aged SAMP8 mice. Li et al. showed that acupuncture improved cognitive deficits according to the MWM test and reduced neuronal loss in the hippocampal CA3 and DG regions (Li et al. 2012a). In addition, acupuncture has been shown to stimulate cell proliferation in the DG, indicating that increasing neurogenesis might improve cognitive ability (Cheng et al. 2008). Patients with AD exhibit abnormal glucose metabolism in the brain, and the rate of glucose metabolism may reflect brain activity and homeostasis (Cunnane et al. 2011). In SAMP8 mice, learning and memory deterioration with aging might reflect lower triose phosphate isomerase (TPI) activity in the hippocampus, an enzyme participating in glycolysis process. Zhao et al. found that acupuncture can increase hippocampal TPI activity, slow cognitive impairment, and regulate the glycolysis process during aging (Zhao et al. 2013). Similar findings have been observed in another study: following EA, the glucose uptake rate was higher in the hippocampus as determined by micro-PET scan and EA treatment improved learning and memory abilities. Although only three acupoints, Baihui (GV20), Shuigou (DU26), and Yintang (EX-NH3) were used in EA manipulation, the therapeutic effects of AD were investigated (Jiang et al. 2015). In aged SAMP10 mice, acupuncture reduces oxidative damage by increasing gene expression, including *Hsp84* and *Hsp86*, and has shown positive effects on transcriptional controls and neuronal activity via Y-box-binding protein (YB-1) upregulation in the hippocampus (Ding et al. 2006; Fu et al. 2009; Ohashi et al. 2011). Moreover, moxibustion intervention significantly increases levels of cerebral neurotransmitters including serotonin (5-HT), dopamine (DA), and norepinephrine (NE) in aged SAMP8 mice compared to non-treated mice. The strength of this effect depends on the doses of moxa smoke and exposure time (Xu et al. 2013). The SAMP mice study shows that both acupuncture and moxibustion produce beneficial effects on neuronal functions including increased cell survival, proliferation, functional activity and neurotransmission, which strongly suggests that acupuncture and moxibustion have potential effectiveness in the anti-aging process and improve age-related cognitive abilities.

10.4.4 AD Animal Model

AD is an irreversible, progressive neurodegenerative disorder characterized by accumulation of β-amyloid peptides and neurofibrillary tangles in the brain area. Patients with AD exhibit dementia, problems with language, loss of communicating and ability to care for themselves. Symptoms worsen over time, ultimately leading to death. The cognitive deficits observed in AD patients are widely believed to result from progressive synaptic dysfunction and neuronal loss, which is probably initiated by the soluble oligomeric form of β-amyloid peptides, in particular the $A\beta_{1-42}$ (Lista et al. 2014). Injection of β-amyloid peptides into the brain region can be used to establish rodent models with AD by to inducing severe neurological damage, as well as learning and memory impairments. However, this animal model did not exhibit neurofibrillary tangles.

Pretreatment of EA and moxibustion at the Baihui (GV20) and Shenshu (BL23) acupoints reduce the cognitive damage induced by β-amyloid peptides intracerebral injection, suggesting that acupuncture and moxibustion have a neuroprotective action in the hippocampus (Zhou et al. 2014). Similar results have also been observed in another study, in which moxibustion performed before Aβ injection alleviated the ultrastructural change of the hippocampus, and neurons had fewer apoptotic features (e.g., pyknosis, nuclear invagination, and karyorrhexis) than non-treated AD rats (Du et al. 2013). The mechanism underlying this beneficial effect may involve the Wnt signaling pathway through regulation of axin and β-catenin expression (Zhou et al. 2014). The notch signaling pathway has also been demonstrated to have a neuroprotective function after EA treatment at the Baihui (GV20) and Shenshu (BL23) acupoints in the Aβ-induced AD rat model. EA treatment decreases neuronal apoptosis and promotes presynaptic protein expression, such as synapsin-1 and synaptophysin in the hippocampus (Guo et al. 2015). According to the above evidence, stimulation of acupoints by EA and moxibustion may potentially be an effective therapy in the prevention and treatment of AD.

10.4.5 Modeling VD in Rats

Patients with VD usually experience brain lesions due to ischemic, ischemic-hypoxic, or hemorrhagic pathological changes. VD is the second cause of dementia after AD (Leys et al. 2005), but there are limited medical or surgical treatments. Recently, investigators have established several models to mimic this cerebrovascular disease. To induce ischemia in the rats, the internal carotid artery was permanently clogged with micrometer-sized blood clot emboli to establish a cerebral multi-infarction model (Li et al. 2015a) or bilateral middle cerebral artery occlusion (MCAO) by double silk suture ligation (Zhu et al. 2012). These models generally exhibit different severe levels of structural and functional dysfunction, and are usually accompanied by cognitive deficits.

Studies have observed that acupuncture stimulation at the Zusanli (ST36) acupoint for 2 weeks significantly improves cognitive deficits in VD rats as assessed by the MWM test and increases pyramidal neurons in the hippocampus CA1 region (Li et al. 2015a). The mechanisms underlying acupuncture treatment may involve inhibition of phosphodiesterase (PDE) activity, which increases cAMP concentration, and activates ERK and the cAMP/PKA/CREB signaling pathway to restore impaired long-term potentiation (LTP) and improve hippocampus cognitive function (Li et al. 2015b). In another study, acupuncture protected hippocampal CA1 neurons from apoptosis by decreasing proapoptotic Bax gene and increasing antiapoptotic gene Bcl-2 expression (Wang et al. 2009). EA at the Baihui (GV20) acupoint reversed the electrical signals of impaired hippocampal LTP, and this was mediated by changes of N-methyl-D-aspartate (NMDA) and transient receptor potential vanilloid subtype 1 (TRPV1) receptors in the MCAO rat model (Lin and Hsieh 2010). Acupuncture can also increase cerebral blood flow and antioxidative enzymatic activities to reduce damage from oxidative stress and hypoperfusion-induced VD (Wang et al.

2004; Zhang et al. 2014). Other acupoints, including the Baihui (GV20), Dazhui (GV14), and bilateral Shenshu (BL23), have been applied in EA treatment. Zhu et al. found that EA stimulation significantly increased the activity of the p70S6 kinase/ribosomal protein S6 signaling pathway in the hippocampus, which correlates with neuronal survival and synaptic plasticity, alleviating memory impairment in MCAO rats (Zhu et al. 2012). Acupuncture intervention also mediates activity of glycometabolic enzymes, such as hexokinase, pyruvate kinase, and glucose 6 phosphate dehydrogenase, to increase glucose utility for improvement of brain function (Zhao et al. 2011). The study evidence shows that acupuncture and EA treatment provide neuroprotective effects against oxidative damage and sustain cell survival and neuronal transmission, to further improve cognitive ability in VD rats.

10.4.6 Other Studies

The hippocampus is considered to be a region involved in learning and memory because of its electric signals, LTP and long-term depression (LTD), cellular correlates of synaptic transmission to modulate long-term activity. He et al. found EA at acupoints Zusanli (ST36) and Sanyinjiao (SP6) significantly enhanced LTP in the rat hippocampus, indicating that EA has the potential to improve electrical activity and alleviate memory loss (He et al. 2012). The DG of the hippocampus continues to generate new neurons throughout adulthood. Adult neurogenesis appears to be a general phenomenon in a wide range of species, including humans, primates, and rodents (Knoth et al. 2010; Leuner et al. 2007; Snyder et al. 2009). Newly generated cells in the hippocampus mature into functional neurons in the adult mammalian brain and play a potential role in learning and memory, because they connect with the original neuronal circuits and evoke electrical activity (van Praag et al. 2002). During the manipulation of acupuncture, neurogenesis is mediated in the hippocampus (Cheng et al. 2008).

Conclusions

Brain aging is a complicated process and individuals are at higher risk of developing AD with age. Nowadays, impaired learning and memory constitute most problems for the elderly, and the total population with dementia worldwide continues to grow, creating a financial burden for society and healthcare. Acupuncture could be an alternative therapy for treating neurodegenerative diseases. In the clinic, acupuncture treatment could help humans to improve their cognitive abilities, however, more evidence is needed to demonstrate the effectiveness of acupuncture in cognitive dysfunction and AD. In contrast, most animal studies demonstrate beneficial effects of acupuncture on cognitive impairment. Acupuncture intervention potentially exerts significantly physiological functions by inhibiting cell apoptosis, increasing the neuroprotective capacity of hippocampal neurons against neurotoxicant damage, regulating gene expression of neurotropic factors and neurotransmitters, promoting adult neurogenesis, and enhancing glucose uptake rate, to ameliorate impaired cholinergic activity during aging. The more promising and successful outcomes from preclinical studies of potential treatments for cognitive impairment could be explored in clinical trials. While aging is a risk factor for the development of neurodegenerative diseases, such as AD, using appropriate animal models with memory impairment and exploring the effects of acupuncture may help us to apply acupuncture as a potential therapeutic approach for prevention and treatment of cognitive impairment worldwide.

Acknowledgment This work was supported by the grants from China Medical University, (CMU103-SR-33) and the National Science Council in Taiwan (NSC 102-2320-B-039-019, MOST 103-2815-C-039-033-B).

References

Allen G, Barnard H, McColl R, Hester AL, Fields JA, Weiner MF, Ringe WK, Lipton AM, Brooker M, McDonald E, et al. Reduced hippocampal functional connectivity in Alzheimer disease. Arch Neurol. 2007;64:1482–7.

Brummelte S, Galea LA. Chronic high corticosterone reduces neurogenesis in the dentate gyrus of adult male and female rats. Neuroscience. 2010;168:680–90.

Burke RE. The relative selectivity of anticholinergic drugs for the M1 and M2 muscarinic receptor subtypes. Mov Disord. 1986;1:135–44.

Bussell J. The effect of acupuncture on working memory and anxiety. J Acupunct Meridian Stud. 2013;6:241–6.

Butterfield DA, Poon HF. The senescence-accelerated prone mouse (SAMP8): a model of age-related cognitive decline with relevance to alterations of the gene expression and protein abnormalities in Alzheimer's disease. Exp Gerontol. 2005;40:774–83.

Cheng H, Yu J, Jiang Z, Zhang X, Liu C, Peng Y, Chen F, Qu Y, Jia Y, Tian Q, et al. Acupuncture improves cognitive deficits and regulates the brain cell proliferation of SAMP8 mice. Neurosci Lett. 2008;432:111–6.

Cunnane S, Nugent S, Roy M, Courchesne-Loyer A, Croteau E, Tremblay S, Castellano A, Pifferi F, Bocti C, Paquet N, et al. Brain fuel metabolism, aging, and Alzheimer's disease. Nutrition. 2011;27:3–20.

De Marco M, Shanks MF, Venneri A. Cognitive stimulation: the evidence base for its application in neurodegenerative disease. Curr Alzheimer Res. 2014;11:469–83.

Ding X, Yu J, Yu T, Fu Y, Han J. Acupuncture regulates the aging-related changes in gene profile expression of the hippocampus in senescence-accelerated mouse (SAMP10). Neurosci Lett. 2006;399:11–6.

Du Y, Liu R, Sun G, Meng P, Song J. Pre-moxibustion and moxibustion prevent Alzheimer's disease. Neural Regen Res. 2013;8:2811–9.

Elgh E, Lindqvist Astot A, Fagerlund M, Eriksson S, Olsson T, Nasman B. Cognitive dysfunction, hippocampal atrophy and glucocorticoid feedback in Alzheimer's disease. Biol Psychiatry. 2006;59:155–61.

Elvander E, Schott PA, Sandin J, Bjelke B, Kehr J, Yoshitake T, Ogren SO. Intraseptal muscarinic ligands and galanin: influence on hippocampal acetylcholine and cognition. Neuroscience. 2004;126:541–57.

Emre M, Ford PJ, Bilgic B, Uc EY. Cognitive impairment and dementia in Parkinson's disease: practical issues and management. Mov Disord. 2014;29:663–72.

Fang J, Jin Z, Wang Y, Li K, Kong J, Nixon EE, Zeng Y, Ren Y, Tong H, Wang P, Hui KK. The salient characteristics of the central effects of acupuncture needling: limbic-paralimbic-neocortical network modulation. Hum Brain Mapp. 2009;30:1196–206.

Feng Y, Bai L, Ren Y, Chen S, Wang H, Zhang W, Tian J. FMRI connectivity analysis of acupuncture effects on the whole brain network in mild cognitive impairment patients. Magn Reson Imaging. 2012;30:672–82.

Flood JF, Morley JE. Learning and memory in the SAMP8 mouse. Neurosci Biobehav Rev. 1998;22:1–20.

Fu Y, Yu JC, Ding XR, Han J. Effects of acupuncture on expressions of the transcription factors NF-E2, YB-1, LRG47 in the SAMP10 mice. J Tradit Chin Med. 2009;29:54–9.

Gamer M. Validity of the concealed information test in realistic mock crime scenarios: comment on Bradley, Malik, and Cullen. Percept Mot Skills. 2012;115:427–31.

Geloso MC, Corvino V, Michetti F. Trimethyltin-induced hippocampal degeneration as a tool to investigate neurodegenerative processes. Neurochem Int. 2011;58:729–38.

Goh YL, Ho CE, Zhao B. Acupuncture and depth: future direction for acupuncture research. Evid Based Complement Alternat Med. 2014;2014:871217.

Guo HD, Tian JX, Zhu J, Li L, Sun K, Shao SJ, Cui GH. Electroacupuncture suppressed neuronal apoptosis and improved cognitive impairment in the AD model rats possibly via downregulation of notch signaling pathway. Evid Based Complement Alternat Med. 2015;2015:393569.

He X, Yan T, Chen R, Ran D. Acute effects of electro-acupuncture (EA) on hippocampal long term potentiation (LTP) of perforant path-dentate gyrus granule cells synapse related to memory. Acupunct Electrother Res. 2012;37:89–101.

Ho TJ, Chan TM, Ho LI, Lai CY, Lin CH, Macdonald I, Harn HJ, Lin JG, Lin SZ, Chen YH. The possible role of stem cells in acupuncture treatment for neurodegenerative diseases: a literature review of basic studies. Cell Transplant. 2014;23:559–66.

Horr T, Messinger-Rapport B, Pillai JA. Systematic review of strengths and limitations of randomized controlled trials for non-pharmacological interventions in mild cognitive impairment: focus on Alzheimer's disease. J Nutr Health Aging. 2015;19:141–53.

Hsieh C. Acupuncture as treatment for nervous system diseases. Biomedicine. 2012;2:51–7.

Iadecola C. The pathobiology of vascular dementia. Neuron. 2013;80:844–66.

Jameison K, Dinan TG. Glucocorticoids and cognitive function: from physiology to pathophysiology. Hum Psychopharmacol. 2001;16:293–302.

Jiang J, Gao K, Zhou Y, Xu A, Shi S, Liu G, Li Z. Electroacupuncture treatment improves learning-memory ability and brain glucose metabolism in a mouse model of Alzheimer's disease: using Morris water maze and micro-PET. Evid Based Complement Alternat Med. 2015;2015:142129.

Jung EY, Lee MS, Ahn CJ, Cho SH, Bae H, Shim I. The neuroprotective effect of gugijihwang-tang on trimethyltin-induced memory dysfunction in the rat. Evid Based Complement Alternat Med. 2013;2013:542081.

Kim J, Yang M, Kim SH, Kim JC, Wang H, Shin T, Moon C. Possible role of the glycogen synthase kinase-3 signaling pathway in trimethyltin-induced hippocampal neurodegeneration in mice. PLoS One. 2013;8:e70356.

Knoth R, Singec I, Ditter M, Pantazis G, Capetian P, Meyer RP, Horvat V, Volk B, Kempermann G. Murine features of neurogenesis in the human hippocampus across the lifespan from 0 to 100 years. PLoS One. 2010;5:e8809.

Kreyberg S, Torvik A, Bjorneboe A, Wiik-Larsen W, Jacobsen D. Trimethyltin poisoning: report of a case with postmortem examination. Clin Neuropathol. 1992;11:256–9.

Kwok T, Leung PC, Wing YK, Ip I, Wong B, Ho DW, Wong WM, Ho F. The effectiveness of acupuncture on the sleep quality of elderly with dementia: a within-subjects trial. Clin Interv Aging. 2013;8:923–9.

Lattanzi W, Corvino V, Di Maria V, Michetti F, Geloso MC. Gene expression profiling as a tool to investigate the molecular machinery activated during hippocampal neurodegeneration induced by trimethyltin (TMT) administration. Int J Mol Sci. 2013;14:16817–35.

Lautenschlager NT, Anstey KJ, Kurz AF. Non-pharmacological strategies to delay cognitive decline. Maturitas. 2014;79:170–3.

Lee B, Shim I, Lee HJ, Yang Y, Hahm DH. Effects of acupuncture on chronic corticosterone-induced depression-like behavior and expression of neuropeptide Y in the rats. Neurosci Lett. 2009;453:151–6.

Lee B, Sur BJ, Kwon S, Jung E, Shim I, Lee H, Hahm DH. Acupuncture stimulation alleviates corticosterone-induced impairments of spatial memory and cholinergic neurons in rats. Evid Based Complement Alternat Med. 2012;2012:670536.

Lee B, Sur B, Shim J, Hahm DH, Lee H. Acupuncture stimulation improves scopolamine-induced cognitive impairment via activation of cholinergic system and regulation of BDNF and CREB expressions in rats. BMC Complement Altern Med. 2014;14:338.

Leuner B, Kozorovitskiy Y, Gross CG, Gould E. Diminished adult neurogenesis in the marmoset brain precedes old age. Proc Natl Acad Sci U S A. 2007;104:17169–73.

Leys D, Henon H, Mackowiak-Cordoliani MA, Pasquier F. Poststroke dementia. Lancet Neurol. 2005;4:752–9.

Li G, Liang JM, Li PW, Yao X, Pei PZ, Li W, He QH, Yang X, Chan QC, Cheung PY, et al. Physiology and cell biology of acupuncture observed in calcium signaling activated by acoustic shear wave. Pflugers Arch. 2011;462:587–97.

Li G, Zhang X, Cheng H, Shang X, Xie H, Yu J, Han J. Acupuncture improves cognitive deficits and increases neuron density of the hippocampus in middle-aged SAMP8 mice. Acupunct Med. 2012a;30:339–45.

Li J, Chen Z, Liang F, Wu S, Wang H. The influence of PC6 on cardiovascular disorders: a review of central neural mechanisms. Acupunct Med. 2012b;30:47–50.

Li F, Yan CQ, Lin LT, Li H, Zeng XH, Liu Y, Du SQ, Zhu W, Liu CZ. Acupuncture attenuates cognitive deficits and increases pyramidal neuron number in hippocampal CA1 area of vascular dementia rats. BMC Complement Altern Med. 2015a;15:133.

Li QQ, Shi GX, Yang JW, Li ZX, Zhang ZH, He T, Wang J, Liu LY, Liu CZ. Hippocampal cAMP/PKA/CREB is required for neuroprotective effect of acupuncture. Physiol Behav. 2015b;139:482–90.

Liang P, Wang Z, Qian T, Li K. Acupuncture stimulation of Taichong (Liv3) and Hegu (LI4) modulates the default mode network activity in Alzheimer's disease. Am J Alzheimers Dis Other Demen. 2014;29:739–48.

Lin JG, Chen WL. Acupuncture analgesia: a review of its mechanisms of actions. Am J Chin Med. 2008;36:635–45.

Lin YW, Hsieh CL. Electroacupuncture at Baihui acupoint (GV20) reverses behavior deficit and long-term potentiation through N-methyl-d-aspartate and transient receptor potential vanilloid subtype 1 receptors in middle cerebral artery occlusion rats. J Integr Neurosci. 2010;9:269–82.

Lista S, Garaci FG, Ewers M, Teipel S, Zetterberg H, Blennow K, Hampel H. CSF Abeta1-42 combined with neuroimaging biomarkers in the early detection, diagnosis and prediction of Alzheimer's disease. Alzheimers Dement. 2014;10:381–92.

Luine V. Recognition memory tasks in neuroendocrine research. Behav Brain Res. 2015;285:158–64.

McEwen BS. Central effects of stress hormones in health and disease: understanding the protective and damaging effects of stress and stress mediators. Eur J Pharmacol. 2008;583:174–85.

Mignini F, Nasuti C, Artico M, Giovannetti F, Fabrizi C, Fumagalli L, Iannetti G, Pompili E. Effects of trimethyltin on hippocampal dopaminergic markers and cognitive behaviour. Int J Immunopathol Pharmacol. 2012;25:1107–19.

Nie K, Yu JC, Fu Y, Cheng HY, Chen FY, Qu Y, Han JX. Age-related decrease in constructive activation of Akt/PKB in SAMP10 hippocampus. Biochem Biophys Res Commun. 2009;378:103–7.

Ohashi S, Moue M, Tanaka T, Kobayashi S. Translational level of acetylcholine receptor alpha mRNA in mouse skeletal muscle is regulated by YB-1 in response to neural activity. Biochem Biophys Res Commun. 2011;414:647–52.

Park HJ, Shim HS, Choi WK, Kim KS, Bae H, Shim I. Neuroprotective effect of Lucium chinense fruit on Trimethyltin-induced learning and memory deficits in the rats. Exp Neurobiol. 2011;20:137–43.

Park HJ, Lee SY, Shim HS, Kim JS, Kim KS, Shim I. Chronic treatment with squid phosphatidylserine activates glucose uptake and ameliorates TMT-induced cognitive deficit in rats via activation of cholinergic systems. Evid Based Complement Alternat Med. 2012;2012:601018.

Rey C, Reinecke HJ, Besser R. Methyltin intoxication in six men; toxicologic and clinical aspects. Vet Hum Toxicol. 1984;26:121–2.

Shi GX, Liu CZ, Li QQ, Zhu H, Wang LP. Influence of acupuncture on cognitive function and markers of oxidative DNA damage in patients with vascular dementia. J Tradit Chin Med. 2012a;32:199–202.

Shi GX, Liu CZ, Wang LP, Guan LP, Li SQ. Biomarkers of oxidative stress in vascular dementia patients. Can J Neurol Sci. 2012b;39:65–8.

Shim HS, Park HJ, Ahn YH, Her S, Han JJ, Hahm DH, Lee H, Shim I. Krill-derived phosphatidylserine improves TMT-induced memory impairment in the rat. Biomol Ther (Seoul). 2012;20:207–13.

Snyder JS, Glover LR, Sanzone KM, Kamhi JF, Cameron HA. The effects of exercise and stress on the survival and maturation of adult-generated granule cells. Hippocampus. 2009;19:898–906.

Takeda T, Hosokawa M, Takeshita S, Irino M, Higuchi K, Matsushita T, Tomita Y, Yasuhira K, Hamamoto H, Shimizu K, et al. A new murine model of accelerated senescence. Mech Ageing Dev. 1981;17:183–94.

Tan CC, Yu JT, Wang HF, Tan MS, Meng XF, Wang C, Jiang T, Zhu XC, Tan L. Efficacy and safety of donepezil, galantamine, rivastigmine, and memantine for the treatment of Alzheimer's disease: a systematic review and meta-analysis. J Alzheimers Dis. 2014;41:615–31.

Tang X, Yang X, Lai G, Guo J, Xia L, Wu B, Xie Y, Huang M, Chen J, Ruan X, et al. Mechanism underlying hypokalemia induced by trimethyltin chloride: inhibition of H+/K+-ATPase in renal intercalated cells. Toxicology. 2010;271:45–50.

Tomobe K, Nomura Y. Neurochemistry, neuropathology, and heredity in SAMP8: a mouse model of senescence. Neurochem Res. 2009;34:660–9.

van Praag H, Schinder AF, Christie BR, Toni N, Palmer TD, Gage FH. Functional neurogenesis in the adult hippocampus. Nature. 2002;415:1030–4.

Wang SJ, Omori N, Li F, Zhang WR, Jin G, Hamakawa Y, Sato K, Nagano I, Shoji M, Abe K. Enhanced expression of phospho-Akt by electro-acupuncture in normal rat brain. Neurol Res. 2002;24:719–24.

Wang L, Tang C, Lai X. Effects of electroacupuncture on learning, memory and formation system of free radicals in brain tissues of vascular dementia model rats. J Tradit Chin Med. 2004;24:140–3.

Wang T, Liu CZ, Yu JC, Jiang W, Han JX. Acupuncture protected cerebral multi-infarction rats from memory impairment by regulating the expression of apoptosis related genes Bcl-2 and Bax in hippocampus. Physiol Behav. 2009;96:155–61.

Wang Z, Nie B, Li D, Zhao Z, Han Y, Song H, Xu J, Shan B, Lu J, Li K. Effect of acupuncture in mild cognitive impairment and Alzheimer disease: a functional MRI study. PLoS One. 2012;7:e42730.

Wang SJ, Zhang JJ, Qie LL. Acupuncture relieves the excessive excitation of hypothalamic-pituitary-adrenal cortex axis function and correlates with the regulatory mechanism of GR, CRH, and ACTHR. Evid Based Complement Alternat Med. 2014a;2014:495379.

Wang Z, Liang P, Zhao Z, Han Y, Song H, Xu J, Lu J, Li K. Acupuncture modulates resting state hippocampal functional connectivity in Alzheimer disease. PLoS One. 2014b;9:e91160.

White A, Ernst E. A brief history of acupuncture. Rheumatology (Oxford). 2004;43:662–3.

WHO. WHO Standard Acupuncture Point Locations in the Western Pacific Region; World Health Organization; 2008.

Wuppen K, Oesterle D, Lewicka S, Kopitz J, Plaschke K. A subchronic application period of glucocorticoids leads to rat cognitive dysfunction whereas physostigmine induces a mild neuroprotection. J Neural Transm. 2010;117:1055–65.

Xu H, Zhao B, Cui Y, Lim MY, Liu P, Han L, Guo H, Lao L. Effects of Moxa smoke on monoamine neurotransmitters in SAMP8 mice. Evid Based Complement Alternat Med. 2013;2013:178067.

Zhang X, Wu B, Nie K, Jia Y, Yu J. Effects of acupuncture on declined cerebral blood flow, impaired mitochondrial respiratory function and oxidative stress in multi-infarct dementia rats. Neurochem Int. 2014;65:23–9.

Zhao K. Acupuncture for the treatment of insomnia. Int Rev Neurobiol. 2013;111:217–34.

Zhao L, Shen P, Han Y, Zhang X, Nie K, Cheng H, Kan B, Li G, Yu J, Han J. Effects of acupuncture on glycometabolic enzymes in multi-infarct dementia rats. Neurochem Res. 2011;36:693–700.

Zhao L, Jia Y, Yan D, Zhou C, Han J, Yu J. Aging-related changes of triose phosphate isomerase in hippocampus of senescence accelerated mouse and the intervention of acupuncture. Neurosci Lett. 2013;542:59–64.

Zhou H, Sun G, Kong L, Du Y, Shen F, Wang S, Chen B, Zeng X. Acupuncture and moxibustion reduces neuronal edema in Alzheimer's disease rats. Neural Regen Res. 2014;9:968–72.

Zhu ZH, Yang R, Fu X, Wang YQ, Wu GC. Astrocyte-conditioned medium protecting hippocampal neurons in primary cultures against corticosterone-induced damages via PI3-K/Akt signal pathway. Brain Res. 2006;1114:1–10.

Zhu Y, Wang X, Ye X, Gao C, Wang W. Effects of electroacupuncture on the expression of p70 ribosomal protein S6 kinase and ribosomal protein S6 in the hippocampus of rats with vascular dementia. Neural Regen Res. 2012;7:207–11.

Acupuncture on Sleep Regulation

11

Fang-Chia Chang, Pei-Lu Yi, and Jaung-Geng Lin

Abstract

Acupuncture or electroacupuncture (EAc) exhibits various therapeutic functions, such as relieving pain, reducing inflammatory responses, and alleviating sleep disruptions. In this chapter, we discuss the neuronal mechanisms involving the electroacupuncture of bilateral Anmian (EX17) acupoints on sleep regulation. We found that administration of 20-min EAc before the beginning of the dark period increases sleep, including rapid eye movement (REM) sleep and non-REM (NREM) sleep. Intraperitoneal injection of a muscarinic receptor antagonist scopolamine attenuates the EAc-induced enhancement of NREM sleep and REM sleep. This signal is relayed to the caudal nucleus tractus solitarius (NTS), since lesion of caudal NTS blocks EAc's effect on sleep. We further determine the role of opioid receptors in the EAc's effect. Our results indicate that low frequency (10 Hz) EAc-induced enhancement of sleep is mediated by the μ-opioid receptor in the NTS, rather than the κ- and δ-opioid receptors, while the κ-opioid

F.-C. Chang
Department of Veterinary Medicine, School of Veterinary Medicine, National Taiwan University, Taipei, Taiwan

Graduate Institute of Brain and Mind Sciences, College of Medicine, National Taiwan University, Taipei, Taiwan

Graduate Institute of Acupuncture Science, College of Chinese Medicine, China Medical University, Taichung, Taiwan

P.-L. Yi
Department of Sport Management, College of Tourism, Leisure and Sports, Aletheia University, Taipei, Taiwan

J.-G. Lin (✉)
School of Chinese Medicine, College of Chinese Medicine, China Medical University, Taichung, Taiwan
e-mail: jglin@mail.cmu.edu.tw

© Springer Nature Singapore Pte Ltd. 2018
J.-G. Lin (ed.), *Experimental Acupuncturology*,
https://doi.org/10.1007/978-981-13-0971-7_11

receptor in the NTS mediates the high frequency (100 Hz) EAC-induced sleep enhancement. The underlying mechanisms of the NTS opioid receptors involved in sleep regulation by EAc are similar to those of EAc-induced analgesia in the spinal cord. This chapter reveals the underlying mechanism of EAc-induced sleep enhancement.

Keywords
Anmian acupoint (EX17) · Cholinergic receptor · Electroacupuncture · Nucleus tractus solitarius (NTS) · Opioid receptors · Vagus nerve

11.1   Introduction

Normal human sleep consists of two different states; non-rapid eye movement (NREM) sleep and rapid eye movement (REM) sleep, which alternate in a sleep episode. The features of these two states are well characterized by the parameters recorded during sleep by polysomnography (PSG), which monitors brain waves on the electroencephalogram (EEG), muscle tone on the electromyogram (EMG), eye movement on the electromyogram (EOG), cardiovascular function on the electrocardiogram (ECG), as well as breathing functions and blood oxygen levels. NREM sleep can be further categorized into three separate stages: stages 1–3, which are followed in order upwards and downwards as sleep cycles progress. Stage 1 is the transitional state between wake and sleep and occurs at the beginning of sleep. Theta waves become dominant in stage 1 of NREM sleep (Kryger et al. 2005). EEGs recorded from stage 2 are characterized by sleep spindles, with relatively unsynchronized brain waves (frequency of 11–15 Hz) and "K-complexes", single, long delta waves that last for only 1 s (Kryger et al. 2005). Stage 3 of NREM sleep is the deepest sleep, dominated by delta waves (Kryger et al. 2005). Brain waves during REM sleep are characterized by low-amplitude and high-frequency EEGs, including theta waves, alpha waves and beta waves, similar to the EEGs acquired from wakeful states (Kryger et al. 2005). Muscle tone is highest during the wakefulness, gradually declines during NREM sleep, and is at its lowest level during REM sleep (Kryger et al. 2005). The most common sleep disorder is insomnia. The manifestations of insomnia include an increased latency to sleep, fail to maintain sleep during nighttime, or the feel of non-refreshment after awake. Primary insomnia is lack of a significantly causative factor, while secondary insomnia is mainly caused by patient's health conditions, such as medications, neurological diseases or mental illness. For example, stress (Cano et al. 2008), depression (Berk 2009), anxiety (Brenes et al. 2009), or health conditions (e.g., pain, arthritis, and fibromyalgia) may cause secondary insomnia (Belt et al. 2009). There are three different types of insomnia: (1) The transient insomnia is normally caused by an acute stressor or a disruption of circadian rhythm, which lasts less than 1 week; (2) The short-term insomnia is related to a long-lasting ongoing stressor, which lasts for 1–4 weeks; (3) The chronic insomnia is usually associated with severely causative factors and lasts for over 4 weeks. Epidemiology indicates that 10–20% of the adult population experience moderate to severe insomnia (Kryger et al. 2005). Especially, a higher percentage (40–70%) of healthy elderly people are suffered from any types of chronic sleep disturbances (Van Someren 2005). The estimated health bills spending in insomnia in the United States is about $30~$107.5 billion each year (Walsh and Engelhardt 1999; Stoller 1994). These expenses mostly spend in the medical treatments (e.g., physician encounters and drug prescriptions), the consumption of medical services, the increased accident risk, and lost workplace productivity. The most common sedatives and hypnotics used for insomnia treatment are benzodiazepines and non-benzodiazepines. However, the currently used sedatives and hypnotics have issues on the inappropriate use, the drug dependence and severe side effects. Therefore, seeking alternative treatments to reduce the economic costs and to reinforce the therapeutic effects have become an important topic in insomnia treatment.

The procedure of acupuncture, in which thin needles are inserted into acupoints to deliver therapeutic effects, has been documented to alleviate pain, reduce inflammation, and treat insomnia. Acupuncture has a success rate of around 90% in the relief of insomnia (Cheng 1985, 1986a, b). Acupoints that are documented in ancient Chinese literature to relieve insomnia include Anmian (EX17), Shenmen (HT7), Sanyinjia (SP6), Zusanli (ST36), Neiguan (PC6), Dazhui (DU40), Taichong (LR3), Tainzhu (BL10), Baihui (DU20), Bishu (BL20) and Zhongwan (RN12) (Cheng 1986a, b; Lu et al. 1993). Although the therapeutic effect on improving insomnia is significant clinically, the theory underling acupuncture remains controversial. The neural mechanisms of acupuncture have been hypothesized in several researches. The spinal gate theory (Melzack and Wall 1965) and activation of particular neuronal circuits, such as the opioidergic and monoaminergic systems (Cheng and Pomeranz 1979), have been hypothesized to involve in the acupuncture function, particularly in analgesia. Acupuncture reduces proinflammatory cytokines in the hypothalamus and subsequently suppresses febrile responses (Son et al. 2002). Furthermore, evidence has demonstrated that the acupuncture effects may be mediated partially by the activation of the vagus nerve (Wang et al. 2002), and it is known that both vagotomy (Noguchi and Hayashi 1996) and blockade of cholinergic activity (Uvnas-Moberg et al. 1992) suppress acupuncture-induced effects. Ascending vagus nerve signals primarily project to the caudal nucleus tractus solitarius (NTS) in the dorsomedial medulla oblongata (Cottle 1964) and then project to the parabrachial nucleus, where located near the junction between pons and midbrain, then to the thalamus, hypothalamus, preoptic area, bed nucleus of the stria terminalis, amygdala and frontal cortex, where commonly belonging to the visceral-limbic forebrain (Norgren 1978; Saper and Loewy 1980). The limbic forebrain regions have been implicated in sleep regulation, rather than the predominant circuits of the NTS via the reticular formation. Low frequency electrical stimulation of the NTS produces the synchronizing slow-wave sleep (SWS) in the cortices (Magnes et al. 1961). In contrast, lesioning of the caudal NTS causes desynchronized EEGs in sleeping animals (Bonvallet and Allen 1963). The opioidergic neurotransmitters in the NTS seem to be involved in the somnogenic effect, since microinjection of morphine into the NTS provokes SWS enhancement, which can be blocked by naloxone (Reinoso-Barbero and de Andres 1995). Based upon the evidence detailed above, we will discuss the hypothesis that the opioidergic circuits in the NTS mediate the effects of acupuncture on sleep regulation.

In order to induce the "de-qi" sensation, the acupuncture needle is inserted into the acupoint and receives different kinds of manipulations, such as spinning, flicking, or moving up and down, constituting acupuncture doses. However, it is difficult to control for uniform acupuncture doses through manual manipulation. Therefore, we used electroacupuncture (EAc), which delivers the continuous electric currents through needles to the acupoints and obtains the therapeutic effect in a same acupuncture dose. Some of the most effective acupoints used for insomnia treatment and well documented in the traditional Chinese literatures include Shenmen (HT17), Sanyinjiao (SP6) and Anmian (EX17). "Anmian" in Chinese means "goodnight sleep"; therefore, the Anmian acupoint is the primary target for investigations into the efficacy and mechanistic neural circuits of acupuncture on sleep regulation.

11.2   Animal Model and Methodology

All the experimental protocols described in this chapter have been approved by the Institutional Animal Care and Use Committee (IACUC) of the National Taiwan University. We used male Sprague-Dawley rats to study acupuncture effects on the sleep-wake activity. In this model, rats are anesthetized and are given analgesic and antibiotic medication to relieve pain and reduce surgical infection. Two EEG electrodes are placed over the frontal and parietal cortices in the right hemisphere and a reference electrode is placed over the cerebellum. Electromyogram (EMG) electrodes are also implanted into the neck muscle. In order to determine the underlying neural mechanism, a microinjection guide cannula is implanted directly into the NTS. The coordinates for the placement of EEG screw electrodes and the microinjection guide cannula were adopted from the Paxinos and Watson rat atlas (Paxinos and Watson 1998). Insulated leads from EEG and EMG electrodes are routed to a Teflon pedestal, which is cemented to the skull with dental acrylic. Rats are allowed to recover and habituated to a 12:12 h cycle of a light:dark rhythm for a week before the experiments. A tether connects the pedestal and the amplifier, and signals from the EEG and EMG electrodes are fed into the amplifier. The output from the EEG signals is routed to an analog bandpass filtering signals between 0.1 and 40 Hz. Gross body movement is also detected by an infrared-based motion detector, and the signal is converted to a voltage output and digitized into 1-s bins. The digitized signals are stored as binary computer files for subsequent analyses. Rats are hosted separately in individual recording cages in an isolated room, and they are freely moving in their cage. Water and food are available *ad libitum*. Determination of the vigilance state is visualized and scored by custom software written in LabView for Windows. The animal's vigilance states are categorized into NREM sleep, REM sleep and wakefulness. In rats, NREM sleep is characterized by synchronized EEG slow waves, a dominant delta frequency band (0.5–4.0 Hz), reduced EMG activity and lack of locomotion before and during entry. During REM sleep, the EEG is desynchronized and amplitude is reduced, the EEG power density is dominant in the theta frequency (6.0–9.0 Hz), EMG activity is minimal, and phasic body twitches could be observed. During wakeful periods, rats are active, with protracted body movements and a high muscle tone, with an EEG amplitude similar to that observed during REM sleep, but power density values in the delta frequency band are generally greater than those in theta frequency band. Detailed methodology covering the acquisition and analysis procedures are supplied in a previously published paper (Yi et al. 2016).

In this chapter, we will discuss the effects on sleep when acupuncture is delivered at the bilateral Anmian (EX17) acupoints. An EAc stimulus is delivered through the stainless needles inserted bilaterally into the Anmian acupoint, with a depth of 2 mm. The electrical stimulation is a train of biphasic pulses with the parameters of 10 (low frequency) or 100 Hz (high frequency), a pulse duration of 150 ms, and a stimulus intensity of 3 mA (Yi et al. 2004; Cheng et al. 2011, 2012). The Anmian acupoint is located at the midpoint between the Yifeng (TH17) and Fengchi (GB20) acupoints. Yifeng (TH17) is on the depression posterior to the ear lobe, between the mandible and mastoid processes. Fengchi (GB20) is on the depression between the upper portion of the musculus sternocleidomastoideus and musculus trapezius. The location of the Anmian in rats is at the relative anatomical location between the sternocleidomastoideus muscle and the splenius capitis muscle (Yi et al. 2004; Cheng et al. 2011, 2012). The manipulation of 20-min of EAc is delivered when rats are lightly anesthetized with ether isoflurane or ketamine/xylazine, and rats are fully awake 20–25 min later. The EAc is given 20 min prior to the beginning of the dark period, and sleep activity is recorded from the onset of the dark period, lasting for 24 h. The rationale for carrying out the experiment in the dark is that manipulation expected to enhance sleep would be easy to observe when the rat is active and sleeping less during the dark period. In contrast, a minimal sleep increase will not be easy to observe when the manipulation is performed during the light period when sleep activity is at its highest level. This method is a general way to fast screen the effect of a particular manipulation on sleep activity. Since we expected to observe sleep enhancement after EAc on the Anmian acupoints, we chose to conduct EAc before the beginning of the dark period and analyzed sleep alterations during the dark period. All of the substances used for pharmacological blockade were administered directly into the NTS.

11.3 Current Results

11.3.1 Effects of Anesthetics on Sleep-Wake Activity

Since the EAc was manipulated when rats were anesthetized, we needed to determine whether the anesthesia affects sleep-wake activity. Our results demonstrated that aerial anesthetization by isoflurane exhibits no change in sleep-wake activity (Yi et al. 2004). Similarly, isoflurane failed to alter any parameter of sleep architecture or slow wave activity during SWS, suggesting that aerial anesthetic does not contribute to the subsequent sleep-wake alteration induced by EAc (Yi et al. 2004). However, anesthetization of rats for 25 min with ketamine/xylazine before the onset of the dark period decreased both NREM and REM sleep during the few hours of the dark period (Cheng et al. 2011). Ketamine is a cyclohexanone derivative, which is clinically used as a dissociative anesthetic and is a non-competitive N-methyl-D-aspartate (NMDA) receptor antagonist to block cation channels (Anis et al. 1983). Administration of the NMDA receptor antagonists ketamine and MK-801 at sub-anesthetic doses produces robust and dose-dependent increases in SWS δ-rhythm (Feinberg and Campbell 1993, 1995). MK-801 induces the enhancement of physiological sleep by increasing the metabolic rate in the hippocampus and other limbic structures, which may cause the suppression of NREM and REM sleep after recovery from the ketamine anesthetization due to homeostatic compensation (Campbell and Feinberg 1999). However, the effect of ketamine on sleep suppression after anesthetic recovery does not mask our observation, because EAc is expected to increase sleep rather than decrease sleep.

11.3.2 Sleep Alterations After 10 Hz EAc Stimuli on Bilateral Anmian Acupoints

A single 20-min 10 Hz EAc stimulation of the bilateral Anmian acupoints did not change the amount of NREM sleep and wakefulness during the dark period. However, REM sleep was increased after the single 20-min 10 Hz EAc stimulation (Yi et al. 2004). When EAc stimulation (for 20 min at 10 Hz) is performed on two consecutive days, NREM and REM sleep increase during the dark period (Yi et al. 2004). In contrast, when rats receive sham EAc on non-acupoints, no effect is observed on sleep-wake activity, which underlines the specificity of EAc upon Anmian acupoints on sleep regulation (Yi et al. 2004). Our results also demonstrate that the slow wave activity during SWS was not altered after the 20-min 10 Hz EAc stimulation on two consecutive days (Yi et al. 2004). These results suggest that 10 Hz EAc enhances the quantity of sleep, rather than the quality of sleep.

11.3.3 Scopolamine Blocks 10 Hz EAc-Induced Sleep Alterations

Activation of vagus nerves mediates the therapeutic effects of acupuncture (Wang et al. 2002), while suppression of vagal activity ether by vagotomy or blockade of cholinergic receptors reduces the effect of acupuncture (Noguchi and Hayashi 1996; Uvnas-Moberg et al. 1992). The caudal NTS primarily receives afferents from the vagus nerves (Cottle 1964) and is involved in sleep-wake regulation (Bonvallet and Allen 1963; Magnes et al. 1961). Previous findings suggest that the NTS mediates the effects of acupuncture (Huang et al. 1991). Therefore, we hypothesized that the effect of 10 Hz EAc-induced sleep enhancement is relayed through the NTS. The NTS contains a high density of muscarinic cholinergic receptors (Hyde et al. 1988). Administration of carbachol directly into the NTS increases REM sleep (Danguir and Saint-Hilaire-Kafi 1988), while electrical stimulation of the NTS increases the amount of NREM sleep and the synchronization of the delta rhythm in EEGs

(Bronzino et al. 1976; Cottle 1964; Golanov and Reis 2001). We first determined whether a cholinergic receptor antagonist blocks the sleep enhancement induced by 10 Hz EAc. Systemic administration of the muscarinic receptor antagonist scopolamine dose-dependently blocks the enhancement of NREM and REM sleep after 10 Hz EAc stimuli (Yi et al. 2004), but does not alter SWA during NREM sleep (Yi et al. 2004). This result suggests the involvement of cholinergic receptors in EAc-induced sleep enhancement. However, pharmacological evidence demonstrates that cholinergic function mediates cortical activation and wakefulness (Domino et al. 1968; Jouvet 1984) and our data have shown enhancement of NREM sleep after intraperitoneal administration of scopolamine in normal rats without EAc (Yi et al. 2004). The effects of scopolamine on sleep have opposite effects upon rats treated with and without EAc, which can be explained by the fact that the muscarinic receptors involved in the action of EAc differ from those that mediate spontaneous sleep. Cholinergic neurons in the basal forebrain are well-known for their involvement in cortical activation and wakefulness (Lo Conte et al. 1982; Stewart et al. 1984), which explains the effect of systemic application of scopolamine on sleep enhancement. Nevertheless, cholinergic neurons in the caudal NTS may mediate sleep and involve EAc-induced sleep alteration. Therefore, we hypothesized that cholinergic neurons in the caudal NTS mediate EAc-induced sleep enhancement.

11.3.4 Bilateral NTS Lesion Blocks 10 Hz EAc-Induced Sleep Enhancement

To test our hypothesis, we lesioned the caudal NTS by applying a 15-s electrical current at 3 mA through two bipolar electrodes placed bilaterally in the caudal NTS. Our findings demonstrate that bilateral electrical lesion of the caudal NTS blocks the enhancement in NREM and REM sleep induced by 10 Hz EAc, but does not alter any parameter of sleep-wake activity in normal rats that do not receive EAc during the dark period (Yi et al. 2004). Since the caudal NTS mediates sleep regulation, it is reasonable to expect that NTS lesioning will not change sleep-wake activity during the active (dark) period when rats are mostly awake. Our results demonstrate that a lesion essentially confined to the caudal NTS markedly blocks the effects of EAc on sleep activity, suggesting the mechanistic involvement of the caudal NTS in EAc.

11.3.5 Effects of Opioid Antagonists on 10 Hz EAc-Induced Sleep Enhancement

EAc increases β-endorphin levels in the arcuate nucleus of the hypothalamus, which mediates the analgesic effects of EAc (Han 2003). There are two anatomically distinct β-endorphin pathways in the brain; the first originates from the arcuate nucleus of the hypothalamus, while the other lies in the caudal NTS (Bronstein et al. 1993). Therefore, it is reasonable to hypothesize that the effect of EAc upon sleep regulation is also caused by the function of endogenous opioid peptides in the caudal NTS. Previous publications have shown that microinjection of morphine into the NTS gives rise to a dose-dependent enhancement of NREM sleep, which is blocked by naloxone, demonstrating the involvement of endogenous opioids in sleep (Reinoso-Barbero and de Andres 1995). Some reports have documented that the endogenous opioid system in the NTS could be activated in response to vagal activation (Ni et al. 1989; Zou et al. 1993). Based on the evidence, the effects of EAc on sleep-wake regulation may be mediated by activation of caudal NTS neurons directly via muscarinic receptors or via cholinergic receptor-mediated increase of endogenous opioids in the caudal NTS. We therefore sought to clarify the involvement of endogenous opioids in the EAc effect.

Our results show that administration of three different doses of the broadspectrum opioid receptor antagonist naloxone into the caudal NTS dose-dependently suppresses 10 Hz EAc-induced sleep enhancement (Cheng et al. 2011). This result implicates the involvement of opioid receptors of the NTS in EAc-induced sleep enhancement. Three main opioid receptors, including μ-, δ-, and κ-opioid receptors, are involved in the underlying mechanisms of EAc-induced analgesia. The endogenous opioids include endomorphin, dynorphin, enkephalin and β-endorphin. Endomorphin is a relatively pure μ-opioid receptor agonist, dynorphin is a κ-opioid receptor agonist, and enkephalin and β-endorphin are mixed μ- and δ-opioid agonists (Han 2004; Waldhoer et al. 2004). Different opioids and receptor subtypes mediate different frequencies of EAc on analgesia (Han 2004). Low-frequency EAc increases enkephalin, but not dynorphin, to induce analgesia, while the effect of high-frequency EAc on analgesia is due to an increase in dynorphin levels (Fei et al. 1987). In addition, it has been demonstrated that both μ- and δ-opioid receptors mediate low-frequency EAc-induced analgesia, and that the analgesic effect of high-frequency EAc is mediated by κ-opioid receptors (Han et al. 1986; Chen and Han 1992). Our investigations explored the involvement of opioid receptors in sleep regulation after 10 Hz EAc. We found that administration of the μ-opioid receptor antagonist, naloxonazine, also dose-dependently blocks EAc-induced NREM sleep enhancement, whereas neither naltrindole (δ-opioid antagonist) nor norbinaltorphimine (κ-opioid antagonist) exhibit effects upon EAc-induced sleep alterations (Cheng et al. 2011). This observation is similar to that observed by Dr. Han and his colleagues, who have reported that the analgesic effect induced by lowfrequency EAc is mediated by μ- and δ-opioid receptors, while analgesia induced by high-frequency EAc is mediated by the κ-opioid receptor (Han et al. 1986; Chen and Han 1992).

11.3.6 Change of β-Endorphin Levels After 10 Hz EAc

Our results demonstrate that β-endorphin levels in the brainstem and hippocampus increase after 10 Hz EAc stimulation, suggesting the involvement of NTS β-endorphins (Cheng et al. 2011). Furthermore, the EAc-induced increase of β-endorphin is blocked by microinjection of scopolamine into the NTS (Cheng et al. 2011), which suggests that the activation of the endogenous opioidergic system by 10 Hz EAc is mediated by cholinergic receptors in the NTS. This result is consistent with the previous finding that the μ-opioid receptor mediates the effects of 10 Hz EAc upon sleep alteration.

11.3.7 Effects of Opioid Antagonists on 100 Hz EAc-Induced Sleep Enhancement

Application of 100 Hz EA stimulation to the bilateral Anmian acupoints augments NREM sleep, with an effect that is similar to that observed after 10 Hz EAc (Cheng et al. 2012). EAc-induced sleep enhancement does not differ between 10 and 100 Hz applications (Cheng et al. 2011, 2012). Naloxone dose-dependently blocks 100 Hz EAc-induced enhancement of NREM sleep when it is administered directly into the caudal NTS (Cheng et al. 2012). To determine the specific involvement of opioid receptors in 100 Hz EAc, three different antagonists for μ-, δ- and κ-opioid receptors were administered directly into the caudal NTS. Our results demonstrate that norbinaltorphimine, a κ-opioid receptor antagonist, exhibited a similar dose-dependent effect on blocking EAc-induced enhancement of NREM sleep as that of naloxone, while naloxonazine (a μ-opioid receptor antagonist) and naltrindole (a δ-opioid receptor antagonist) had no such effect (Cheng et al. 2012). This result suggests that the effect of 100 Hz EAc on NREM sleep enhancement is mediated by the κ-opioid receptors, rather than the μ- and δ-opioid receptors.

These findings elucidate that distinct opioid receptors in the NTS mediate the NREM sleep enhancement through different opioid receptors; NREM sleep enhancement induced by 10 Hz EAc is mediated by μ-opioid receptors, while the sleep increase caused by 100 Hz EAc is the consequence of κ-opioid receptors. The underlying mechanisms of the NTS opioid receptors involved in sleep regulation by EAc are similar to those of EAc-induced analgesia in the spinal cord as reported by Han and his colleagues (Han et al. 1986; Chen and Han 1992). A diagram elucidating one hypothetical mechanism by which different frequencies of EA at Anmian (EX17) alter sleep is depicted in the Fig. 11.1.

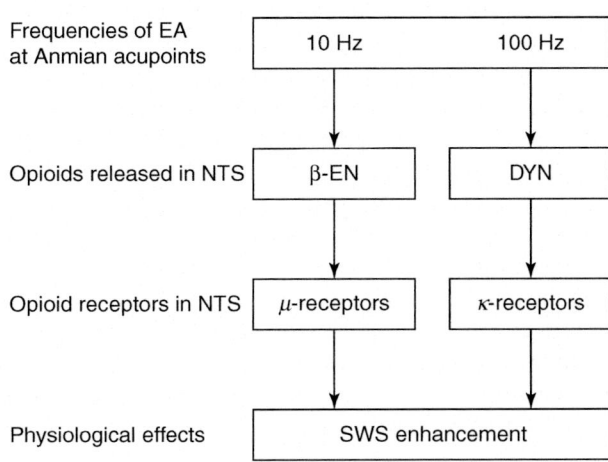

Fig. 11.1 *EA* electroacupuncture, *NTS* nucleus tractus solitarius, *β-EN* β-endorphin, *DYN* dynorphin, *SWS* slow-wave sleep

11.4   Future Directions for Acupuncture Study

In our previous studies, we found that both 10 and 100 Hz EAc stimulation of Anmian acupoints before the beginning of the dark period increased NREM sleep during the dark (active) period in rats. Furthermore, we have found that EAc may activate the vagus nerve and relay the signals to the caudal NTS, as lesioning of the NTS blocks the effect induced by EAc. We also demonstrate that the opioid receptors in the caudal NTS mediate the EAc-induced sleep alterations; the μ-opioid receptors are involved in the effects of 10 Hz EAc upon sleep, while the κ-opioid receptors mediate NREM sleep enhancement induced by 100 Hz EAc. All of these findings suggest that EAc low- or high-frequency stimulation on the bilateral Anmian (EX17) acupoints before the active period of the light:dark cycle increases sleep during the dark period in rats. Although we performed EAc before the active period and observed sleep alterations in the active period, this is the most efficient way to screen for the manipulation that is expected to exhibit a somnogenic effect, as according to the rationale that we mentioned earlier. Future research is needed to further confirm the effect of EAc upon the bilateral Anmian acupoints in an insomniac animal model. Our unpublished data and other researchers have established insomniac rat models by employing psychological stress, such as the cage exchange procedure (personal unpublished data; Cano et al. 2008). EAc will be given either before or after stress-induced insomnia.

Sleep can be easily disturbed by many medical and health conditions. For example, it has been well documented that epilepsy and sleep reciprocally affect each other. Epilepsy is often accompanied by co-morbid sleep disruptions (Malow et al. 1997; Stores et al. 1998). Notably, epilepsy-induced sleep disruptions further deteriorate and worsen seizure control (Bazil 2002). Furthermore, different stages of sleep influence epilepsy differently; REM sleep suppresses seizure activity, while NREM sleep facilitates epileptogenesis (Kumar and Raju 2001; Shouse et al. 2000). A therapy that possesses both epilepsy suppression and improvement of sleep disturbance will become the most appropriate therapy for seizure control. Another example is Parkinson's disease. The excessive somnolence in Parkinsonian rats induced by MG-132 and rotenone is mediated, respectively, by the pro-inflammatory cytokines, tumor-necrosis factor-α (TNF-α) and interleukin-1β (IL-1β) (Lu et al. 2010; Yi et al. 2007). The involvement of pro-inflammatory cytokines in the pathogenesis of epilepsy and Parkinson's disease has been documented and discussed (Huang et al. 2016; Li et al. 2011; Nagatsu and Mogi 1998). Furthermore, acupuncture or electroacupuncture exhibits anti-inflammatory effects in the peripheral and central nervous systems (McDonald et al. 2013; Lan et al. 2013). Based on the evidence, acupuncture or EA seems to be an appropriate therapy to improve sleep disruptions induced by neurological disease. Our previous results also demonstrate that the opioid receptors in the caudal NTS mediate effects on epileptogenesis and epilepsy-induced sleep alterations (Yi et al. 2013, 2013, 2015).

In this chapter, we have discussed the role of opioid receptors in the caudal NTS in mediating EAc-induced sleep alterations. Our results conclude that the enhancement of NREM sleep induced by 10 Hz EAc is mediated by μ-opioid receptors, while the increase in sleep caused by 100 Hz EAc is the consequence of κ-opioid receptors. The underlying mechanisms of the NTS opioid receptors involved in sleep regulation by EAc are similar to those of EAc-induced analgesia in the spinal cord as reported by Han and his colleagues (Han et al. 1986; Chen and Han 1992). Furthermore, acupuncture or EA not only improve sleep *per se* but are also associated with benefits in epileptogenesis and epilepsy-induced sleep alteration.

References

Anis NA, Berry SC, Burton NR, Lodge D. The dissociative anaesthetics, ketamine and phencyclidine, selectively reduce excitation of central mammalian neurones by N-methyl-aspartate. Br J Pharmacol. 1983;79:565–75.

Bazil CW. Sleep and epilepsy. Semin Neurol. 2002;22:321–7.

Belt NK, Kronholm E, Kauppi MJ. Sleep problems in fibromyalgia and rheumatoid arthritis compared with the general population. Clin Exp Rheumatol. 2009;27:35–41.

Berk M. Sleep and depression—theory and practice. Aust Fam Physician. 2009;38:302–4.

Bonvallet M, Allen MB Jr. Prolonged spontaneous and evoked reticular activation following discrete bulbar lesions. Electroencephalogr Clin Neurophysiol. 1963;15:969–88.

Brenes GA, Miller ME, Stanley MA, Williamson JD, Knudson M, McCall WV. Insomnia in older adults with generalized anxiety disorder. Am J Geriatr Psychiatry. 2009;17:465–72.

Bronstein DM, Day NC, Gutstein HB, Trujillo KA, Akil H. Pre- and posttranslational regulation of beta-endorphin biosynthesis in the CNS, effects of chronic naltrexone treatment. J Neurochem. 1993;60:40–9.

Bronzino JD, Stern WC, Leahy JP, Morgane PJ. Power spectral analysis of EEG activity obtained from cortical and subcortical sites during the vigilance states of the cat. Brain Res Bull. 1976;1:285–94.

Campbell IG, Feinberg I. Comparison of MK-801 and sleep deprivation effects on NREM, REM, and waking spectra in the rat. Sleep. 1999;22:423–32.

Cano G, Mochizuki T, Saper CB. Neural circuitry of stress-induced insomnia in rats. J Neurosci. 2008;28:10167–84.

Chen XH, Han JS. Analgesia induced by electroacupuncture of different frequencies is mediated by different types of opioid receptors: another cross-tolerance study. Behav Brain Res. 1992;47:143–9.

Cheng G. Treatment of 55 cases of insomnia by acupuncture. Chin Acupunct Moxibustion. 1985;5:26.

Cheng LG. Observation of the therapeutic effect on treatment of 2485 cases of insomnia by needling Shenmen point. Chin Acupunct Moxibustion. 1986a;6:18–9.

Cheng XN. Traditional Chinese acupuncture and moxibustion. Beijing: People's Hygiene Press; 1986b.

Cheng RSS, Pomeranz B. Electroacupuncture analgesia could be mediated by at least two pain-relieving mechanisms: endorphin and nonendorphin system. Life Sci. 1979;25:1957–62.

Cheng CH, Yi PL, Lin JG, Chang FC. Endogenous opiates in the nucleus tractus solitarius mediate electroacupuncture-induced sleep activities in rats. Evid Based Complement Alternat Med. 2011;2011:159209.

Cheng CH, Yi PL, Chang HH, Tsai YF, Chang FC. Kappa-opioid receptors in the caudal nucleus tractus solitarius mediate 100 Hz electroacupucture-induced sleep activities in rats. Evid Based Complement Alternat Med. 2012;2012:715024.

Cottle MK. Degeneration studies of primary afferents of IXth and Xth cranial nerves in the cat. J Comp Neurol. 1964;122:329–45.

Danguir J, Saint-Hilaire-Kafi S. Somatostatin antiserum blocks carbachol-induced increase of paradoxical sleep in the rat. Brain Res Bull. 1988;20:9–12.

Domino EF, Yamamoto K, Dren AT. Role of cholinergic mechanisms in states of wakefulness and sleep. Prog Brain Res. 1968;28:113–33.

Fei H, Xie GX, Han JS. Low and high frequency electroacupuncture stimulation release [Met^5] enkephalin and dynorphin A in rat spinal cord. Sci Bull China. 1987;32:1496–501.

Feinberg I, Campell IG. Ketamine administration during waking increases delta EEG intensity in rat sleep. Neuropsychopharmacology. 1993;9:41–8.

Feinberg I, Campell IG. Stimulation of NREM delta EEG by ketamine administration during waking: demonstration of dose dependence. Neuropsychopharmacology. 1995;12:89–90.

Golanov EV, Reis DJ. Neurons of nucleus of the solitary tract synchronize the EEG and elevate cerebral blood flow via a novel medullary area. Brain Res. 2001;892:1–12.

Han JS. Acupuncture: neuropeptide release produced by electrical stimulation of different frequencies. Trends Neurosci. 2003;26:17–22.

Han JS. Acupuncture and endorphins. Neurosci Lett. 2004;361:258–61.

Han JS, Ding XZ, Fan SG. The frequency as the cardinal determinant for electroacupuncture analgesia to be reversed by opioid antagonists. Acta Physiol Sin. 1986;38:475–82.

Huang Z, Liu N, Zhong S, Lu J, Zhang N. The role of nucleus tractus solitarii (NTS) in acupuncture inhibition of visceral-somatic reflex (VSR). Zhen Ci Yan Jiu. 1991;16:43–7.

Huang TR, Jou SB, Chou YJ, Yi PL, Chen CJ, Chang FC. Interleukin-1 receptor (IL-1R) mediates epilepsy-induced sleep disruption. BMC Neurosci. 2016;17:74.

Hyde TM, Gibbs M, Peroutka SJ. Distribution of muscarinic cholinergic receptors in the dorsal vagal complex and other selected nuclei in the human medulla. Brain Res. 1988;447:287–92.

Jouvet M. Neuromédiateurs et facteurs hypnogenes. Rev Neurol (Paris). 1984;140:389–400.

Kryger MH, Roth T, Dement WC, editors. Principles and practice of sleep medicine. Philadelphia: Elsevier; 2005.

Kumar P, Raju TR. Seizure susceptibility decreases with enhancement of rapid eye movement sleep. Brain Res. 2001;922:299–304.

Lan L, Tao J, Chen A, Xie G, Huang J, Lin J, Peng J, Chen L. Electroacupuncture exerts anti-inflammatory effects in cerebral ischemia-reperfusion injured rats via suppression of TLR4/NF-B pathway. Int J Mol Med. 2013;31:75–80.

Li G, Bauer S, Nowak M, Norwood B, Tackenberg B, Rosenow F, Knake S, Oertel WH, Hamer HM. Cytokines and epilepsy. Seizure. 2011;20:249–56.

Lo Conte G, Casamenti F, Bigl V, Milaneschi E, Pepeu G. Effect of magnocellular forebrain nuclei lesions on acetylcholine output from the cerebral cortex, electrocorticogram and behavior. Arch Ital Biol. 1982;120:176–88.

Lu JS, He SH, Geng SH. Selection of treatment experience by single acupoint needling. Beijing: People's Hygiene Press; 1993.

Lu CY, Yi PL, Tsai CH, Cheng CH, Chang HH, Hsiao YT, Chang FC. TNF-NF-B signaling mediates excessive somnolence in hemiparkinsonian rats. Behav Brain Res. 2010;208:484–96.

Magnes J, Moruzzi G, Pompeiano O. Synchronization of the EEG produced by low-frequency electrical stimulation of the region of the solitary tract. Arch Ital Biol. 1961;99:33–41.

Malow BA, Bowes RJ, Lin X. Predictors of sleepiness in epilepsy patients. Sleep. 1997;20:1105–10.

McDonald JL, Cripps AW, Smith PK, Smith CA, Xue CC, Golianu B. The anti-inflammatory effects of acupuncture and their relevance to allergic rhinitis: a narrative review and proposed model. Evid Based Complement Alternat Med. 2013;2013:591796.

Melzack R, Wall PD. Pain mechanisms: a new theory. Science. 1965;150:971–9.

Nagatsu T, Mogi M. Cytokines in Parkinson's disease. In: Fisher A, Hanin I, Yoshida M, editors. Progress in Alzheimer's and Parkinson's disease. New York: Springer; 1998.

Ni H, Jing LX, Shen S. The role of medial medulla in the depressive responses in pulmonary and carotid arteries to injection of acetylcholine at fourth ventricle. Sheng Li Xue Bao. 1989;41:291–8.

Noguchi E, Hayashi H. Increase in gastric acidity in response to electroacupuncture stimulation of the hindlimb of anesthetized rats. Jpn J Physiol. 1996;46:53–8.

Norgren R. Projections from the nucleus of solitary tract in the rat. Neuroscience. 1978;3:207–18.

Paxinos G, Watson C. The rat brain in stereotaxic coordinates. 4th ed. San Diego: Academic Press; 1998.

Reinoso-Barbero F, de Andres I. Effects of opioid microinjections in the nucleus of the solitary tract on the sleep-wakefulness cycle states in cats. Anesthesiology. 1995;82:144–52.

Saper CB, Loewy DD. Efferent connections of the parabrachial nucleus in the rat. Brain Res. 1980;197:291–317.

Shouse MN, Farber PR, Staba RJ. Physiological basis: how NREM sleep components can promote and REM sleep components can suppress seizure discharge. Clin Neurophysiol. 2000;111:S9–S18.

Son YS, Park HJ, Kwon OB, Jung SC, Shin HC, Lim S. Antipyretic effects of acupuncture on the lipopolysaccharide-induced fever and expression of interleukin-6 and interleukin-1 beta mRNA in the hypothalamus of rats. Neurosci Lett. 2002;319:45–8.

Stewart DJ, MacFabe DF, Vanderwolf CH. Cholinergic activation of the electrocorticogram: role of the substantia innominate and effects of atropine and quinuclidinyl benzilate. Brain Res. 1984;322:219–32.

Stoller MK. Economic effects of insomnia. Clin Ther. 1994;16:873–97.

Stores G, Wiggs L, Campling G. Sleep disorders and their relationship to psychological disturbances in children with epilepsy. Child Care Health Dev. 1998;24:5–19.

Uvnas-Moberg K, Lundeberg T, Bruzelius G, Alster P. Vagally mediated release of gastrin and cholecystokinin following sensory stimulation. Acta Physiol Scand. 1992;146:349–56.

Van Someren EJW. Circadian and sleep disturbances in the elderly. Exp Gerontol. 2005;35:1229–37.

Waldhoer M, Bartlett S, Whistler J. Opioid receptors. Annu Rev Biochem. 2004;73:953–90.

Walsh JK, Engelhardt CL. The direct economic costs of insomnia in the United States for 1995. Sleep. 1999;22:S386–93.

Wang JD, Kuo TB, Yang CC. An alternative method to enhance vagal activities and suppress sympathetic activities in humans. Auton Neurosci. 2002;100:90–5.

Yi PL, Tsai CH, Lin JG, Liu HJ, Chang FC. Effects of electroacupuncture at 'Anmian (extra)' acupoints on sleep activities in rats: the implication of the caudal nucleus tractus solitarius. J Biomed Sci. 2004;11:579–90.

Yi PL, Tsai CH, Lu MK, Liu HJ, Chen YC, Chang FC. Interleukin-1 mediates sleep alteration in rats with rotenone-induced parkinsonism. Sleep. 2007;30:413–25.

Yi PL, Lu CY, Cheng CH, Tsai YF, Lin CT, Chang FC. Amygdala opioid receptors mediate the electroacupuncture-induced deterioration of sleep disruptions in epilepsy rats. J Biomed Sci. 2013;20:85.

Yi PL, Lu CY, Jou SB, Chang FC. Low-frequency electroacupuncture suppresses focal epilepsy and improves epilepsy-induced sleep disruptions. J Biomed Sci. 2015;22:49.

Yi PL, Jou SB, Wu YJ, Chang FC. Manipulation of epileptiform electrocorticograms (ECoGs) and sleep in rats and mice by acupuncture. J Vis Exp. 2016;118:e54896.

Zou CJ, Gu YH, Chang YZ. Roles of vagal projection area afferents on vagal input-evoked depressor response. Sheng Li Xue Bao. 1993;45:561–7.

High-Tech Acupuncture Research: Laser Acupuncture

12

Gerhard Litscher

Abstract

Basic and clinical research on high-tech acupuncture has been performed at the Research Unit of Biomedical Engineering in Anesthesia and Intensive Care Medicine and the TCM Research Center at the Medical University of Graz in cooperation with partners in Asia since 1997. This book chapter focuses on the latest innovative aspects that underline the further enhancement and development of acupuncture. Special emphasis is given to totally new methodological and technical investigations, e.g. results obtained from teleacupuncture and violet as well as yellow laser acupuncture. In addition a summary and recent result of auricular medicine including auricular acupuncture will be reported briefly.

Keywords

High-tech acupuncture network · Teleacupuncture · Laser acupuncture · Violet laser acupuncture · Yellow laser acupuncture · Auricular medicine · Auricular acupuncture

G. Litscher
TCM Research Center Graz, Research Unit of Biomedical Engineering in Anesthesia and Intensive Care Medicine, and Research Unit for Complementary and Integrative Laser Medicine, Medical University of Graz, Graz, Austria

China Medical University, Taichung, Taiwan
e-mail: gerhard.litscher@medunigraz.at

© Springer Nature Singapore Pte Ltd. 2018
J.-G. Lin (ed.), *Experimental Acupuncturology*,
https://doi.org/10.1007/978-981-13-0971-7_12

183

12.1 Transcontinental High-Tech Acupuncture Network

High-tech acupuncture, that is the demystification of acupuncture by modern technical methods, is an important bridging in transcontinental research projects.

Basic research on high-tech acupuncture has been successfully performed in Graz since 1997 (http://litscher.info) using a broad spectrum of methods (Fig. 12.1). Main goal of this innovative project is to combine basic research on the topic of high-tech acupuncture with necessary further experimental and clinical pilot studies (age-related diseases including metabolic syndrome, chronic diseases, lifestyle-related diseases etc.) in Asia and Europe for the first time.

Acupuncture has been used for medical treatment for thousands of years. A large number of empirical data is available but the technical quantification of effects was not possible up to now. Using needle, electro acupuncture or laser needle stimulation and modern biomedical techniques, it was possible to quantify changes in biological activities caused by acupuncture (Litscher G. 2002, 2006a, b, c, d, e, 2007a, b, 2008, 2009, 2010a, b, c; Litscher G. and Schikora 2002; Litscher G. et al. 1999, 2009; Zhang et al. 2008).

The patient is in Asia—the analysis for the efficacy of acupuncture is performed by experts in Europe (Graz). This *"transcontinental teleacupuncture"* is a way which promises and brought already new results in acupuncture research and was realized within one of our projects (Gao et al. 2012; Litscher G. 2010d, e; Wang and Litscher G. 2010). Firstly, this research has been performed on healthy volunteers in Graz, now within the last years the investigations are carried out over thousands of

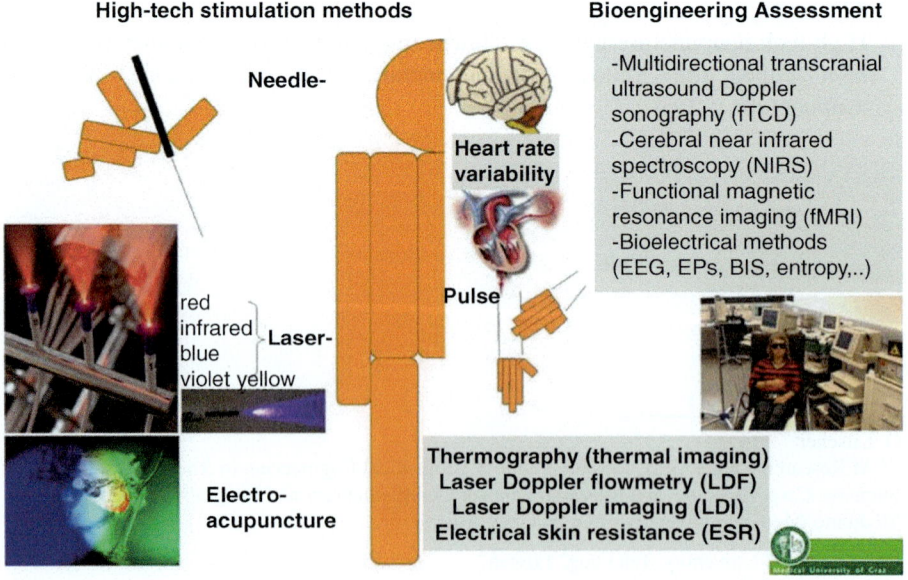

Fig. 12.1 Modernization of acupuncture

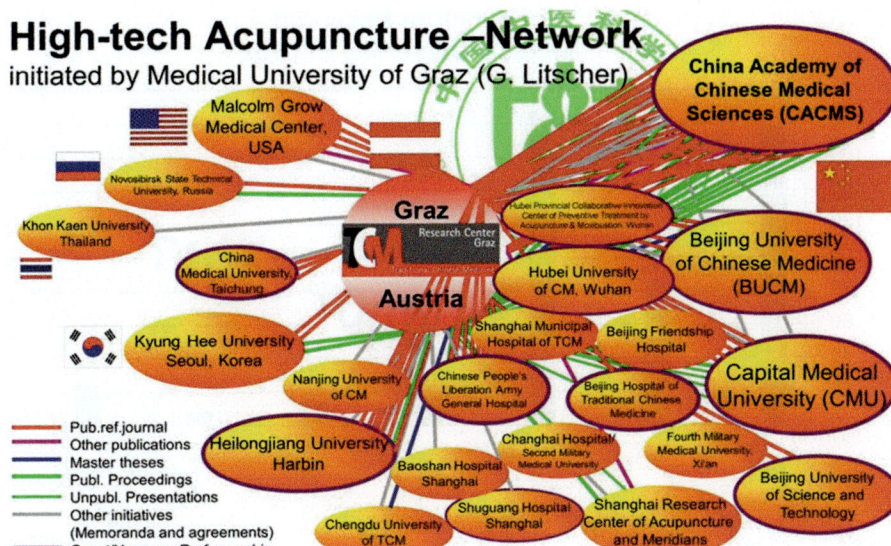

Fig. 12.2 The network of high-tech acupuncture initiated by the TCM Research Center Graz

kilometres: 24-h-electrocardiograms from patients are registered in China, and the data are transferred directly after the acupuncture treatment to an analysis computer at the Medical University of Graz. The acupuncturists in Asia are informed about the results immediately based on the analysis protocol. This innovation was introduced in several meetings and high level publications (Shu et al. 2016). Apart from the China Academy of Chinese Medical Sciences in Beijing, there are important cooperations with the Beijing University of Chinese Medicine, the Capital Medical University in Beijing, the Heilongjiang University of Chinese Medicine in Harbin, the Hubei University of Chinese Medicine in Wuhan and the China Medical University in Taichung which is partly already reflected in many publications on the topic (see Fig. 12.2). Another important column is the completion of master theses, all of which are based on data acquired in Asia and Europe by the medical students. A special emphasis is also put on public relations, which is reflected by participation in important exhibitions and press reports.

The scientific output of the last 10 years of the acupuncture research at the TCM Research Center Graz at Medical University of Graz is shown in Fig. 12.3.

Within the last 10 years, altogether 186 first order outputs (publications in refereed journals) have been published together with our colleagues in Asia. In addition, 85 conference papers and proceedings have been published. Seventeen master theses and dissertations from the Medical University of Graz were supervised in cooperation with partners in Asia. One important point was the use of partners' research infrastructure and equipment: seven different types of equipment were used in China and Austria respectively. The project—the high-tech acupuncture network— is interacting with several other teams in Austria, Europe, Asia and the USA.

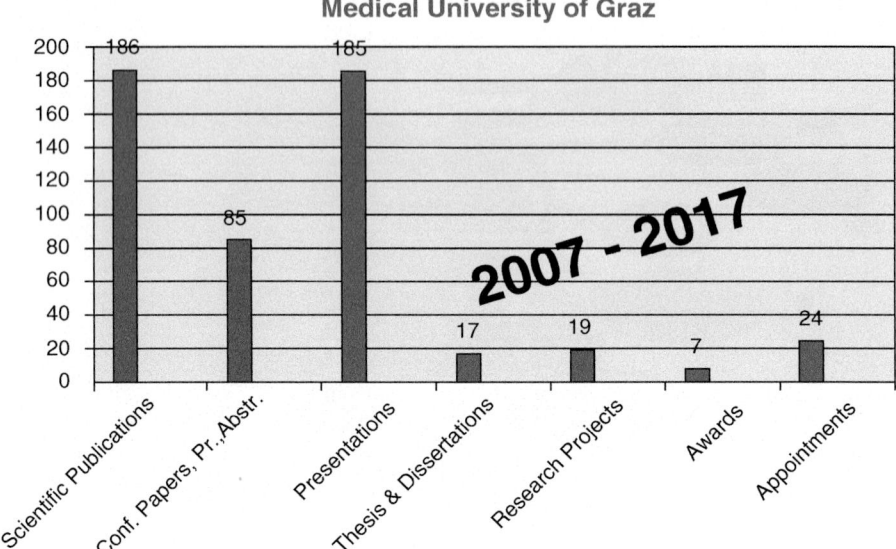

Fig. 12.3 Scientific output of the acupuncture research at the TCM Research Center, Medical University of Graz (Head Prof. Gerhard Litscher)

12.2 Traditional Chinese Medicine (TCM) Research Center Graz

There are different applications of the laser in medicine. The invention of the laser celebrated its 55th anniversary in 2015, but there are still some areas especially in traditional medicine that require intensive innovative laser research. One of these research field is laser acupuncture.

TCM is booming and is effective: It has been practiced with great success for thousands of years, and interest to complement classical Western medicine has been increasing for many years. Graz has a central role in the study of TCM in the world. In 2007 the Research Center of TCM was established, and a global network of high-tech acupuncture has been developed (see Fig. 12.2), which integrates the various national and international activities in research and teaching. The Medical University of Graz and the University Graz are the two Austrian universities doing research in the forefront.

The Research Unit of Biomedical Engineering in Anaesthesia and Intensive Care Medicine and the Research Unit of Complementary and Integrative Laser Medicine both at the Medical University of Graz have been dealing with acupuncture research for a long period. In this case, evidence-based, scientific work is the foundation. Consequently, all research is carried out on the basis of scientific methods (see also Fig. 12.1).

The interest of TCM in Europe has also grown in recent years. More than 70% of the Austrians want conventional Western medicine to be supplemented by complementary medicine. Similar data exist in Germany and Switzerland. The acceptance of TCM is very high, with an approval rate of 80%. However, not only the patients, even the doctors show a growing interest. For the city of Graz the establishment of the competence center will have long-term positive impacts: already existing cooperations with institutions that perform research in the field of TCM will be multiplied, and the know-how transfer between Austria and Asia will also be intensified.

12.3   Violet Laser Acupuncture

The first results concerning the 'violet laser needle acupuncture', were presented in 2010 and 2011. Significant effects such as increases in blood flow in small vessels with the violet wavelength of 405 nm (Fig. 12.4) and a specially focused beam at the acupuncture point, despite low penetration depth were obtained.

Within joint research projects between Austria and Asia, first scientific results on this violet laser acupuncture method were published (Litscher G. et al. 2010; Wang et al. 2011). The violet laser is able to trigger a deqi feeling, which is usually typical only for needle acupuncture. This often manifests itself as a mild electric tingling.

For people in Asia, this deqi feeling is necessary for a successful treatment with acupuncture. With a red or infrared laser the stimulus is not immediately felt. This is different using the violet laser needle. Chinese adult volunteers reported a stimulus, similar to a deqi feeling evoked by a metal needle. The acupoint Neiguan was stimulated and there was a significant decrease in heart rate associated with a pleasant, stress-reducing feeling. This acupoint (Pericard 6) is located near the wrist crease should have a circulatory-regulating effect. This effect did not occur in a control study in which the violet laser was switched off. Further investigations, concerning the question whether this effect is also present in Europeans have to be performed.

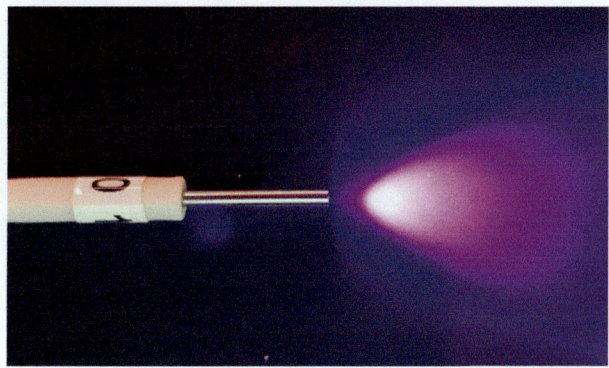

Fig. 12.4 Example of a violet laser acupuncture 'needle'

12.4   Yellow Laser Acupuncture

Many different kinds of lasers have been used in acupuncture and integrative medicine within the last years. The first yellow laser for medical purposes was constructed in Germany in 2014 after several years of research and development. This
system is available for example for non-invasive acupuncture treatment at the
Medical University of Graz, where it is being used for evidence-based medical
research at the Research Center for Traditional Chinese Medicine (Fig. 12.5)
(Litscher D. et al. 2015a). Yellow laser represents a new option, e.g. in the field of
laser acupuncture, in addition to the already existing red, near infrared, green and
violet lasers. First evidence suggests that the yellow laser may be able to stimulate
the mitochondrial respiratory chain at complex III (cytochrome) (Litscher D. et al.
2015a).

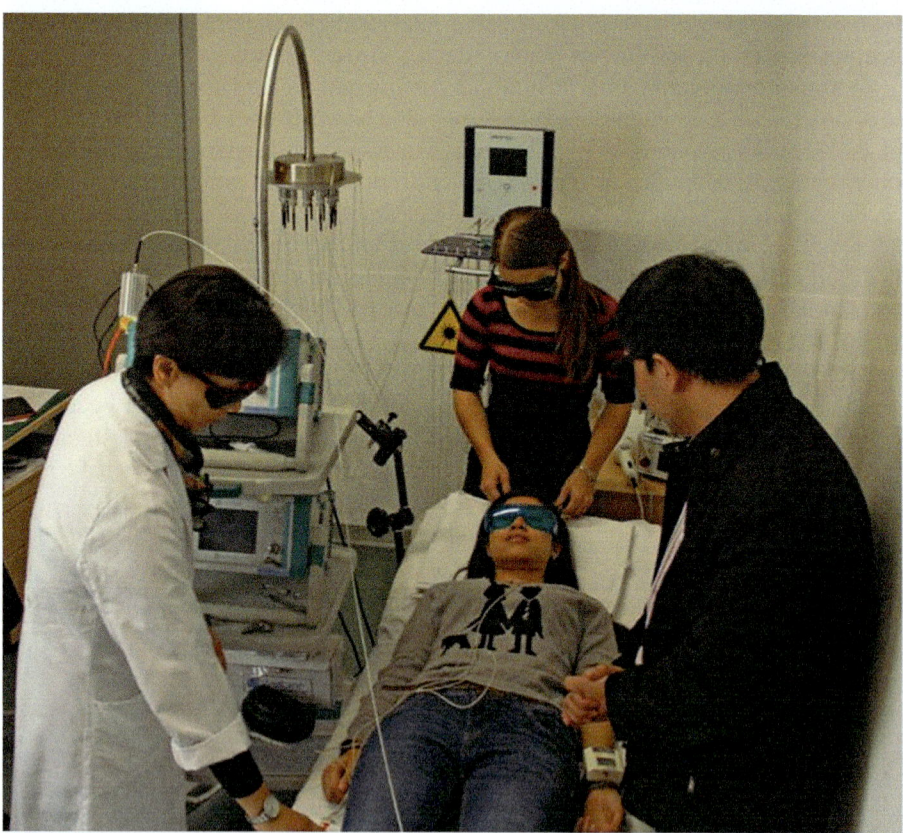

Fig. 12.5 Yellow laser stimulation at the Medical University of Graz

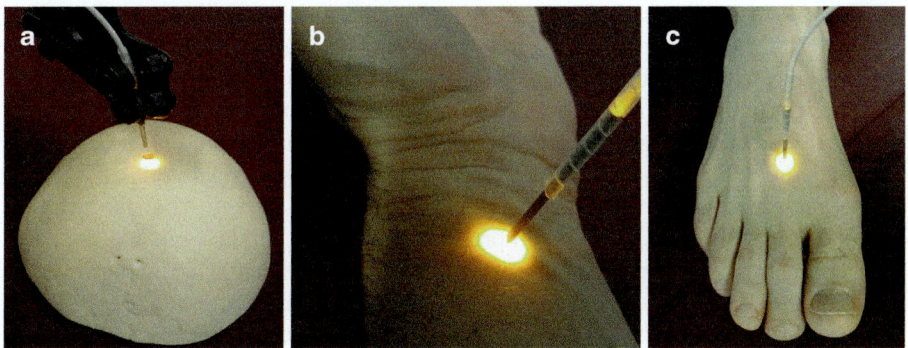

Fig. 12.6 Acupoints used in the first yellow laser acupuncture study. (**a**) Baihui, (**b**) Neiguan, (**c**) Taichong

> "Lifestyle-related diseases are a big problem in our society. For example stroke is one of the leading causes of death worldwide. But not only the elderly population is affected by this kind of diseases, also more and more young people are among the patients. A previous study from our research team had proven that the yellow laser could penetrate the skull, and therefore might be a promising new approach for the noninvasive stroke therapy. Also dementia is a big problem for our population. Mainly because of the movement in the age pyramid, experts assume that the incidence of dementia will show an enormous increase worldwide in the coming decades." (Litscher D. et al. 2015a).

Another big problem, which is related to many of those lifestyle-related diseases, is hypertonic blood pressure (BP). In a study performed by our team (Litscher D. et al. 2015a), which was the first trial worldwide using yellow laser acupuncture, the effects of yellow laser on BP were investigated in volunteers. A significant decrease of the systolic BP was found. This might be an effect of the combination of all acupoints used. Therefore one can assume that stimulation with yellow laser on the acupoints Baihui, Neiguan and Taichong (Fig. 12.6), applied one after another, could be useful in the treatment of hypertonic patients. We also compared the difference between female and male volunteers. In women the systolic BP decreased significantly, but not in men. This could appear because women might be more sensitive to the effects of yellow laser. Diastolic BP also decreased, but not significantly (Litscher D. et al. 2015a).

One of the future aims of our research is to investigate whether simultaneous yellow laser stimulation of the acupoints mentioned above results in more pronounced decreases in BP than the successive stimulation and to compare these findings to those of the pilot study (Litscher D. et al. 2015a). Other goals are to demonstrate possible effects of yellow laser, applied transcranially, on mean blood flow velocity in the middle cerebral artery. This is a very important topic in the field of laser therapy and might have promising positive effects in the treatment of lifestyle-related diseases.

The yellow laser works with a wavelength of 589 nm and an output power of 50 mW, and the fiber diameter is 500 μm. The one-channel Weberneedle yellow Endolaser system (Weber Medical, Lauenförde, Germany) is currently available at the Medical University of Graz. From the technical point of view, it is not easy to produce yellow laser light. Usually, a laser consists of an infrared laser diode and a so-called combo crystal. This pair of crystals produces the visible laser light. In this process, the combo crystal receives the necessary energy from the infrared diode. For a green laser, one crystal produces laser light of 1064 nm and the other one doubles the frequency, which means that the wavelength is divided in half, resulting in 532 nm, i.e. green light. For yellow laser light to be produced, 1340 nm is necessary. If these were simply frequency-doubled, the emitted laser light would be red, but if red and green light is mixed, the result is yellow light. It is, however, a disadvantage that at 1340 nm only very little light is emitted, so the infrared diode needs to have a large power. Moreover, special filters have to be used in order for the correct ratio of 1064 and 1340 nm to permeate. This makes the production expensive and complex, which is why yellow lasers are very expensive and accordingly rare (Litscher D. et al. 2015a).

Baihui is located at electroencephalographic (EEG) electrode position C_z, on the continuation of the line connecting the lowest and highest points of the ear, on the median line of the head, and it is thought to be a very effective point, with a general sedative and harmonizing effect. The acupoint Baihui serves as acupuncture point, but is also used as transcranial stimulation area. It could be shown in a previous study (Litscher G. et al. 2015b) that the yellow laser is able to penetrate the human skull (Fig. 12.7).

Neiguan is located at the wrist, between the tendons of m. palmaris longus and m. flexor carpi radialis, 2 cun (1 cun = width of a person's thumb at the knuckle)

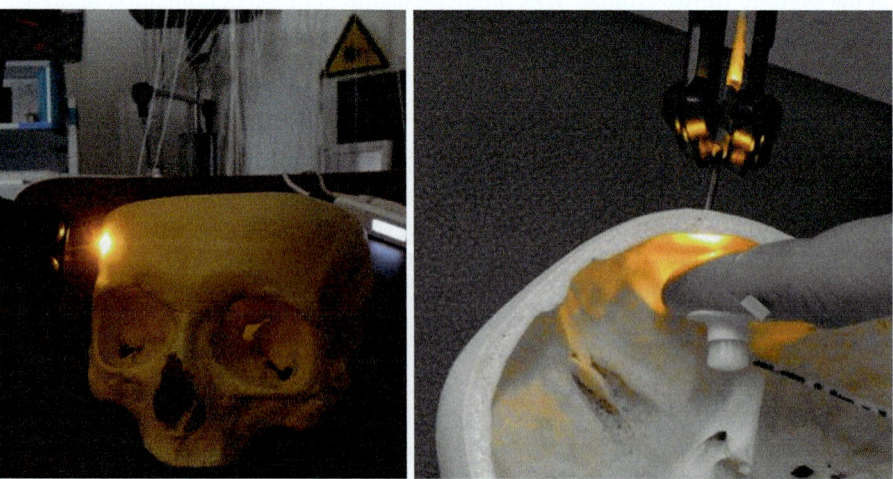

Fig. 12.7 Yellow laser (589 nm) can penetrate the human skull

proximal to the transverse crease of the wrist, and it is a very important point in disorders of the upper abdomen and for heart disorders. Taichong is located on the dorsum of the foot, between the first and second metatarsal bones, 2 cun proximal to the margin of the web; it should be a very important point in the treatment of hypertension.

Laser in general and acupuncture and transcranial laser therapy in particular are exciting, future-oriented topics in the field of TCM and biomedical research. A large number of empirical data is available for needle acupuncture stimulation, but only few evidence-based data can be found for the different kinds of laser stimulation. Up to now, only one study concerning yellow laser acupuncture is published (Litscher D. et al. 2015a). Using optical stimulation and modern biomedical techniques like blood pressure investigations, heart rate variability measurements and transcranial Doppler sonographic recordings, changes in different parameters can now be objectified under laser stimulation.

12.5   Teleacupuncture: Patient is in Asia, the Analysis in Europe

The so-called 'transcontinental teleacupuncture' is even more spectacular. First studies have been carried out successfully: 24-h registrations of the heart beat were recorded in patients in Asia with a system developed in Graz. Immediately after the treatment the heart beat data were sent from bedside computers in Beijing, Harbin and Wuhan over a distance of more than 7000 km for computer analysis at the Medical University of Graz (Gao et al. 2012, Litscher G. 2010d, e; Shi et al. 2013). Computer-based heart rate and heart rate variability measurements are important variables in this content.

Already the ancient medical expert Wang Shu-He (~220 BC.) stated: "If the heartbeat becomes as regular as the beating of the woodpecker or the dripping of rain on the roof the patient will be dead within four days." A variable heart rate as a good sign of health is therefore already very well known. HRV represents percentage changes of consecutive ventricular complexes in the electrocardiogram, and is modulated by the blood-pressure control system, influences from the hypothalamus and especially by the vagal part of centres in the lower brain stem.

Figure 12.8 shows the improvement in health (sleep-wake cycle) of a 31-year-old female patient from Beijing over the course of more than 2 months. At the beginning of treatment the sleep-wake cycle is not clearly marked. After ten acupuncture treatments the pattern has clearly changed. The therapeutic effect of acupuncture can be visualized not only subjectively, as described by the patient, but with computer-based objective data (Litscher G. 2010d).

The innovative research on laser acupuncture (telecacupuncture) between Europe and Asia shows one thing clearly: Bridging the gap between Eastern and Western medicine has become reality thanks to modern technology.

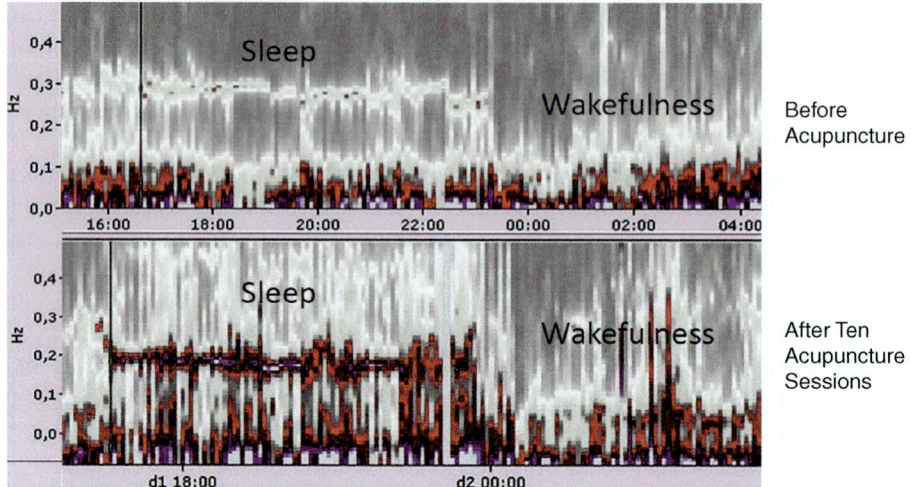

Fig. 12.8 Transcontinental teleacupuncture measurements between Europe (Graz) and Asia (Beijing). Sympathetic and vagal activity is shown during sleep and in the awake state

12.6   Innovative Research on Auricular Medicine

Auricular therapy has a long history. Ear acupoint research has been advancing step by step worldwide. Within our research center new developments and results from innovative research on auricular medicine have been published recently (Litscher D. and Litscher G. 2016; Litscher G. et al. 2011a, b; Niemtzow et al. 2009; Rong et al. 2015; Round et al. 2013; Széles and Litscher G. 2004). The introduction of lasers into medicine brought besides the already existing stimulation with needles, electricity, pressure and liquids an additional technique to auricular acupuncture. The latest scientific findings on auricular acupuncture with laser (infrared, red, blue, green and yellow) have been discussed in these publications in context to the evidence to clinical applications. Furthermore a new system for ear vibration stimulation and the resulting acute effects of vibration and manual ear acupressure on heart rate, heart rate variability, pulse wave velocity, and the augmentation index using new non-invasive recording methods has also been developed.

The reflex auriculo-cardiac (RAC; also vascular autonomic signal) is an important method in auricular medicine. New methodological approaches for the detection and quantification of the RAC from the Medical University of Graz have been developed. A new high-resolution imaging technique for the registration of pulsatory surface changes might allow the RAC to be quantified reproducibly for the first time. The methods combine innovative microscope systems, video analysis software, special image processing software and visualization of biologically active ear points (Litscher G. et al. 2011a; Navrotsky et al. 2015). Even small, pulse-dependent alterations of the skin surface can be clearly visualized.

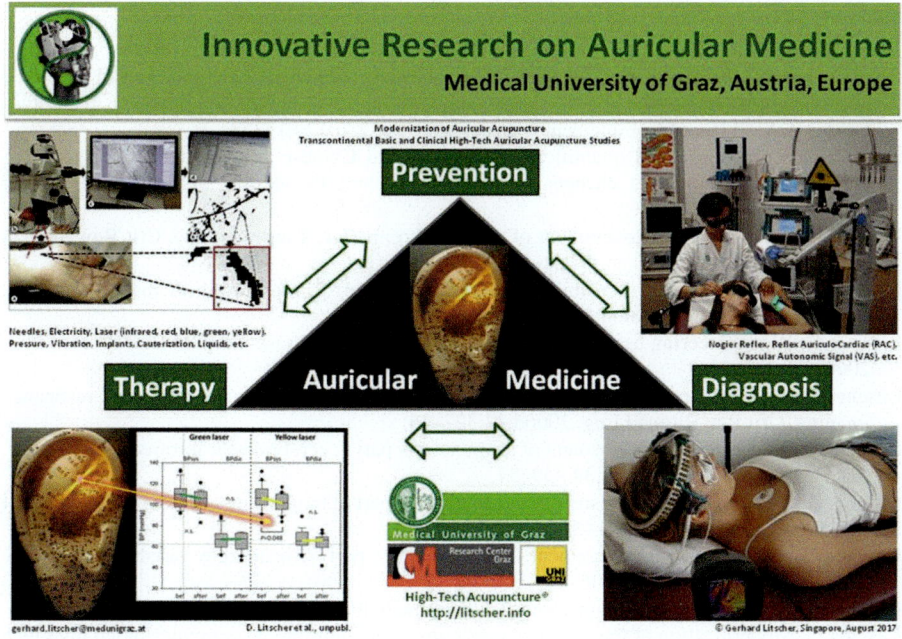

Fig. 12.9 Auricular medicine research at Medical University of Graz

European-Asian transcontinental basic and clinical high-tech auricular acupuncture studies demonstrate the modernization of auricular acupuncture and the scientific way from auricular therapy to auricular medicine (Fig. 12.9).

Conclusion

Since 1997 the Research Unit of Biomedical Engineering in Anesthesia and Intensive Care Medicine and in succession the TCM Research Center Graz at the Medical University of Graz has been dealing with the demystification of acupuncture and examining, using non-invasive methods, how different stimulation modalities (manual needle acupuncture, laser needle acupuncture, electro acupuncture) affect peripheral and central functions. However, as already mentioned several times, all aspects concerning the medical application of yellow laser stimulation are completely new, and only very few basic research on this topic exists up to now. Therefore basic research on this topic is absolutely necessary to obtain evidence-based data before such systems can be used in clinical practice.

Acknowledgements The studies were supported by the Austrian Federal Ministry of Education, Science and Research and the German Academy of Acupuncture (DAA).

The author thanks Ms. Lu Wang, MD LA, and Ms. Daniela Litscher, MSc PhD for their valuable help, for performing acupuncture, data registration and analysis (both Research Unit of Biomedical Engineering in Anesthesia and Intensive Care Medicine and TCM Research Center Graz, Medical University of Graz).

References

Gao XY, Liu K, Zhu B, Litscher G. Sino-European transcontinental basic and clinical high-tech acupuncture studies—part 1: auricular acupuncture increases heart rate variability in anesthetized rats. Evid Based Complement Alternat Med. 2012;2012:817378.

Litscher G. Computer-based quantification of traditional Chinese-, ear- and Korean hand acupuncture: needle-induced changes of regional cerebral blood flow velocity. Neurol Res. 2002;24:377–80.

Litscher G. Bioengineering assessment of acupuncture, part 1. Thermography. Crit Rev Biomed Eng. 2006a;34:1–22.

Litscher G. Bioengineering assessment of acupuncture, part 2: monitoring of microcirculation. Crit Rev Biomed Eng. 2006b;34:273–94.

Litscher G. Bioengineering assessment of acupuncture, part 3: ultrasound. Crit Rev Biomed Eng. 2006c;34:295–326.

Litscher G. Bioengineering assessment of acupuncture, part 4: functional magnetic resonance imaging. Crit Rev Biomed Eng. 2006d;34:327–45.

Litscher G. Bioengineering assessment of acupuncture, part 5: cerebral near infrared spectroscopy. Crit Rev Biomed Eng. 2006e;34:439–57.

Litscher G. Bioengineering assessment of acupuncture, part 6: monitoring—neurophysiology. Crit Rev Biomed Eng. 2007a;35:1–38.

Litscher G. Bioengineering assessment of acupuncture, part 7: heart rate variability. Crit Rev Biomed Eng. 2007b;35:183–95.

Litscher G. High-tech laser acupuncture is Chinese medicine. Med Acupunct. 2008;20:245–54.

Litscher G. Modernization of traditional acupuncture using multimodal computer-based high-tech methods—recent results of blue laser and teleacupuncture from the Medical University of Graz. J Acupunct Merid Stud. 2009;2:202–9.

Litscher G. Biomedical engineering meets acupuncture—development of an innovative miniaturized 48-channel skin impedance measurement system for needle and laser acupuncture and preliminary results. Biomed Eng Online. 2010a;9:78.

Litscher G. Bioengineering assessment of acupuncture, part 8: innovative moxibustion. Crit Rev Biomed Eng. 2010b;38:117–26.

Litscher G. Ten years evidence-based high-tech acupuncture, part 3: a short review of animal experiments. Evid Based Complement Alternat Med. 2010c;7:151–5.

Litscher G. Translational research in acupuncture—teleacupuncture bridges science and practice. Health. 2010d;2:16–9.

Litscher G. Transcontinental and translational high-tech acupuncture research using computer-based heart rate and 'fire of life' heart rate variability analysis. J Acupunct Meridian Stud. 2010e;3:156–64.

Litscher D, Litscher G. The history of liquid ear acupuncture and the current scientific state of the art. J Pharmacopuncture. 2016;19:109–13.

Litscher G, Schikora D. Cerebral vascular effects of non-invasive laserneedles measured by transorbital and transtemporal Doppler sonography. Lasers Med Sci. 2002;17:289–95.

Litscher G, Wang L, Yang NH, Schwarz G. Ultrasound-monitored effects of acupuncture on brain and eye. Neurol Res. 1999;21:373–7.

Litscher G, Zhang WB, Yi SH, Wang L, Huang T, Gaischek I, Tian YY, Wang GJ. The future of acupuncture moxibustion—a transcontinental three-center pilot study using high-tech methods. Med Acupuncture. 2009;21:115–21.

Litscher G, Huang T, Wang L, Zhang WB. Violet laser acupuncture—part 1: effects on brain circulation. J Acupunct Meridian Stud. 2010;3:255–9.

Litscher G, Bahr F, Litscher D, Min LQ, Rong PJ. A new method in auricular medicine for the investigation of the Nogier reflex. Integr Med Int. 2011a;1:205–10.

Litscher G, Bauernfeind G, Gao XY, Müller-Putz G, Wang L, Anderle W, Gaischek I, Litscher D, Neuper C, Niemtzow RC. Battlefield acupuncture and near-infrared spectroscopy—

miniaturized computer-triggered electrical stimulation of battlefield ear acupuncture points and 50-channel near-infrared spectroscopic mapping. Med Acupuncture. 2011b;23:263–70.

Litscher D, Wang GJ, Gaischek I, Wang L, Wallner-Liebmann S, Petek E. Yellow laser acupuncture—a new option for prevention and early intervention of lifestyle-related diseases: a randomized, placebo-controlled trial in volunteers. Laser Ther. 2015a;24:53–61.

Litscher G, Min LQ, Passegger CA, Litscher D, Li M, Wang M, Ghaffari-Tabrizi-Wizsy N, Stelzer I, Feigl G, Gaischek I, Wang GJ, Sadjak A, Bahr F. Transcranial yellow, red, and infrared laser and LED stimulation—changes of vascular parameters in a chick embryo model. Integr Med Int. 2015b;2:80–9.

Navrotsky LG, Blokhin AA, Belavskaya SV, Lisitsyna LI, Lyutkevich AA, Poteryaeva EL, Yudin VI, Litscher G. Patterns of skin luminescence resulting from the visualization of active acupuncture points using optical stimulation. Integr Med Int. 2015;2:1–8.

Niemtzow RC, Litscher G, Burns SM, Helms JM. Battlefield acupuncture: update. Med Acupuncture. 2009;21:43–6.

Rong PJ, Zhao JJ, Li YQ, Litscher D, Li SY, Gaischek I, Zhai X, Wang L, Luo M, Litscher G. Auricular acupuncture and biomedical research—a promising Sino-Austrian research cooperation. Chin J Integr Med. 2015;21:887–94.

Round R, Litscher G, Bahr F. Auricular acupuncture with laser. Evid Based Complemen Alternat Med. 2013;2013:984763.

Shi X, Litscher G, Wang H, Wang L, Zhao Z, Litscher D, Tao J, Gaischek I, Sheng Z. Continuous auricular electroacupuncture can significantly improve heart rate variability and clinical scores in patients with depression: first results from a transcontinental study. Evid Based Complement Alternat Med. 2013;2013:894096.

Shu Q, Wang H, Litscher D, Wu S, Chen L, Gaischek I, Wang L, He W, Zhou H, Litscher G, Liang F. Acupuncture and moxibustion have different effects on fatigue by regulating the autonomic nervous system: a pilot controlled clinical trial. Sci Rep. 2016;25:37846.

Széles JC, Litscher G. Objectivation of cerebral effects with a new continuous electrical auricular stimulation technique for pain management. Neurol Res. 2004;26:797–800.

Wang L, Litscher G. Modern technology for acupuncture research: a short review from the Medical University of Graz. Chinese Med. 2010;1:59–62.

Wang L, Huang T, Zhang W, Litscher G. Violet laser acupuncture—part 2: effects on peripheral microcirculation. J Acupunct Meridian Stud. 2011;4:24–8.

Zhang WB, Wang LL, Huang T, Tian YY, Xu YH, Wang L, Litscher G. Laser Doppler perfusion imaging for assessment of skin blood perfusion after acupuncture. Med Acupuncture. 2008;20:109–18.

Acupuncture Regulation of Gastrointestinal Function by Selection of Homotopic and Heterotopic Acupoints

13

Kun Liu, Shu-Ya Wang, Xiang Cui, Xiao-Xue Li, Shu Han, Xun He, Xin-Yan Gao, and Bing Zhu

Abstract

Functional gastrointestinal (GI) disorders, especially motor dysfunction of the GI tract are common in general population. Acupuncture has been widely adopted in the treatment of GI symptoms in China for thousands of years. During the last decades, the effects and mechanisms of acupuncture on gastrointestinal function have been investigated by numerous studies. In this chapter, we review studies on acupuncture regulating GI functions under normal or pathological conditions, including clinical observations and basic researches in experimental animals and put forward neurophysiological mechanisms. The concept of homotopic and heterotopic acupoints is raised by our research team to illustrate how to select acupoints for visceral disorders. In addition we clarify that stimulation of homotopic and heterotopic acupoints may produce sympathomimetic and parasympathomimetic regulations on GI motilities, thus providing a potential discipline on acupoints selection for GI dysfunctions.

Keywords

Gastrointestinal disorders · Acupuncture · Autonomic nervous system

Kun Liu, Shu-Ya Wang, and Xiang Cui contributed equally to this work.

K. Liu · S.-Y. Wang · X. Cui · X.-X. Li · S. Han · X. He
Department of Physiology, Institute of Acupuncture and Moxibustion, China Academy of Chinese Medical Sciences, Beijing, People's Republic of China

X.-Y. Gao (✉) · B. Zhu
Department of Physiology, Institute of Acupuncture and Moxibustion, China Academy of Chinese Medical Sciences, Beijing, People's Republic of China

The Innovation Research Institution of Acupuncture and Chinese Medicine, Shaanxi University of Chinese Medicine, Xi'an, People's Republic of China
e-mail: gaoxy@mail.cintcm.ac.cn

© Springer Nature Singapore Pte Ltd. 2018
J.-G. Lin (ed.), *Experimental Acupuncturology*,
https://doi.org/10.1007/978-981-13-0971-7_13

13.1   Introduction of Acupuncture Treatment of Gastrointestinal (GI) Disorders

Gastrointestinal (GI) disorders are commonly observed in clinical practices, including variety of functional diseases in GI tract. Functional gastrointestinal disorders (FGIDs) are composed of a group of disorders with gastrointestinal (GI) symptoms: disturbance motility, visceral hypersensitivity, altered mucosal and immune function, gut microbiota, and signal processes in the central nervous system (CNS) (Drossman 2016). The most widely recognized FGIDs are functional dyspepsia (FD) and irritable bowel syndrome (IBS) (Oshima and Miwa 2015). GI diseases bring a large economic burden to societies. In 2004, it was estimated that GI diseases affected about 60–70 million United States citizens, and to take up probably $142 billion in direct and indirect costs (Everhart and Ruhl 2009). Also previous studies have shown that the prevalence of FGIDs were 26.2% in Taiwan (Chang et al. 2012), 62% in Canada (Thompson et al. 2002) and 36.1% in Australia (Boyce et al. 2006). Modern medicine considers the development of the FGIDs to be associated with a variety of factors, as inflammation, eating disorders, emotional distress, and genetics. The pathogenic mechanism of FGIDs is still not completely understood, and thus there is currently no specific treatment available (Drossman 2016; Ji et al. 2016).

Many patients seek complementary and alternative medicine to treat GI diseases as conventional medical therapies either produce unsatisfactory results or have side effects (Michelfelder et al. 2010). Several lines of clinical (Li et al. 1992; Lin et al. 1997; Lux et al. 1994) and animal (Chen et al. 2008; Ouyang et al. 2002; Tatewaki et al. 2003) studies prove that acupuncture has positive effects on GI disorders (Table 13.1). This chapter will summarize the existing evidence on the therapeutics and mechanisms of acupuncture for FGIDs. Among them, series of studies have been conducted in our laboratory to verify the hypothesis that the neural mechanisms of acupuncture on GI function are based on selection of homotopic and heterotopic acupoints, which will be also introduced in detail in this chapter.

13.2   Acupuncture on Gastric Function

Coordinated gastric motility is so important to the gut that dietary digestion and absorption of nutrients cannot take place without it. The gastrointestinal tract needs to generate not only simple contractions but coordinated contractions to produce peristalsis to transit luminal contents in order to complete the gut functions effectively. Accommodation, pacemaking activity (myoelectrical activity), contractions and accommodation constitute gastric motility functions. Functional dyspepsia (FD) and gastroparesis are common gastric motility disorders. The characteristic symptoms of FD is postprandial fullnesss, early satiation, epigastric pain and burning without a readily identifiable organic cause (Tack et al. 2006). Gastroparesis, which is classified as diabetic, postoperative and idiopathic ones due to etiology, is

Table 13.1 Effects of acupuncture on GI motility

Segments	Subjects	Methods	Results	References
Stomach	Normal rats	EA at ST36 or ST37	Increase	Gao et al. (2012); Gao et al. (2016); Li et al. (2006, 2007); Sun (2017)
	Normal rats	EA at ST25 or RN12	Decrease	Gao et al. (2016); Li et al. (2006, 2007); Sun (2017)
	Dogs with impaired gastric motility	EA at ST36	Increase	Chen et al. (2008)
Jejunum	Normal rats Constipated rats Diarrheal rats	MA at LI11 and ST37	Increase	Qin et al. (2014)
	Normal rats Constipated rats Diarrheal rats	MA at ST25	Decrease	Qin (2013)
	Normal kunming mice	MA at ST36	Increase	Yuxue et al. (2015)
	Normal kunming mice	MA at ST25	Inhibit	
	Normal rats	EA at ST25	Inhibit	Wang et al. (2014); Yu et al. (2016)
Colon	Rats with stress	EA at ST36	Inhibit	Iwa et al. (2006)
	Normal kunming mice	MA at ST36	Increase	Yuxue et al. (2015)
	Normal kunming mice	MA at ST25	Increase	
	Normal rats, Constipated rats Diarrhea rats	MA at LI11, ST37, ST25 and BL25	Increase	Gao et al. (2015); Qin (2013)

Animals in this study was treated in strict accordance with the Guide for the Care and Use of Laboratory Animals of the National Institutes of Health. The protocol was approved by the Committee on the Ethics of Animal Experiments of China Academy of Chinese Medical Sciences (Approval Number: AE20110510-001)

defined as severely delayed gastric emptying without mechanical obstruction (Abell et al. 2006).

Adequate clinical evidences suggest that acupuncture has curative effect on FD (Jin et al. 2015; Liu et al. 2008; Takahashi 2006; Xu et al. 2006) and diabetic gastroparesis (Chang et al. 2001; Wang 2004). Acupuncture at ST36 and PC6 enhanced gastric migrating motor complex (MMC) in conscious dogs (Qian et al. 1999) and in anesthetized rats (Sato et al. 1993). Reversely, manual acupuncture on abdominal acupoint inhibited gastric motility (Sato et al. 1993) and induced gastric relaxation through the somato-sympathetic pathway in anesthetized rats (Tada et al. 2003). The neural pathways and transmitters mediating acupuncture effects via regulation of autonomic system has been explored in our group during the last decade.

We put an intrapyloric balloon to monitor gastric motility in anesthetized rats, and to detect the effects of acupoint or combined acupoints of different locations on gastrointestinal motility. (Li et al. 2006, 2007). The intragastric pressure was adjusted at 100 mm H_2O by modulating the volume of the balloon via a T tube system filled with warm water. The pressure was recorded with a data acquisition system and bridge amplifier through a transducer connected to the intragastric balloon. This intraluminal balloon paradigm was commonly used in our study for gastrointestinal functioning recording. Subdiaphragmatic gastric vagus nerves or sympathetic nerves innervating the stomach were dissected from peripheral tissue under microscope. Bipolar platinum electrodes were used to record activities of the vagal or sympathetic nerves. Discharges of the vagal or sympathetic nerves which amplified by a microelectrode amplifier were read through the data acquisition system. Laminectomy was performed in C8-T1 spinal cord in some rats for animal spinalization. A reversible cold block was produced by frozen physiological saline or chordotomy was conducted.

Results of our studies, systemically observed in anaesthetized rats, demonstrated that effects of acupuncture stimulation at homotopic (segmental) acupints or heterotopic (non-segmental) acupoints from different parts of the body produced quite different regulations on gastric motility. Heterotopic acupoints to the stomach (T6–10) which located at head, neck, upper limbs, upper chest-dorsum and lower dorsum, hindlimb and non-acupoin on tail enhanced gastric peristalsis during stimulation period (20–40s). Whereas homotopic acupoints to the stomach at abdominal and middle dorsum suppressed the gastric tonic motility with a rapid onset and the rhythmic wave of contractions (Li et al. 2007). The inhibitory effect of acupuncture on gastric motility was abolished after sympathectomy but with vagus nerve intact while the facilitative effect of acupuncture was destroyed after vagotomy but with entire sympathetic nerve. The facilitative effect of acupuncture at ST36 on gastric motility disappeared completely after spinalization, but the inhibitory effect was reserved (Li et al. 2007) (Fig. 13.1). Also according to Noguchi et al., electroacupuncture stimulation to a hindpaw facilitate duodenal motility, which is a supraspinal reflex response involving vagal excitatory nerves. This enhanced duodenal response by electroacupuncture is not affected by splanchnic nerve cutting. (Noguchi et al. 2003).

The facilitative or inhibitory effects of heterotopic or homotopic acupoints were dependent on electroacupuncture (EA) intensity. High intensity of EA to activate Aδ/C fibers and low intensity to activate Aβ fibers were performed on the ipsilateral sural nerve (heterotopic acupoint). High intensity stimulation over Aδ/C fibers threshold inhibited gastric activity via activation of sympathetic nerves, whereas low intensity below Aδ fiber threshold had unapparent effect (Kametani et al. 1979). Su et al. explored the "intensity-response" relationship between EA and gastric motility in rats. In his study, the half maximal facilitative or inhibitory intensity at ST36 or CV12 was 2.1–2.3 mA or 2.8 mA of EA in male adult Sprague-Dawley rats (Su et al. 2013).

Additional investigations suggested that EA regulation on gastric motility involved TRPV1 receptor, whereas effects of either heterotopic acupupoints or homotopic acupoints in ASIC3−/− mice were not of statistical significance (Su et al. 2013). Moreover, NMDA receptors (NMDARs) in dorsal motor nucleus of

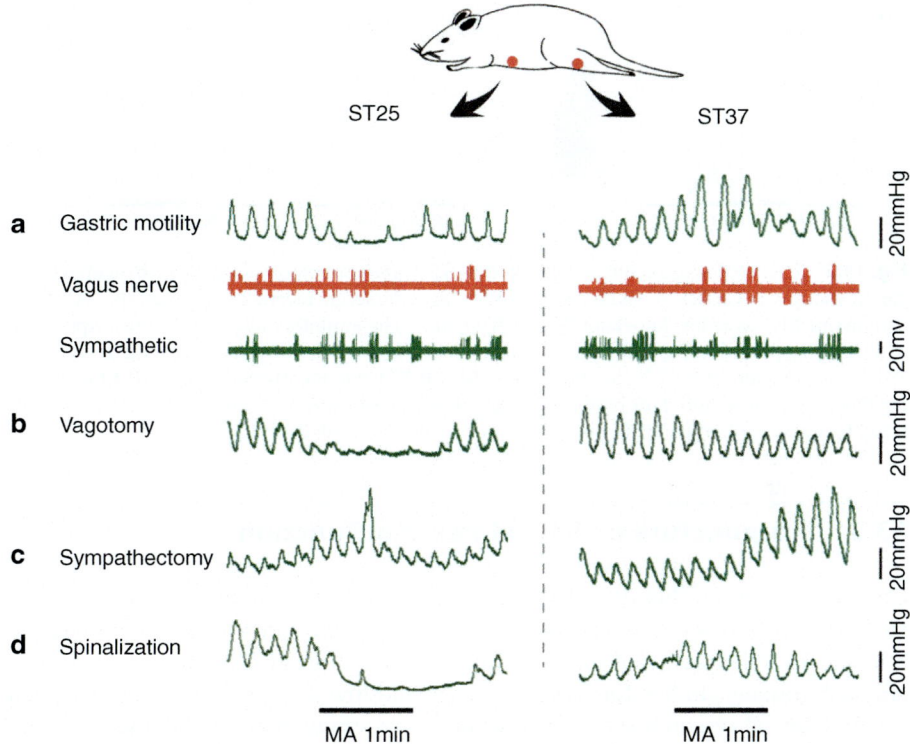

Fig. 13.1 Effect of acupuncture stimulation on gastric motility in rats with intact autonomic nervous system (**a**, Normal); and after sympathectomy of bilateral splanchnic nerves but vagi intact (**b**); or after bilateral subdiaphragmatic vagotomy but sympathetic nerve intact (**c**), or after spinalization at C8-T1 (**d**). It shows that in rats with autonomic nervous system intact, acupuncture at hindlimb (ST37, L5), heterotopic acupoint to stomach, had increased gastric motility by exciting parasympathetic nerve activity; this effect remained after sympathectomy, but was damaged after vagotomy. Whereas acupuncture at abdomen (ST25, T10), homotopic acupoint, inhibited gastric peristalsis by exciting sympathetic nerve discharge; this inhibition was consistent after vagotomy, but attenuated after sympathectomy. The effect of homotopic acupoint remained while the effect of heterotopic acupoint disappeared after spinalization at C8-T1 (Li et al. 2007; Sun 2017)

the vagus nerve (DMV) gastric projecting neurons played a critical role in electroacupuncture at ST36 enhancing gastric motility in anesthetized rats. Stimulating ST36 enhanced NMDAR-mediated synaptic transmission through inhibiting presynaptic μ-opioid receptors (Gao et al. 2012). Still in another study, we revealed that $M_{2/3}$ receptors binding with acetylcholine released from cholinergic neuronal endings were required for enhanced gastrointestinal transition produced by acupuncture at heterotopic acupoints, whereas $\beta_{1/2}$ receptors affinity to norepinephrine from catecholaminergic ones were required for inhibitory gastrointestinal motility processes by acupuncture at homotopic acupoints (Gao et al. 2016) (Fig. 13.2).

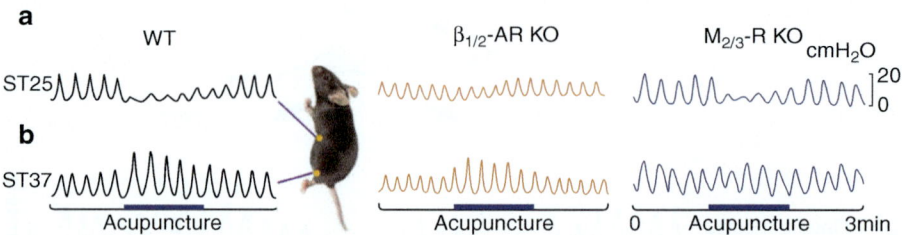

Fig. 13.2 Effects of acupuncture at heterotopic (ST 37) (**a**) or homotopic (ST25) (**b**) acupoints on gastric motility in C57BL/6 wild type mice (WT), $\beta_{1/2}$ adrenergic receptors knockout ($\beta_{1/2}$-AR KO), cholinergic $M_{2/3}$ receptors knockout ($M_{2/3}$-R KO) mice. The inhibitory effect in WT by acupuncture at ST25 disappeared in $\beta_{1/2}$-AR KO, but remained in $M_{2/3}$-R KO; however, the excitatory effect in WT by acupuncture at ST 37 was abolished in $M_{2/3}$-R KO, but not affected in $\beta_{1/2}$-AR KO, indicating that $\beta_{1/2}$-AR is required for inhibitory effect of homotopic acupoint, whereas $M_{2/3}$-R was recognized for excitatory influence of heterotopic acupoint (Gao et al. 2016)

13.3   Acupuncture on Small Intestinal Function

Gastrointestinal motility disorders also attribute to lots of small intestinal diseases, such as impaired accommodation, dumping syndrome, constipation and diarrhea. Somatic stimulation, as an effective treatment method for GI disorders, has been adopted in many studies for its convenience and low-cost property (Yin and Chen 2010). Clinical research shows that acupuncture stimulation on abdomen is effective for eliminating diarrhea and abdominal pain syndromes, which suggesting that acupuncture may inhibit GI motility or alleviate gastrospasms (Anastasi et al. 2009; Huang et al. 2014; Zhou et al. 2013)

Previous studies displayed that stimulation at homotopic acupoints, reduced intraluminal pressure in rats with or without spinalization, while acupuncture at heterotopic acupoints, covering different segmental innervations in the spinal cord to visceral organs, induced GI facilitation only in complete spinal rats (Li et al. 2007). Qin et al. (2014) observed that acupuncture at heterotopic acupoints Quchi (LI11, containing afferents to C5 spinal dorsal horn) and Shangjuxu (ST37, L5), increased the amplitude of peristalsis waves and enhanced jejunal motility in normal rats, constipated and diarrheic rats. Homotopic acupoints, such as Tianshu (ST25, T10), reduced jejunal motility regardless of its original basic value. In addition, acupuncture on Dachangshu (BL25) caused no significant change on jejunal motility in normal, constipated, and diarrheic rats (Fig. 13.3).

Small intestinal motility exhibits two distinct motor patterns: fasting and feeding. The typical manifestation in the fasting state is the migrating motor complex (MMC) as in stomach. Intestinal dysmotility includes absence of the MMC, impairment of the MMC, such as impaired propagation of the MMC along the gut, postprandial hypomotility and hypermotility. In purpose of exploring acupuncture's mechanism underlying regulation of intestinal function, Wang et al. observed the effect of acupuncture stimulation of ST25 on electrical and mechanical activities of

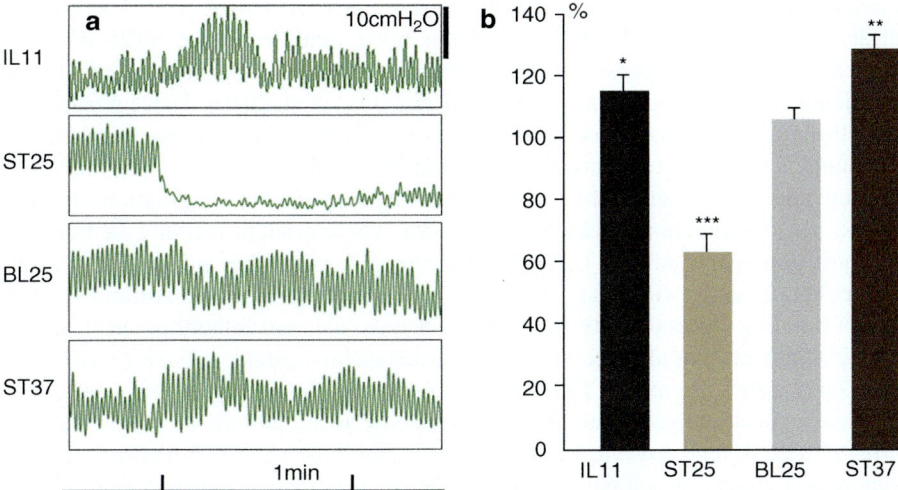

Fig. 13.3 Effects of manual acupuncture at homotopic and heterotopic acupoints on jejunal motility in normal rats. Chart **a** is raw trace of jejunal motility and chart **b** is data statistics. Acupuncture at forelimb LI11 (C5) and hindlimb ST37 (L5), both heterotopic acupoints to small intestine, increased the amplitude of peristalsis waves. While acupuncture at abdomen homotopic acupoint ST25 (T10), decreased jejunal motility. BL25 (L3), also heterotopic acupoint did not have an apparent effect (Qin et al. 2014) (Reprint with permission from PLoS ONE)

jejunum smooth muscle at different phases of inter-digestive MMC in normal SD rats and in rats with detached jejunum in *vivo*. The results in both normal SD rats and rats with detached jejunum showed that acupuncture could inhibit the jejunum activities at three phases of MMC (Su et al. 2014; Wang et al. 2014).

Based on previous studies, Qin et al. used an A fiber selective demyelination agent and a C fiber blocker to determine the type of afferent fibers take effects during acupuncture regulation of jejunal motility. Results showed that Aδ fibers mediated the regulation of jejunal motility by manual acupuncture; whereas the role of C fiber was more significant in the regulation of jejunal motility by the same intervention. They also observed that acupuncture at heterotopic acupoints (LI11, ST37 and BL25) led to excitatory effects on jejunal motility whereas homotopic acupoints (ST25) caused an opposite inhibitory effect on it, depending on the conditions of intestine, as normal, hypomotile, or hypermotile (Qin et al. 2014).

Parasympathetic nerves played a critical role in the excitatory regulation of intestinal motility via acupuncture at heterotopic acupoints such as ST36, ST37 and Quchi (Luo et al. 2008; Yoshimoto et al. 2012). Acetylcholine(ACh), released by parasympathetic terminals, exerts excitatory effects on smooth muscle tissues by binding to muscarinic receptors (Goyal and Hirano 1996). Among the five distinct subtypes of muscarinic receptors, M_2 and M_3 receptors are preferentially expressed in gastrointestinal smooth muscle tissues (Eglen et al. 1996). Studies involving the recent utilization of mutant mouse strains lacking specific muscarinic receptor subtypes suggested that both M_2 and M_3 receptors played direct roles in generating contraction in gastric and ileal smooth muscle tissues (Stengel et al. 2000; Unno et al. 2005, 2006). In $M_{2/3}$-R knocked out mice, acupuncture at ST25 not only decreased intragastric pressure and contraction frequency, but also reduced both intrajejunal pressure and contraction frequency (Gao et al. 2016). These phenotypes are attributed to the hallmark homotopic connection of ST25 to the stomach and jejunum, as well as ectopic connection to the distal colon.

Activation of Aδ and C fibers contributes to acupuncture's regulation on autonomic nervous function (Uchida et al. 2000). The capsaicin receptor or transient receptor potential vanilloid-1 (TRPV1) receptor is a member of the TRP-cation-channel superfamily (Rahmati 2012), and is mainly expressed on Aδ and C fiber. TRPV1 endings receptor acts as a sensor for heat, pH, and inflammation (Caterina et al. 2000), and it has also been shown to participate in mechanosensation (Bielefeldt and Davis 2008). Therefore, TRPV1 channels can be affected by the physical stimulation associated with acupuncture, thus producing an autonomic response (Wu et al. 2014). Yu et al. reported 2 mA and 4 mA EA stimulation at ST25 had significantly suppressed effects on jejunal motility in TRPV1−/− mice compared with that for wild type mice, suggesting that TRPV1 receptor may serve as one of the afferent pathway underlying the EA stimulation in regulating jejunal motility (Yu et al. 2016).

13.4   Acupuncture on Colonic Motility

Colon, as a storage organ, mainly plays a role in the absorption of water, electrolytes, and nutrients at same time. The motility of colon compromises individual phasic contractions and giant migrating contractions. The individual phasic contraction, happening during the fasting and feeding states, is the basic unit of contractile activity and contains short-duration and long-duration contraction. In detail, short-duration contractions last less than 15 s, long-duration contractions for 40–60 s in dog and human colon (Huizinga et al. 1985; Sarna et al. 1982, 1984; Sarna 1991). The motility of colon is activated by the ingestion of meal (gastro-colonic reflex), while it goes to sleep during sleeping. The pattern of individual phasic contractions is complicated with a lack of specific dominant frequencies, which probably is related to the functions of the colon: storage. The giant migrating contractions play a vital role in the bowel movement (Torsoli et al. 1971; Williams et al. 1987). Proximal colon is the main part that plays spontaneous mass movements and related giant migrating contractions. Previous study reported the mean migration distance is about 13 cm in dog colon (Sarna 1991). Numerous functional diseases are associated with disrupted colonic motility, such as irritable bowel syndrome (IBS), constipation and diarrhea. In a randomized controlled trial (RCT), 448 participants with Diarrhea-predominant irritable bowel syndrome (IBS-D) and functional diarrhea (FD) were recruited. Among them, 336 subjects were treated with EA (15 Hz, continuous-wave mode, 30 min, 4 weeks) at LI11, ST37, ST25 and BL25. The results showed that the stool frequency was significantly decreased after 4 week therapy (Zheng et al. 2016). The author supposed that the effect of EA was through a positive regulation of gastrointestinal motility, brain-gut axis, and visceral hypersensitivity (Ma et al. 2014). The other similar RCTs showed that EA at bilateral ST25, SP14, and ST37 (10/50 Hz, 30 min, 30 min, 8 weeks) alleviated symptoms and improved quality of life in patients with chronic severe functional constipation (CSFC) (Liu et al. 2016). The efficacy of EA on CSFC was considered to be in correlation with the improvement of intestinal motility via parasympathetic activation, induced by the acupoint stimulation (Gao et al. 2015; Li et al. 2007). Moreover, in 17 children with chronic constipation, needling at ST36, LI12 and LI4 gradually elevated the frequency of intestinal motility during the period of 10-week treatment (Broide et al. 2001). According to the acupoints used by them and in our previous study (Gao et al. 2016; Qin et al. 2014), we concluded that parasympathetic system activated by acupuncture application played the role in the positive results. Additional, the other randomized clinical trial reported that EA can obviously improve stress urinary incontinence in women via stimulating BL33 and BL35 (Liu et al. 2017). It was indicated that the role of segmental parasympathetic nerve system played a role in acupuncture effect. Previous studies showed that EA could stimulate S3 via BL33 and the pudendal nerve via BL35 at the lumbosacral region. Thus, EA at the lumbosacral region could cause muscle contraction and stimulate pelvic floor muscle training (Wang and Zhang 2012), and improve the dysfunction of intrinsic urethral sphincter and pelvic floor muscles (Yoshimura and Miyazato 2012). Their studies on stress urinary incontinence also indicated that segmental excitatory regulation of parasympathetic tone by acupuncture could be also effective on constipation, which is consistent with our later clinical trials in patients with constipation.

In recent years, our group investigated the mechanism of acupuncture efficacy on colonic motility. We observed the effect of manual acupuncture on the colonic motility by stimulating acupoints LI11, ST37, ST25 and BL25 at normal, constipated and diarrheal rats respectively. It is known that the distal colon was innervated by the sacral parasympathetic nerve, which mainly originated from S1 spinal segment in rats, while the spinal segment of acupoints LI11, ST37, ST25 and BL25 are C5, L5, T10 and L3 respectively, indicating non-segmental innervations to colon. The results showed that needling at heterotopic acupoints augmented colonic motility in all rats, had nothing to do with the physiological or pathological state of the gastrointestine (Fig. 13.4). Besides, we also confirmed that acupuncture at

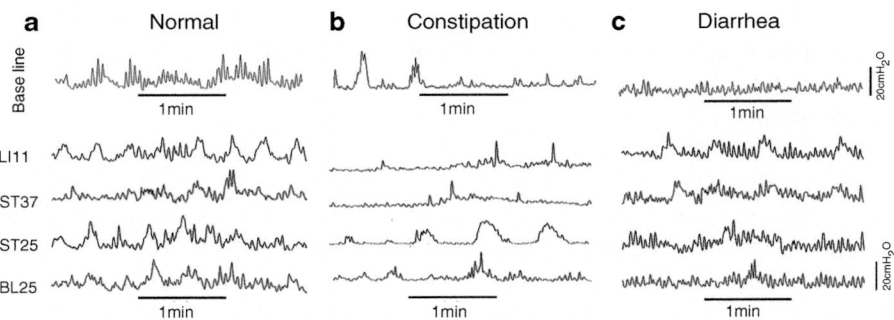

Fig. 13.4 Effects of acupuncture at different heterotopic acupoints on distal colonic motility in normal (**a**), constipation (**b**) and diarrhea rats (**c**). Acupuncture stimulation at forelimb (LI11), hindlimb (ST37), abdomen (ST25) and low back (BL25) are all heterotopic acupoints to colon, and either under normal condition or pathological conditions, acupuncture could promote colonic activities (Gao et al. 2016) (Reprint with permission from PLoS ONE)

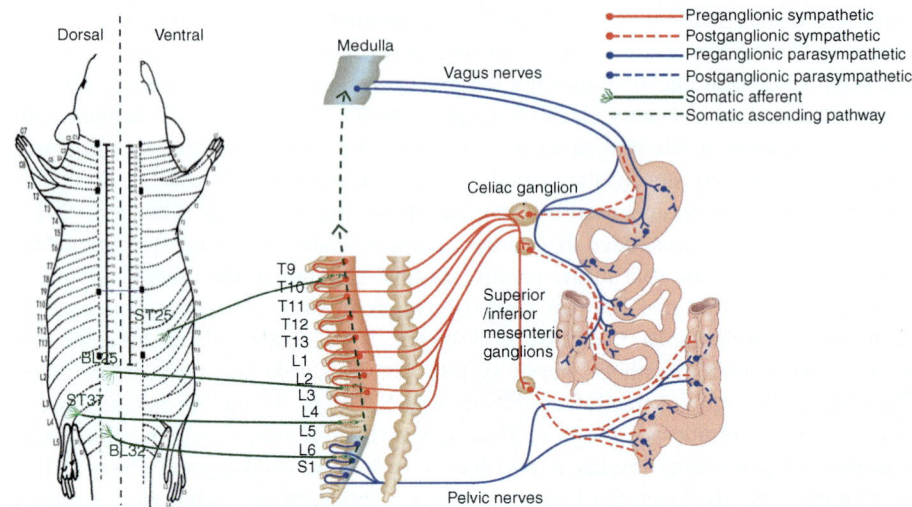

Fig. 13.5 The spinal and supraspinal mechanisms underlying somato-visceral reflex. Activities of stomach (T6–10) and small intestine (T9–12) are inhibited through sympathetic efferent at spinal level when acupuncture conducted at ST25 (T10). ST37 (L5) and BL25 (L3) activate gastric, intestinal and colonic motility through parasympathetic pathway when the somatic afferent ascend to supraspinal levels. Acupuncture at BL32 (S2) increases colonic motility via sacral parasympathetic tone

heterotopic acupoints promoted colonic motility via C-fibers, and M_3 muscarinic receptors played a vital role in this process. M_3 muscarinic receptors are mainly distributed in colon and bond by ACh (Stengel et al. 2000). Based on the results above, we further explored outputs of sympathetic and parasympathetic system in acupuncture-induced enhancement on colonic motility using $\beta_{1/2}$ receptor-knockout mice and $M_{2/3}$ receptor-knockout mice (Gao et al. 2016). The findings verified that $M_{2/3}$ receptor played a direct role in the improvement of colonic motility via stimulating heterotopic acupoints, while there was no relationship between $\beta_{1/2}$ receptor-knockout and acupuncture effect on colonic function whatever acupoints were stimulated. Therefore, it is quite clear that parasympathetic nerve plays an important role in acupuncture-induced enhancement on colonic motility.

Conclusions

Based on the evidences from our laboratory as well as others, in both animals and humans, EA is effective in eliminating GI functional disorders. Acupoints and viscera innervated by the same spinal segment organize as a homotopic structure-functional unit via sympathetic control. Contrarily, acupoints innervated by the other spinal segment (non-segment) organize with the viscus as a heterotopic-unit via parasympathetic dominant. The neurologic mechanisms underlying acupuncture are related to segmental or non-segmental innervation of acupoint with that of the gut.

The facilitative effects of heterotopic acupoints on GI motility attribute to the somato-parasympathetic reflex pathway, while the inhibitory effects of homotopic acupoints on GI function via the somato-sympathetic one (Fig. 13.5). The underlying molecular mechanism refers to cholinergic M receptors and catecholaminergic β receptors on smooth muscles. NMDARs in the DMV of the brainstem are also involved as supraspinal regulation. Additionally, dominant innervations of autonomic nervous system for different viscera should be taken into consideration. Both homotopic- and heterotopic-unit acupoints establish a homeostasis condition that somatic input regulates visceral functions to a balance. Our doctrine of heterotopic and homotopic acupoints sets up a novel explanation for acupuncture like somatic therapy and propose directions in acupuncture clinic for acupoints selection.

Acknowledgments This short review includes works in our laboratory supported by the following grants: National Basic Research Program of China (No. 2005CB523308, 2011CB50520, 2014CB543103), National Natural Science Foundation of China (No. 81173345, 81130063, 81273831, 30772706, 30371804, C30100245) and Intramural Program of Institute of Acupuncture and Moxibustion (No. ZZ12006). Kun Liu, Shu-Ya Wang, Xiang Cui contributed equally to this article. Related studies have been conducted by Dr. Qing-Guang Qin, Dr. Hai-Ping Wang, Dr. Chang-Xiang Cui, Dr. Yu-Xue Zhao, Dr. Yang-Shuai Su, M.M.S. Hao Liu, and M.M.S. Guang Sun.

References

Abell TL, Bernstein RK, Cutts T, Farrugia G, Forster J, Hasler WL, McCallum RW, Olden KW, Parkman HP, Parrish CR, et al. Treatment of gastroparesis: a multidisciplinary clinical review. Neurogastroenterol Moti. 2006;18:263–83.
Anastasi JK, McMahon DJ, Kim GH. Symptom management for irritable bowel syndrome: a pilot randomized controlled trial of acupuncture/moxibustion. Gastroenterol Nurs. 2009;32:243–55.
Bielefeldt K, Davis BM. Differential effects of ASIC3 and TRPV1 deletion on gastroesophageal sensation in mice. Am J Physiol Gastrointest Liver Physiol. 2008;294:G130–8.
Boyce PM, Talley NJ, Burke C, Koloski NA. Epidemiology of the functional gastrointestinal disorders diagnosed according to Rome II criteria: an Australian population-based study. Intern Med J. 2006;36:28–36.
Broide E, Pintov S, Portnoy S, Barg J, Klinowski E, Scapa E. Effectiveness of acupuncture for treatment of childhood constipation. Dig Dis Sci. 2001;46:1270–5.
Caterina MJ, Leffler A, Malmberg AB, Martin WJ, Trafton J, Petersen-Zeitz KR, Koltzenburg M, Basbaum AI, Julius D. Impaired nociception and pain sensation in mice lacking the capsaicin receptor. Science. 2000;288:306–13.
Chang CS, Ko CW, Wu CY, Chen GH. Effect of electrical stimulation on acupuncture points in diabetic patients with gastric dysrhythmia: a pilot study. Digestion. 2001;64:184–90.
Chang FY, Chen PH, Wu TC, Pan WH, Chang HY, Wu SJ, Yeh NH, Tang RB, Wu L, James FE. Prevalence of functional gastrointestinal disorders in Taiwan: questionnaire-based survey for adults based on the Rome III criteria. Asia Pac J Clin Nutr. 2012;21:594–600.
Chen J, Song GQ, Yin J, Koothan T, Chen JD. Electroacupuncture improves impaired gastric motility and slow waves induced by rectal distension in dogs. Am J Physiol Gastrointest Liver Physiol. 2008;295:G614–20.
Drossman DA. Functional gastrointestinal disorders: history, pathophysiology, clinical features and Rome IV. Gastroenterology. 2016;150(6):1262–79.
Eglen RM, Hegde SS, Watson N. Muscarinic receptor subtypes and smooth muscle function. Pharmacol Rev. 1996;48:531–65.
Everhart JE, Ruhl CE. Burden of digestive diseases in the United States part I: overall and upper gastrointestinal diseases. Gastroenterology. 2009;136:376–86.

Gao X, Qiao Y, Jia B, Jing X, Cheng B, Wen L, Tan Q, Zhou Y, Zhu B, Qiao H. NMDA receptor-dependent synaptic activity in dorsal motor nucleus of vagus mediates the enhancement of gastric motility by stimulating ST36. Evid Based Complement Alternat Med. 2012;2012:438460.

Gao X, Qin Q, Yu X, Liu K, Li L, Qiao H, Zhu B. Acupuncture at heterotopic acupoints facilitates distal colonic motility via activating M3 receptors and somatic afferent C-fibers in normal, constipated, or diarrhoeic rats. Neurogastroenterol Motil. 2015;27:1817–30.

Gao X, Zhao Y, Su Y, Liu K, Yu X, Cui C, Yang Z, Shi H, Jing X, Zhu B. β1/2 or M2/3 receptors are required for different gastrointestinal motility responses induced by acupuncture at heterotopic or homotopic acupoints. PLoS One. 2016;11:e0168200.

Goyal RK, Hirano I. The enteric nervous system. N Engl J Med. 1996;334:1106–15.

Huang R, Zhao J, Wu L, Dou C, Liu H, Weng Z, Lu Y, Shi Y, Wang X, Zhou C, Wu H. Mechanisms underlying the analgesic effect of moxibustion on visceral pain in irritable bowel syndrome: a review. Evid Based Complement Alternat Med. 2014;2014:895914.

Huizinga JD, Stern HS, Chow E, Diamant NE, El-Sharkawy TY. Electrophysiologic control of motility in the human colon. Gastroenterology. 1985;88:500–11.

Iwa M, Nakade Y, Pappas TN, Takahashi T. Electroacupuncture elicits dual effects: stimulation of delayed gastric emptying and inhibition of accelerated colonic transit induced by restraint stress in rats. Dig Dis Sci. 2006;51:1493–500.

Ji J, Huang Y, Wang XF, Ma Z, Wu HG, Im H, Liu HR, Wu LY, Li J. Review of clinical studies of the treatment of ulcerative colitis using acupuncture and moxibustion. Gastroenterol Res Pract. 2016;2016:1–10.

Jin Y, Zhao Q, Zhou K, Jing X, Yu X, Fang J, Liu Z, Zhu B. Acupuncture for functional dyspepsia: a single blinded, randomized, controlled trial. Evid Based Complement Alternat Med. 2015;2015:904926.

Kametani H, Sato A, Sato Y, Simpson A. Neural mechanisms of reflex facilitation and inhibition of gastric motility to stimulation of various skin areas in rats. J Physiol. 1979;294:407.

Li Y, Tougas G, Chiverton SG, Hunt RH. The effect of acupuncture on gastrointestinal function and disorders. Am J Gastroenterol. 1992;87:1372–81.

Li YQ, Zhu B, Rong PJ, Ben H, Li YH. Effective regularity in modulation on gastric motility induced by different acupoint stimulation. World J Gastroenterol. 2006;12:7642–8.

Li YQ, Zhu B, Rong PJ, Ben H, Li YH. Neural mechanism of acupuncture-modulated gastric motility. World J Gastroenterol. 2007;13:709–16.

Lin X, Liang J, Ren J, Mu F, Zhang M, Chen JD. Electrical stimulation of acupuncture points enhances gastric myoelectrical activity in humans. Am J Gastroenterol. 1997;92:1527–30.

Liu S, Peng S, Hou X, Ke M, Chen JD. Transcutaneous electroacupuncture improves dyspeptic symptoms and increases high frequency heart rate variability in patients with functional dyspepsia. Neurogastroenterol Motil. 2008;20:1204–11.

Liu Z, Yan S, Wu J, He L, Li N, Dong G, Fang J, Fu W, Fu L, Sun J. Acupuncture for chronic severe functional constipation: a randomized trial. Ann Inter Med. 2016;165:761.

Liu Z, Liu Y, Xu H, He L, Chen Y, Fu L, Li N, Lu Y, Su T, Sun J. Effect of electroacupuncture on urinary leakage among women with stress urinary incontinence: a randomized clinical trial. JAMA. 2017;317:2493.

Luo D, Liu S, Xie X, Hou X. Electroacupuncture at acupoint ST-36 promotes contractility of distal colon via a cholinergic pathway in conscious rats. Dig Dis Sci. 2008;53:689–93.

Lux G, Hagel J, Backer P, Backer G, Vogl R, Ruppin H, Domschke S, Domschke W. Acupuncture inhibits vagal gastric acid secretion stimulated by sham feeding in healthy subjects. Gut. 1994;35:1026–9.

Ma XP, Hong J, An CP, Zhang D, Huang Y, Wu HG, Zhang CH, Meeuwsen S. Acupuncture-moxibustion in treating irritable bowel syndrome: how does it work? World J Gastroenterol. 2014;20:6044–54.

Michelfelder AJ, Lee KC, Bading EM. Integrative medicine and gastrointestinal disease. Prim Care. 2010;37:255–67.

Noguchi E, Ohsawa H, Tanaka H, Ikeda H, Aikawa Y. Electro-acupuncture stimulation effects on duodenal motility in anesthetized rats. Jpn J Physiol. 2003;53:1–7.

Oshima T, Miwa H. Epidemiology of functional gastrointestinal disorders in Japan and in the world. J Neurogastroenterol Motil. 2015;21:320–9.

Ouyang H, Yin J, Wang Z, Pasricha PJ, Chen JD. Electroacupuncture accelerates gastric emptying in association with changes in vagal activity. Am J Physiol Gastrointest Liver Physiol. 2002;282:G390–6.

Qian L, Peters LJ, Chen JD. Effects of electroacupuncture on gastric migrating myoelectrical complex in dogs. Dig Dis Sci. 1999;44:56–62.

Qin Q, Haiping W, Liu K, Zhao Y, Ben H, Gao X, Zhu B. Effect of acupuncture at ST25 on intestinal motility in normal, diarrhea and constipation model rats. World J Tradit Chin Med. 2013;8:245–9.

Qin QG, Gao XY, Liu K, Yu XC, Li L, Wang HP, Zhu B. Acupuncture at heterotopic acupoints enhances jejunal motility in constipated and diarrheic rats. World J Gastroenterol. 2014;20:18271–83.

Rahmati R. The transient receptor potential vanilloid receptor 1, TRPV1 (VR1) inhibits peristalsis in the mouse jejunum. Arch Iran Med. 2012;15:433–8.

Sarna SK. Physiology and pathophysiology of colonic motor activity (1). Dig Dis Sci. 1991;36:827.

Sarna S, Latimer P, Campbell D, Waterfall WE. Electrical and contractile activities of the human rectosigmoid. Gut. 1982;23:698–705.

Sarna SK, Condon R, Cowles V. Colonic migrating and nonmigrating motor complexes in dogs. Am J Phys. 1984;246:355–60.

Sato A, Sato Y, Suzuki A, Uchida S. Neural mechanisms of the reflex inhibition and excitation of gastric motility elicited by acupuncture-like stimulation in anesthetized rats. Neurosci Res. 1993;18:53–62.

Stengel PW, Gomeza J, Wess J, Cohen ML. M(2) and M(4) receptor knockout mice: muscarinic receptor function in cardiac and smooth muscle in vitro. J Pharmacol Exp Ther. 2000;292:877–85.

Su YS, He W, Wang C, Shi H, Zhao YF, Xin JJ, Wang XY, Shang HY, Hu L, Jing XH, Zhu B. "Intensity-response" effects of electroacupuncture on gastric motility and its underlying peripheral neural mechanism. Evid Based Complement Alternat Med. 2013;2013:535742.

Su YS, Yang ZK, Xin JJ, He W, Shi H, Wang XY, Hu L, Jing XH, Zhu B. Somatosensory nerve fibers mediated generation of De-qi in manual acupuncture and local moxibustion-like stimuli-modulated gastric motility in rats. Evid Based Complement Alternat Med. 2014;2014:673239.

Sun G, L Hao., Liu K, Wang HF, Zhi MJ, Gao XY, Zhu B. Effect of grouped ST36 or RN12 on gastric motility and sensation. World J Tradit Chin Med (English). 2017; 1.

Tack J, Talley NJ, Camilleri M, Holtmann G, Hu P, Malagelada JR, Stanghellini V. Functional gastroduodenal disorders. Gastroenterology. 2006;130:1466–79.

Tada H, Fujita M, Harris M, Tatewaki M, Nakagawa K, Yamamura T, Pappas TN, Takahashi T. Neural mechanism of acupuncture-induced gastric relaxations in rats. Dig Dis Sci. 2003;48:59–68.

Takahashi T. Acupuncture for functional gastrointestinal disorders. J Gastroenterol. 2006;41:408–17.

Tatewaki M, Harris M, Uemura K, Ueno T, Hoshino E, Shiotani A, Pappas TN, Takahashi T. Dual effects of acupuncture on gastric motility in conscious rats. Am J Physiol Regul Integr Comp Physiol. 2003;285:R862–72.

Thompson WG, Irvine EJ, Pare P, Ferrazzi S, Rance L. Functional gastrointestinal disorders in Canada: first population-based survey using Rome II criteria with suggestions for improving the questionnaire. Dig Dis Sci. 2002;47:225–35.

Torsoli A, Ramorino ML, Ammaturo MV, Capurso L, Paoluzi P, Anzini F. Mass movements and intracolonic pressures. Am J Dig Dis. 1971;16:693–6.

Uchida S, Kagitani F, Suzuki A, Aikawa Y. Effect of acupuncture-like stimulation on cortical cerebral blood flow in anesthetized rats. Jpn J Physiol. 2000;50:495–507.

Unno T, Matsuyama H, Sakamoto T, Uchiyama M, Izumi Y, Okamoto H, Yamada M, Wess J, Komori S. M(2) and M(3) muscarinic receptor-mediated contractions in longitudinal smooth muscle of the ileum studied with receptor knockout mice. Br J Pharmacol. 2005;146:98–108.

Unno T, Matsuyama H, Izumi Y, Yamada M, Wess J, Komori S. Roles of M2 and M3 muscarinic receptors in cholinergic nerve-induced contractions in mouse ileum studied with receptor
knockout mice. Br J Pharmacol. 2006;149:1022–30.

Wang L. Clinical observation on acupuncture treatment in 35 cases of diabetic gastroparesis. J
Tradit Chin Med. 2004;24:163–5.

Wang S, Zhang S. Simultaneous perineal ultrasound and vaginal pressure measurement prove the
action of electrical pudendal nerve stimulation in treating female stress incontinence. BJU Int.
2012;110:1338–43.

Wang HP, Gao XY, Liu K, Qin QG, Zhu B. Effects of acupuncture at "Tianshu" (ST 25) on electro-
activity and mechanical motility of migrating motor complex during jejunal digestion period in
rats with detached jejunum. Zhongguo Zhen Jiu. 2014;34:469–74.

Williams CL, Peterson JM, Villar RG, Burks TF. Corticotropin-releasing factor directly mediates
colonic responses to stress. Am J Phys. 1987;253:G582–6.

Wu SY, Chen WH, Hsieh CL, Lin YW. Abundant expression and functional participation of
TRPV1 at Zusanli acupoint (ST36) in mice: mechanosensitive TRPV1 as an "acupuncture-
responding channel". BMC Complement Altern Med. 2014;14:96.

Xu S, Hou X, Zha H, Gao Z, Zhang Y, Chen JD. Electroacupuncture accelerates solid gastric
emptying and improves dyspeptic symptoms in patients with functional dyspepsia. Dig Dis
Sci. 2006;51:2154–9.

Yin J, Chen JD. Gastrointestinal motility disorders and acupuncture. Auton Neurosci Basic Clin.
2010;157:31.

Yoshimoto S, Babygirija R, Dobner A, Ludwig K, Takahashi T. Anti-stress effects of transcutaneous
electrical nerve stimulation (TENS) on colonic motility in rats. Dig Dis Sci. 2012;57:1213–21.

Yoshimura N, Miyazato M. Neurophysiology and therapeutic receptor targets for stress urinary
incontinence. Int J Urol. 2012;19:524.

Yu Z, Zhang N, Lu CX, Pang TT, Wang KY, Jiang JF, Zhu B, Xu B. Electroacupuncture at ST25
inhibits jejunal motility: role of sympathetic pathways and TRPV1. World J Gastroenterol.
2016;22:1834–43.

Yuxue Z, Changxiang C, Qingguang Q, Hui B, Junhong G, Xiaochun Y, Bing Z. Effect of manual
acupuncture on bowel motility in normal kunming mouse. J Tradit Chin Med. 2015;35:227–33.

Zheng H, Li Y, Zhang W, Zeng F, Zhou SY, Zheng HB, Zhu WZ, Jing XH, Rong PJ, Tang
CZ. Electroacupuncture for patients with diarrhea-predominant irritable bowel syndrome or
functional diarrhea: a randomized controlled trial. Medicine. 2016;95:e3884.

Zhou S, Zeng F, Liu J, Zheng H, Huang W, Liu T, Chen D, Qin W, Gong Q, Tian J, Li Y. Influence of
acupuncture stimulation on cerebral network in functional diarrhea. Evid Based Complement
Alternat Med. 2013;2013:975769.

Printed by Printforce, the Netherlands